Ethical Dimensions of Health Policy

Ethical Dimensions of Health Policy

Edited by

MARION DANIS, M.D.
Head, Section on Ethics and Health Policy
Department of Clinical Bioethics
Warren G. Magnuson Clinical Center
National Institutes of Health
Bethesda, MD

CAROLYN CLANCY, M.D.
Director, Center for Outcomes and Effectiveness Research
Agency for Healthcare Research and Quality
Rockville, MD

LARRY R. CHURCHILL, PH.D.
Professor of Social Medicine
Co-Director, Center for Health Ethics and Policy
University of North Carolina at Chapel Hill
Chapel Hill, NC

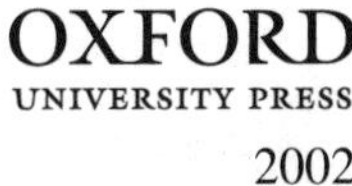

OXFORD
UNIVERSITY PRESS
2002

OXFORD
UNIVERSITY PRESS

Oxford New York
Auckland Bangkok Buenos Aires Cape Town Chennai
Dar es Salaam Delhi Hong Kong Istanbul Karachi Kolkata
Kuala Lumpur Madrid Melbourne Mexico City Mumbai Nairobi
São Paulo Shanghai Singapore Taipei Tokyo Toronto

and an associated company in Berlin

Published by Oxford University Press, Inc.
198 Madison Avenue, New York, New York 10016
http://www.oup-usa.org
1-800-334-4249

Library of Congress Cataloging-in-Publication Data
Ethical dimensions of health policy /
[edited by] Marion Danis, Carolyn Clancy, Larry R. Churchill.
p. cm. Includes bibliographical references and index.
ISBN 0-19-514070-2
1. Medical policy—Moral and ethical aspects.
2. Medical policy.
I. Danis, Marion. II. Clancy, Carolyn M. III. Churchill, Larry R., 1945–
RA395.A3 E846 2002
174'.2—dc21 2001036414

2 3 4 5 6 7 8 9

Printed in the United States of America
on acid-free paper

Dedicated to our spouses, Roger, Bill, and Sande

Foreword

EZEKIEL J. EMANUEL

This book makes an important contribution to a fledgling conversation between bioethics and health policy. This conversation has not been easy, but it is much needed.

More than 40 years ago, in his famous Rede Lectures, C. P. Snow identified two distinct cultures, each of which were

> comparable in intelligence, identical in race, not grossly different in social origin, earning about the same incomes, who had almost ceased to communicate at all, who in intellectual, moral and psychological climate had so little in common that . . . one might have crossed an ocean.
>
> Snow, 1959, 2

He claimed that

> between the two [had emerged] a gulf of mutual incomprehension—sometimes (particularly among the young) hostility and dislike, but most of all a lack of understanding. They have a curious distorted image of each other. Their attitudes are so different that, even on the level of emotion, they can't find much common ground
>
> Snow, 1959, 4–5

Snow, of course, was referring to the chasm between scientists and what he called literary intellectuals, or humanists. And he thought this chasm a serious "problem of the entire West" and for practical as well as intellectual life.

But Snow might have been referring to the two cultures of health policy and bioethics. There has been a long history of mutual incomprehension between these two groups. Health policy makers have frequently been skeptical and suspicious of bioethics. Some of their apprehension may stem from the training of many health policy makers. Many have been educated in a manner that emphasizes a kind of fact–value distinction. So they see themselves as presenting the facts, while the bioethicists deal with the values. The facts are objective and open to rational discussion, while values are subjective and not amenable to rational deliberation.

Even beyond intellectual habits generated and reinforced by different training are other substantive differences. Health policy makers see bioethics as preoccupied with the doctor–patient relationship, informed consent, and sensational cases revolving around terminating respirators, euthanasia, and Baby Does. And discussions of these topics by bioethicists occur isolated—sometimes even consciously and explicitly—from their resource implications. Health policy makers further see that the value dominating discussions of bioethics is autonomy. These issues and autonomy do not readily appear to have any serious import for the major resource allocation issues confronting health policy. More importantly, when bioethicists discuss issues related to health coverage or insurance, they can sound naive and simplistic to policy makers. Bioethicists often do not distinguish between health care finance and delivery systems or understand more subtle complexities of the finance system in the United States. Consequently, when philosophers have commented on issues related to coverage, they applaud themselves for arguing persuasively about the importance of allocating resources on the basis of "need" rather than ability to pay, or making a case for a "decent minimum" without specifying anything about the content of the minimum (Walzer, 1983; Williams, 1997). These "insights" may be helpful, but they do not go far in the current health care debate (Emanuel, 1991).

It is not just naivete that alienates health policy makers from bioethics. They view the elaboration of the principle of justice in bioethics—the single principle that might enrich health policy discussions—as vague, abstract, even vacuous. After all, how helpful is the principle of "treating equals equally" when considering the justice of health benefits provided by managed care organizations? Indeed, the charge that the principle of justice is empty is one leveled by many bioethicists themselves, and this has only reinforced health policy makers' wariness of bioethics' conceptual tools. Health policy makers will thus frequently ask, in a skeptical tone, "what help or insight does considering this issue from the ethical perspective make?" And, when leading bioethicists contend that "a comprehensive and unified theory of justice that captures our diverse conceptions [for health care] may be impossible," health policy types feel vindicated in dismissing bioethics (Beauchamp and Childress, 1994, 327). The result has been a lack of interest by health policy makers in even using the term *ethics*, let alone discussing ethical issues.

From their perspective, bioethicists think health policy makers are too dismissive and unreflective. They contend that the fact–value distinction relied upon by health policy makers is not so entrenched. Indeed, it has been widely discredited in the social sciences. More importantly, it seems untenable to claim that when issues revolve around allocating scarce medical resources or determining what services to cover, values are not critically implicated. After all, the decision about whether to manage pharmacy benefits by using a three-tiered co-payment system, a quarterly cap on covered drugs, or step therapy entails questions not just about efficiency and cost-savings but also about ethics—what values are pharmacy benefits to realize? What is the justification for the different burdens on patients, physicians, etc.?

Similarly, attempts by many managed care companies to distinguish health from "lifestyle" pharmaceuticals and cover only the former are hardly value neutral (Titlow et al, 2000). Neither health nor lifestyle are self-defining terms; determining what legitimately constitutes "lifestyle" is infused with values. Is trying to stop smoking a health or a lifestyle issue? Is alcoholism a health or a lifestyle issue? Are impotence, birth control, and abortions health or lifestyle issues? More importantly, why is this a relevant distinction for allocating pharmaceutical benefits? Invoking this distinction to determine coverage decisions requires some justification—or in more neutral terms, explanation—that will surely be infused with value claims about why the costs of "health" drugs should be socially shared while the cost of "lifestyle" drugs should be the responsibility of the individual. Indeed, bioethicists find reliance on this fact–value distinction in health policy an obfuscation. They feel vindicated in this judgment when studies demonstrate that health policy recommendations have little to do with the facts and much more to do with policy makers' values and political leanings (Fuchs, 1996). Bioethicists begin to wonder whether dismissing the importance of ethics in health policy is not just a way of surreptitiously smuggling in values without having to reveal or defend them.

Finally, bioethicists believe that debates about managed care affirm the importance of ethics in health policy debates. The public's vocal concerns about the confidentiality of medical records, physicians' conflicts of interest related to reimbursement policies, coverage of experimental therapies, appeals and grievance procedures, and choice of health plan all point to the importance of ethical issues in health policy (Randel et al, 2001). Indeed, managed care organizations and health policy makers may have disregarded the importance of these issues until repeatedly emphasized by public opinion precisely because of the failure of these agents to appreciate the ethical underpinnings of their policies.

This book constitutes an important landmark. It literally connects the two hitherto separate and antagonistic cultures of health policy and bioethics. Symbolically, its editors—and conference hosts—come from the worlds of health policy and bioethics, and represent some of the federal government's primary initiatives in these areas. In addition, the book began as a conference that brought together some of the nation's leading health policy makers and political philosophers and bioethicists. The conference required bioethicists to engage health policy makers and vice versa.

There are two additional substantive elements that bode well for linking health policy and bioethics more closely. The first, and probably more important, is the fact that the bioethicists who contributed to this work went beyond abstract principles. They are bioethicists who have begun to understand the complexities of the health care system; they have first-hand experience of working with managed care organizations, pharmacy benefits management companies, and other key health system actors, and they have conducted case studies of actual allocation decisions. Consequently, they have begun to address real allocation problems that arise on both the finance and delivery sides of the system—the kinds of questions that confront chief medical officers, benefits managers, and purchasers. While their work may still strike some health policy makers as too abstract and philosophical in the pejorative sense, it is grounded in the facts of the real world. In this way, the ethics-related work connects more closely to actual problems of the system. It is hard for the work to be dismissed as merely armchair philosophizing. Similarly, the health policy makers were asked to look beyond the facts and reason about the underlying values and how they affect policies. They explore not only the "is" but also the "ought."

Fifteen years ago the well-known health economist Rashi Fein argued that

> the federal budget is not only an economic but a social document through which [our shared] values are expressed. The expenditure and revenue numbers in the budget represent our collective decision about programs and priorities.
>
> Fein, 1986, 220

Similarly, all decisions about the allocation of resources involve setting priorities that inevitably express values. Ultimately, this book is an attempt to clarify how values affect both the process and the content of health care policy decisions. By beginning to bridge the gap between health policy makers and bioethicists, the book should foster better health policy and better bioethics.

REFERENCES

Beauchamp TL and Childress JF (1994) *Principles of Biomedical Ethics, 4th Edition.* New York: Oxford University Press.

Emanuel E (1991) *The Ends of Human Life*. Cambridge, MA: Harvard University Press.

Fein R (1986) *Medical Care, Medical Costs*. Cambridge, MA: Harvard University Press.

Fuchs VR (1996) Economics, values, and health care reform. American Economic Review. 86:1–24.

Randel L, Pearson SD, Hyams TR, Sabin J, Emanuel E (2001) How managed care can be ethical. *Health Affairs* 20:43–56.

Snow CP (1959) *The Two Cultures and the Scientific Revolution. Lecture I.* Cambridge: Cambridge University Press.

Titlow K, Randel L, Clancy CM, Emanuel EJ (2000) Drug coverage decisions: The role of dollars and values. *Health Aff (Millwood)* 19:240–7.

Walzer M (1983) *Spheres of Justice*. New York: Basic Books.

Williams B (1997) The idea of equality. In: Goodin R and Pettit P (eds) *Contemporary Political Philosophy: An Anthology*. Oxford: Blackwell Publishers.

Acknowledgments

To appreciate those who helped in the development of this volume requires some insight into its evolution. In 1997 we first explored the possibility of collaborating to study and strengthen the connections between ethics and health policy. Our efforts were wholeheartedly supported by John Eisenberg at the Agency for Healthcare Research and Quality and Ezekiel Emanuel at the Department of Clinical Bioethics in the Clinical Center of the National Institutes of Health. Their excitement about the potential to expand the opportunities for collaboration among those interested in health care policy and ethics was a critical inspiration for this work. Without their endorsement the effort would not have been possible. We also approached Lew Sandy at the Robert Wood Johnson Foundation, whose support was equally indispensable.

We began with a planning meeting in June of 1998 to which we invited a group of about 20 leaders in ethics and health policy to help us formulate a research agenda and plans for a larger conference. Victor Fuchs was helpful in laying the groundwork for the discussion through his opening remarks. The advice of this group helped us formulate a list of key issues that needed to be addressed. This initial work determined the preliminary outline for the book. In October of 1999 we held a conference, "Connecting Ethics and Health Policy," at which many of the contributors to this volume spoke.

As we focused our attention on developing this book, Donald Patrick suggested that we contact Jeff House at Oxford University Press. We are grateful for his recommendation and for Jeff House's enthusiastic response. We appreciate the comments of several anonymous reviewers who suggested that the volume would have a fuller perspective if various participants in the process of health care policy contributed to it. Hence the addition of the third part of the book.

We particularly appreciated the editorial help of Amy Sepinwall, who served as a research assistant while she was a graduate student in the philosophy department at Georgetown University. We also thank Becky Chen for her administrative support and Terri Jacobs for her secretarial support.

Finally, we are indebted to John Gallin, whose vision created the Department of Clinical Bioethics at the National Institutes of Health. He has given the department unswerving support for pursuing the highest scholarship regarding all aspects of bioethics and the intellectual exchanges reflected in this book.

While we thank those individuals who provided their support, the opinions expressed in this book are those of the contributing authors exclusively and do not reflect the policies of the National Institutes of Health, the Agency for Healthcare Research and Quality, or the Department of Health and Human Services.

Contents

Ethical Considerations of Health Services Research

Contributors

M. Gregg Bloche, J.D.
Georgetown University Law School
Georgetown University
Washington, D.C.

Jo Ivey Boufford, M.D.
Robert F. Wagner Graduate School of Public Service
New York University
New York, NY

Dan W. Brock, Ph.D.
Department of Philosophy
Brown University
Providence, RI

Lawrence D. Brown, Ph.D.
Department of Health Policy and Management
Columbia University
New York, NY

Stuart Butler, PhD
Heritage Foundation
Washington, DC

Daniel Callahan, Ph.D.
The Hastings Center
Garrison, NY

Christine K. Cassel, M.D.
Department of Geriatrics
Mount Sinai Medical Center
New York, NY

Larry R. Churchill, Ph.D.
Department of Social Medicine
Center for Health Ethics and Policy
University of North Carolina at Chapel Hill
Chapel Hill, NC

Carolyn Clancy, M.D.
Center for Outcomes and Effectiveness Research
Agency for Healthcare Research and Quality
Rockville, MD

NORMAN DANIELS, PH.D.
Department of Philosophy
Tufts University
Medford, MA

MARION DANIS, M.D.
Section on Ethics and Health policy
Department of Clinical Bioethics
Warren G. Magnuson Clinical Center
National Institutes of Health
Bethesda, MD

EZEKIEL J. EMANUEL, M.D., PH.D.
Department of Clinical Bioethics
National Institutes of Health
Bethesda, MD

ELI GINZBERG, PH.D.
The Eisenhower Center for the Conservation of Human Resources
Columbia University
New York, NY

STANLEY B. GREENBERG, PH.D.
Greenberg Quinlin Rosner Research
Washington, DC

AMY GUTMANN, PH.D.
University Center for Human Values
Princeton University
Princeton, NJ

LISA I. IEZZONI, M.D., MSC
Division of General Medicine and Primary Care
Harvard Medical School
Boston, MA

ICHIRO KAWACHI, M.D., PH.D.
Center for Society and Health
Harvard School of Public Health
Boston, MA

BRUCE KENNEDY, PH.D.
Center for Society and Health
Harvard School of Public Health
Boston, MA

JOHN W. KINGDON, PH.D.
University of Michigan
Ann Arbor, MI

PHILIP R. LEE, M.D.
Stanford University Program in Human Biology
Stanford University
Stanford, CA

BERNARD LO, M.D.
Program in Medical Ethics
University of California at San Francisco
San Francisco, CA

HAROLD S. LUFT, PH.D.
Institute for Health Policy Studies
University of California at San Francisco
San Francisco, CA

RUTH E. MALONE, PH.D., R.N.
Institute for Health Policy Studies and Department of Physiological Nursing
University of California at San Francisco
San Francisco, CA

ELAINE MCPARLAND, M.D., J.D.
Rye, NY

JONATHAN OBERLANDER, PH.D.
Department of Social Medicine
University of North Carolina at Chapel Hill
Chapel Hill, NC

DONALD L. PATRICK, PH.D.
Department of Health Services
University of Washington
Seattle, WA

LEWIS G. SANDY, M.D.
Robert Wood Johnson Foundation
Princeton, NJ

DENNIS THOMPSON, PH.D.
Program in Ethics and the Professions
Harvard University
Cambridge, MA

Introduction

MARION DANIS,
CAROLYN CLANCY, AND
LARRY R. CHURCHILL

Among the hardest of societies' challenges in determining health policies is to identify the values and goals that frame them. Making policies in legitimate ways so they are a fair expression of a society's constituents is a monumental task. Without attention to these values and legitimate processes, nations are likely to have health policies that do not meet their expectations.

The purpose of this book is to explore how to develop health policies that fairly represent the views and needs of all stakeholders. We examine what goals to strive for in setting health policy and consider how stakeholders might negotiate differences, how various key participants in society contribute to making policy, and how some of the more contentious policy issues might be approached. The exploration of these ethical dimensions of health policy should kindle the interest of anyone who is seriously concerned with how a society goes about planning for the health of its residents.

Several dramatic forces have influenced health policy during the past 15 to 20 years. Striking increases in health-care spending have stimulated many stakeholders to question the return for substantial investments in health-care and have reinforced their interest in accountability. Changes in demographics and the growing prevalence of chronic diseases have altered the health-care needs of the population. Dramatic changes in the structure of health-care delivery, such as consolidation of health-care organizations and the move to managed care, have shifted the locus of decision making and have exacerbated concern about its fairness. Shifting views about the proper balance between the public and private sector and about the balance of power between federal and state governments have changed the locus and responsibility for planning and implementing policies.

Concerns about the quality and safety of health care and the status of the health of the public have not gone unaddressed. Efforts to assure the quality and outcomes of health care have included multiple attempts at legislation to regulate health care and many court cases that have considered the locus of responsibility for treatment decisions. What has received far less attention is how individual and societal values can be incorporated into framing, shaping, and implementing health policy. Demand for a patients' bill of rights is a clear manifestation of an unresolved debate about the values underlying health-care policy. In short, changes in health-care financing and delivery make the need to connect ethics and health policy even more apparent.

Along with the dramatic changes in health-care delivery has come another revolutionary change. Unprecedented information technology and access to data make it possible for health services researchers to examine the outcomes of health-care practices and policies in ways that were never possible before. This expanded research capacity creates sharp ethical tensions between the right to privacy of personal health information and the potential for developing knowledge that can benefit large numbers of individuals. In addition, an understanding of the goals of health care is crucial to the conduct of well-focused research. Part of the agenda for this book thus pertains to the recognition that deciding which outcomes to measure in research can influence which issues receive priority in health-care delivery and financing.

While particular policy developments are specific to the moment, the focus of the book is intended to be more enduring. We hope to provide a perspective that stimulates thought about how the ethical dimensions of health-care policy can be more explicitly engaged. The focus is thus intended to be attentive to but transcendent of the particulars. We explore questions that constantly need to be addressed and readdressed about who should be given authority and responsibility for making policy decisions, and how the benefits of limited resources should be distributed.

Of course, the health status of a population is determined by more than the health-care delivery system alone. Access to food and shelter, income distribution, the management of natural resources, the provision of education, and the safety of transportation and the workplace all have important influences on a population's health status. While these factors have not been considered traditionally under the domain of health policy, health-care decision makers cannot ignore the reality that the health status of the population is not exclusively within their purview. To maximize health thus requires that those responsible for health policy work with other public policy makers. The tension between what is known about the broad determinants of health and what is focused upon in the health policy arena may be apparent to readers as they progress through the book. While the authors who focus on goals at the beginning of the volume recognize the broad determinants, those authors who address roles in policy making take a narrower focus on health care. This tension reflects the state of health-care policy making and points to the need of the field to evolve in the future.

Attention to the challenges we address is growing, particularly in the international arena. The identification and use of benchmarks for fair health-care reform have begun to occur in several countries (Daniels et al, 1996). Efforts to set societal priorities for guaranteeing health and access to health care is a concern of many national governments and international organizations, from the World Health Organization to the International Society for Priority Setting in Health (Coulter and Ham, 2000). If this book contributes to scholarship focused on the ethical dimensions of health policy, then it will serve the larger purpose of facilitating the exploration of worthwhile goals for health policy and promoting the accomplishment of these goals.

The skeptic might argue that discussion of the ethics of health-care policy is a futile endeavor because we cannot agree about the goals for health-care delivery. Radically different philosophies exist about how to prioritize the delivery of health-care services equitably and efficiently to whole populations, how to balance equity and efficiency with individual choice, and how great a role government should play in the funding and delivery of health care. For example, in response to cost containment pressures, market driven health care has stimulated demands for information on the cost effectiveness of alternative interventions. Explicit quantification of costs and benefits highlights previously obscured tensions between individual and population benefits. For instance, how do we value maintaining function for a disabled individual compared with providing preventive care to children? How do we address the preferences of individuals with no effective or cost-effective treatment options? Lack of a coherent framework that can incorporate principles of equity with economic concerns presents a formidable barrier to the use of cost-effectiveness analysis to inform decision making in the 21st century.

Yet, despite the difficulty of the questions and the disparity in philosophical views, the identification of goals and priorities cannot wait indefinitely and need not aim at unanimity of opinion. If we can find clear grounds for discussion and an ethical framework for assessing the implications of policy options, we will have taken a substantial and helpful step forward. Even more important than integrating the work of ethicists and clinicians or identifying approaches for making the health policy–making process inclusive, then, is the goal of determining just what the aims and content of health policies ought to be. This book is thus an effort to examine the ethical dimensions of health policy. Such an examination involves consideration of who makes policy, what goals they wish to achieve, how they negotiate differences, and how these goals get translated into effective strategies for health-care delivery.

Ethical Dimensions of Health Policy is organized in four parts. The first part focuses on identifying the goals of health care. Daniel Callahan provides a clear discussion of what the goals of health care ought to be. He builds on his long history of thinking about health-care goals, particularly those for the international arena. He argues that the goals of medicine should be tempered by concern for their sustainability and considers whether goals should vary with circumstances or ought to be immutable. Following this consideration of the goals of health-care, Norman Daniels, Bruce Kennedy, and Ichiro Kawachi discuss how we should attend to the growing realization that health care is far from the major determinant of health status. In light of this reality, how should health policy experts attend to the other important determinants of health? They suggest that, to the extent that the rationale for providing health care lies in attempting to provide equal opportunities through efforts to achieve species typical function for members of society, we cannot ignore those factors that, in addition to health care, contribute to health status.

After this discussion of the goals of health care, the second part of the book focuses on how we can proceed to connect ethical considerations with the making of health policy. Larry Churchill discusses at greater length the rationale for connecting ethics and health policy, emphasizing much of the reasoning that we have suggested in these introductory remarks. Having established some arguments for connecting ethics and health policy, the book turns to a historical perspective. Eli Ginzberg highlights aspects of health-care policy making in 20th century U.S. history and examines some of the ethical assumptions that lay more or less explicitly behind these policies. After this retrospective look, Amy Gutmann and Dennis Thompson consider how we could proceed in order to develop policies in the fairest way possible. Building on their prior work on deliberative democracy, they discuss how we might use such a deliberative process to make rationing decisions in managed care and other health-care organizations. Their approach is useful for developing policy in the face of existing disagreements.

Many parties and stakeholders contribute to health policy. In the third part of the book we consider the ethical ramifications of their efforts. We examine the role of legislative politics, public opinion, the courts, federal and state policy makers, and the private sector. John Kingdon, who has studied how policy in fact, gets made, writes the first chapter in this part. The insights from his empirical research as a political scientist offer those interested in making policy an invaluable understanding of the process. He highlights the need to be prepared to take advantage of opportunities for making policy by having well-developed solutions ready for opportune moments. Stan Greenberg and Marion Danis write about the role of public opinion in making health policy and the role of opinion polling in incorporating the public's views into policy making. They consider how polling compares to other strategies for incorporating the public's views into decision making. Gregg Bloche writes about the role of ethical reasoning in court decisions concerning the provision of health care. He argues that institutional constraints limit judges' freedom to draw upon ethical analysis but that ethics can contribute much more than it has. Next the book focuses on the balance of power between the federal and state governments in the United States. Jo Ivey Boufford and Phillip Lee consider the role the federal government plays in the complex mosaic of health care in the United States, while Jonathan Oberlander and Larry Brown explore the role of state governments. Oberlander and Brown examine the way state governments control the cost of public insurance programs, the role of the marketplace in delivering care in publicly funded programs, and the responsibility of government in shaping the medical marketplace. Finally, in this part, Stuart Butler writes about the role the private sector plays in making health policy and how legislation can facilitate more or less effective participation of the private sector in just health-care delivery.

In Part IV some of the key areas of ethical controversy intrinsic to making policy are addressed. The authors explore ethical approaches to policy questions about resource allocation, accountability, the needs of vulnerable populations, and the conduct of health services research. This part begins with Ezekiel Emanuel's exploration of an ethical approach for resolving the tension between individual and population-based needs. In their chapter on accountability, Christine Cassel and Elaine MacParland propose that the practice of medicine has become so complex, with so many competing perspectives and goals, that it is best to view medicine as a public good. As such, the best way to oversee its functions may be akin to the way we oversee the functions of various utilities. They thus suggest the possibility of regulating medicine as a public good, accountable to the public.

Ruth Malone and Harold Luft address questions of accountability in the more circumscribed arena of the doctor–patient relationship. In this context they suggest a set of criteria to which this relationship should be held accountable. They then propose a model of accountability that suggests that health-care services be centered around groups of clinicians who join together on the basis of shared philosophies of medical practice. When strong scientific evidence is available on which to base standards of care, practice should adhere to the standard approach. When less evidence is available, accountability would permit providers more leeway so that their philosophy and paitent preferences would have more influence on treatment decisions.

Daniel Brock explores, from the standpoint of moral philosophy, whether we owe vulnerable individuals special attention when we set priorities in health-care delivery. Adopting an egalitarian argument for equality of opportunity based on Daniels's theory of just health care, Brock argues for special attention to the vulnerable. He explores what the limits of this priority should be.

Marion Danis and Donald Patrick take a different approach to vulnerability. They argue that vulnerability is a universal phenomenon. While some populations are more at risk or vulnerable than others, in their view philosophical arguments for fair attention to vulnerability are most soundly based on a universal conception of vulnerability because it leads to less partisanship in understanding and discussing what is owed to whom. Based on this argument, policy for allocating health-care resources that takes into account health status, age, and socioeconomic status is developed.

Lisa Iezzoni and Bernard Lo each tackle pressing ethical issues in health services research that arise as it functions to provide a scientific basis for health-care delivery. Lisa Iezzoni delineates features of health services research that differ from more traditional research and argues that these differences have several ethical implications. In particular, individuals may never be aware of their inclusion in population-based data collection. The distinction between research and monitoring of patient care is thus often blurred. Given this reality, investigators may be obliged to more scrupulously justify the need for person-specific information, clarify who owns the data, and account for the possibility that seemingly unobtrusive studies may affect on clinically important outcomes. Bernard Lo explores strategies for setting research priorities in health services research. He considers the ethical implications of how we define health services research, and how our values shape the agenda and methods of health services research.

The contributors to this book do not all agree with one another. While Amy Gutmann and Dennis Thompson argue for making issues explicit, John Kingdon warns that doing so can make commonly agreeable plans hard to achieve. The strategies that Luft and Malone suggest might be considered antithetical to those that Cassel and MacParland propose. But they may also be viewed as complementary. To the extent that medicine is practiced through private arrangements but also serves the good of all, various models of accountability may be worthwhile.

We hope that this book will contribute to the growth of a lively and fruitful body of interdisciplinary scholarship in ethics and health policy that will prepare us to find equitable ways to address health-care needs and health-related priorities that perennially seem to outstrip resources. If we can accomplish this goal, we will be better equipped to anticipate the pressing priority questions about health and health care in the early decades of this century.

REFERENCES

Coulter A, Ham C (2000) *The Global Challenge of Health Care Rationing*. Buckingham: Open University Press.

Daniels N, Light D, Caplan R (1996) *Benchmarks for Fairness in Health Care Reform*. New York: Oxford University Press.

I

Identifying the goals of health care

1

Ends and means: the goals of health care

DANIEL CALLAHAN

Pluralistic societies, reflecting diversity and a love of freedom, have characteristically been wary of efforts to achieve agreement on goals and ends. Often enough, this wariness occurs even in ethics. Yet if ethics is to make a serious contribution to health policy, it must focus its attention as much on the substantive ends of medicine and health care as on the moral means of attaining them. The current ends of medicine and health care ensure not only that health policy will face intractable resource dilemmas and economic unsustainability, they ensure no less that the prevention of illness and the care of the sick will have no reflective goals. In particular, if justice is a primary aspiration for health care, then what kind of health care will be most conducive to making that possible? A health policy such as we have now, which has indiscriminately declared all-out war on death and disease, cannot be a sustainable policy.

To speak at all sensibly on a topic as sweeping as "the goals of health care" requires beginning at the beginning and working out from there. And a common way to start such a venture is to define one's terms. Yet while it is possible to have endless debates on most of the terms used in this chapter, I will simply stipulate my meanings, hoping that they come reasonably close to common usage (Nordenfeldt, 1999).

The goal of health care is that of health. The means to pursue health are socioeconomic change, medicine, and public health. Socioeconomic conditions are important for the preservation and improvement of health and should surely enter into any broad scheme of health care, but I will touch upon that topic only lightly here, defining health care for the purposes of this chapter a little more narrowly: Health care consists of the organized methods used by a society to promote the health of its members, ordinarily encompassing the fields of public health and medicine. A society's health policy will be the organization of those methods into some overall financial and distributional structure designed to pursue the general goals of health care and, ultimately, of health. Health might best and most simply be defined as an individual's experience of well-being and integrity of mind and body. It is characterized by an acceptable absence of malady and consequently by a person's ability to pursue his or her vital goals and to function in ordinary social and work contexts. This definition puts to one side the famous World Health Organization (WHO) definition of health as encompassing "complete social well-being," an implausible and hazardous health care aim.

The WHO definition would, in principle, make medicine and health care responsible for all human welfare. That is an impossible task for them, and, even worse, it invites distraction from the wide range of causes of social ills such as poverty, injustice, and poor government.

My definition is also meant to make room for age-relative standards of health, out of a recognition that, with aging, there will be a decline in many physical and some mental capabilities but that a person can be considered in "good health" for his or her years despite that decline. It would make no sense to have the same health expectations for someone 90 years of age as one would have for that same person at age 9. To do so would be to act as if the process of aging simply did not exist.

Why should we give any special thought at all to the goals of health care? Don't we already know what they are? Not necessarily. It is reasonable to expect that the next few decades will witness enormous gains in biomedical knowledge and technological development. These gains will force a reexamination of many, if not most, features of current medicine and health care, including the priorities among its goals. They will also force a scrutiny of the penumbra of issues and assumptions surrounding them—namely, our understanding of health, the role of medicine, the extent of the social obligation to provide health care, and the place of health in relation to other social goods. Shaping the contents of a health policy that embodies the shifting priorities and often subtle changes in the interpretation of health-care goals will raise many inescapable ethical problems.

I begin, then, with three premises. First is that the ends of health care ought to be as much a part of the ethical enterprise as the means chosen to achieve them. Second is that the ends of health care should embody some larger view of the human condition and the place the pursuit of health should have in promoting human welfare. Third is that, while pluralism and a diversity of visions should command respectful deference, it will be important to achieve at least a rough political consensus on the appropriate goals of health care, without which there can be no effective policy.

My purpose is to lay out the ingredients necessary to devise morally defensible goals for health care and then use my own approach as one illustration of the way content may be given to the framework I have set forth. If I am minimally successful, I will have presented a plausible general direction in which to proceed in thinking about goals. If I am maximally successful, my specifications for giving the general framework some detailed content might just seem plausible, as well.

While I will attempt to show why a discussion of goals is insistently necessary now, mention should be made of some problems in pursuing the subject. A perennial problem seems to be the American temperament, which is much more comfortable in fashioning health policy, or any kind of policy, using the language of management techniques and economic efficiency, of money and incentives, and of practical matters of making policies work, than with the articulation of clear health-care goals.

A second problem is that the Supreme Court has historically resisted reaching final decisions about constitutionality, preferring to resolve legal crises at lower levels. So also, analogously, there is resistance to public debate about the meaning of life and death, of suffering, of the definition of health, and other old, complex questions that run as deep, often underground rivers through all health policy. Those topics appear to make many people nervous. They are perceived to be too religious, too philosophical, too general, too controversial, too boring, or too abstract. Nonetheless, those risks have to be run with health care, and I will do my best to avoid the twin dangers of other-worldly abstraction, on the one hand, and a tiresome array of distinctions and qualifications, on the other.

SOME NECESSARY DISTINCTIONS

Some preliminary distinctions are necessary, not all of which I will follow through on in detail, but all of which need to be mentioned as part of the larger task of defining the goals of health care. I begin by defining my topic more precisely: It is to specify the goals of health care, the relationship of those goals to the fashioning of the goals of health policy, and the way ethics might best fit into such deliberations. Why not, however, simply specify the goals of health policy? Now for the first distinction: It makes no sense to talk of the goals of health policy without, as a prior step, taking on the goals of health care; and, for that matter, going one level deeper and asking what we should mean by *health* and why it is an important human good.

The second necessary distinction is this: When we speak of health care and its ends, should those ends be determined by an inductive effort to discover the de facto ends of American health care—what we do as opposed to what we say—or should we move at once to the normative level, aiming to determine what those ends ought to be? A direct move to the latter level, which might initially seem most obvious if ethics is the focus, runs the risk of ignoring deeply imbedded tacit values of health care that remain forceful because of the various reinforcements they provide for the more explicit values.

A third distinction is that between the goals of medicine and the goals of health care. Medicine is the historically prior institution, and its goals in practice determined for many centuries what health care became available (and long before the concept of health care was devised). With the advent of a public health perspective much later, and then of organized social and political systems designed to improve health by deploying both medicine and public health, it became possible to speak of health care as the generic category for all efforts, medical and otherwise, to protect and foster good health. Nonetheless, even if medicine can now be subsumed under the broader category of health care, its scientific knowledge and ability to determine (usually, if not always) the biological pathways of disease give it a central role in health care. Medicine remains the fundamental discipline of health care.

The most recent addition to this array of nested concepts has been that of the socioeconomic determinants of health and illness and their implications for the improvement of health (Evans et al, 1984). They should surely be understood as demanding a role in health policy, even though they are outside health care systems as customarily understood.

A fourth distinction turns on the debate about whether medicine as a profession and discipline has inherent ends endemic to its practice or whether it is a social construct, ever open to reconstruction (Pellegrino, 1999). It is surely the case that, almost by definition, the provision of health care is a social practice, and the policies that shape those practices are social constructs. Many ways of organizing health-care systems exist, and, in that respect, they are malleable political artifacts. Yet this malleability might complicate our search for health care ends. For, if we think of medicine as having inherent ends, then we have one type of institution, with more fixed goals, placed inside another type of institution, a health care system, with variable and readily reconstructed goals.

The fifth and final distinction is that between our current and future concerns regarding health-care allocation. We need to consider how to divide the scientific and technological knowledge, skills, and therapies now available to health care and those that could and should be made available in the future through biomedical, behavioral, and socioeconomic research. Research produces those goods (to speak generically) that have the potential not only to change health profiles in the future, but also, as an indirect consequence, to change cultural concepts of health and the role of medicine. It also has provided different understandings of the ends of health care and its shaping policies.

MOTIVATING INQUIRY INTO THE GOALS OF HEALTH CARE AND MEDICINE

Why is a reconsideration of the goals of health care and medicine now necessary? The likely impact of new biomedical knowledge and technological innovation, already mentioned, is surely one reason, but there are others as well. Most health-care systems in the world are facing steadily heavier economic pressures, forcing a variety of reforms that require (usually covert) rationing and other restrictions on the provision of health care. A turn to the market is one consequence in many places, and a consideration of priority-setting is still another (Callahan, 1999). Changes of the kind just described can affect the formal goals of health care (e.g., a strong market approach can make choice rather than health the aim of a health-care system), while a move to setting priorities will set up a hierarchy of subgoals within some general framework of goals.

The goals of health care need reconsideration, then, because of the part they play within the broader goals of health policy. A market approach in health policy will have a potent impact on the doctor–patient relationship, as will any rationing policy that forces physicians to deny some forms of medical care to their patients. The rise of chronic disease as a corollary of aging societies requires a reexamination of the relative priority to be given to curing and caring in research and resource allocation. The fact of aging societies and the possibility of competition among different age groups for scarce resources suggest an urgent need to ask whether the goals of medicine for the elderly should be the same as those for the young, with policy age-blind in its resource allocation.

The growing attraction of a medicine that could enhance human capacities and capabilities rather than simply restore or maintain some traditional level of health obviously raises questions about what the most appropriate goals are for health care (Parens, 1999). The so-called medicalization of many problems once considered nonmedical, such as substance abuse (explained only in part by a possible biological basis to addiction), leads to the question of the scope of medicine in responding to human suffering not obviously biological in origin, and that question, in turn, forces consideration of the scope of health care. Changing cultural attitudes toward the reduction of heath risks and constant improvement of medical outcomes aiming for a kind of medical utopia are no less important in motivating a fresh inquiry into goals.

A final motivation for a reexamination of the goals of health care would be to take better account of the increasing knowledge of the socioeconomic determinants of health. As matters now stand, medical treatments and cures are sought for many health conditions that might be greatly reduced by such nonmedical strategies as improvements in education, employment, and the environment. The traditional medical goal of treating the sick would remain, but a greater emphasis would fall not only on public health but also on improving those social conditions known to affect health. The aim would be (as it has been put) to intervene in the "upstream" sources of disease and illness and, by changing them, avert the need for medical interventions "downstream" (Daniels et al, 1999).

SPECIFYING THE GOALS OF HEALTH CARE

Having provided that set of prefatory clarifications, I believe the best place to begin an examination of the goals of health care is with the goals of medicine, for not only do those goals have historical priority, they have also focused on those conditions of an individual's body and mind that have occasioned the abiding interest in health. Accordingly, I will begin with the goals of medicine and then expand those goals to encompass public health. Together, they encompass the goals of health care. The borderlines among these different focal points are not clear cut, however, and I would not want to be understood as suggesting anything close to air-tight compartments. Like all typologies, this one is meant to put the world into some kind of order; and the world, as always, is not nearly so accommodating as are our invented categories.

Medicine as a discipline arose in response to the finitude of the human body. It is a body subject to disease and illness, to aging and decay, to accidents and frailty. Along with the maladies of the body, there are an array of mental and emotional aberrations capable of producing miseries competitive with those imposed by a dysfunctional body. It is at least imaginable that one or more, or many more, of these bodily and mental burdens can and will be cured or effectively relieved in the future, but it is only in the realm of science fiction that there could exist bodies or minds totally free of such maladies or their threats. It is thus the broad aim of medicine to find ways of dealing with those maladies, by cure or amelioration.

To specify the goals of medicine is to seek the right fit between (*1*) the human desire to avoid illness, suffering, and death and (*2*) the capacity of medicine as a combination of science and clinical skills to do something, within the boundaries of its professional competence and integrity, about those evils.

There are a variety of possible ways, of specifying those goals, but I will here draw upon a three-year project of which I was a part and whose purpose was to specify those goals (The Hastings Center, 1996). Our method was to examine the historical goals, to identify present practices that embodied different goals and practices (we identified at least 40), and then to seek a plausible blend of the old and the new. Characteristically, the goals distilled by this process were, in keeping with the most ancient traditions, focused on the care and treatment of individuals, not of populations. Indeed, the continuity with the past was most strikingly singled out by the absence of population-oriented goals in contemporary expressions of appropriate goals. I will now turn to the four goals that emerged from our examination as the most plausible, reflecting both the past and the present.

The Prevention of Disease and Injury and the Promotion of Health

While it is sometimes thought that this is a relatively modern goal, the writings of Hippocrates give it a strong place, one that was carried down through the generations, though with varying degrees of intensity. Its purpose as a formal goal of medicine is to serve the overarching good of health, recognizing that it is as valuable to prevent threats of illness as to relieve those threats once they manifest themselves.

The Relief of Pain and Suffering

Typically, the first manifestations of physical or mental disease are physical pain and psychological distress, often to the point of suffering. Pain and suffering are not identical, since each can exist without the other, but they commonly move in tandem. It is pain and/or suffering that usually brings patients to physicians and, if nothing else can be accomplished, their diminishment or relief are basic goals to be sought.

The Care and Cure of Those with a Malady and the Care of Those Who Cannot Be Cured

This goal is stated in the form of a tension embodying two ideals. One ideal, more modern than ancient in its feasibility and intensity, is to find the biological or other cause of pain and suffering and to eliminate or otherwise neutralize that cause, that is, to cure the patient. The other ideal is to provide comfort, rehabilitation, or other means whereby an illness or disability can be tolerated and the highest possible degree of accommodation with ordinary functioning achieved. A tension exists between these two ideals because cure cannot always be achieved but ought always initially to be sought, and must, when not found, give way to the ancient caring function of medicine.

The Avoidance of a Premature Death and the Pursuit of a Peaceful Death

This goal also is expressed as a tension, here between the aim of preventing a premature death in an individual and the realization that, since death comes eventually to everyone, the physician should strive to make that death as peaceful as possible. The tension comes from the uncertainty, intensified by contemporary medicine, of knowing when death should be accepted. Technological progress has rendered the line between living and dying ever more tenuous, in great part because a growing number of ways exist to give a critically ill patient a few more hours, or days, or weeks of life. The ideal of prolonging life and the ideal of a peaceful death are both strong. The difficulty, which shows no sign of abatement, comes in knowing when to invoke one rather than the other.

SETTING PRIORITIES AMONG THE GOALS

While much more could be said of each of these goals, three comments are in order, each in answer to a question. First, should there be a context-free set of priorities among these goals? Second, are there some de facto biases in the current priorities given to the four goals? Third, what are some of the obstacles and threats to devising a reasonable set of priorities in different historical contexts?

While it might seem attractive, and even necessary, to set permanent priorities among the goals of medicine, that effort turns out to be generally unwise. Health promotion and disease prevention make little sense as goals for patients who are terminally ill, nor is cure a meaningful goal if a patient is well. Instead, while it can be said that the goals of medicine as specified above are ultimate, their deployment in particular historical contexts is best understood as proximate and contingent.

The question always to be asked is this: What is the appropriate priority with this patient at this time? There are a number of advantages of this approach: It forces a careful examination of individual patient needs, it allows for a change in goals as the patient's condition changes, and it helps to neutralize the constant and familiar hazard of rote, or automatic, treatment patterns that would otherwise be offered regardless of patient needs. Even the goal of relieving pain and suffering, which is important for all patients, could admit of a temporary lower priority in the case of a treatment that would bring time-limited pain for an eventual health gain (such as a bone marrow transplant that aimed to preserve life).

The same way of thinking is appropriate for specifying the goals of health policy, in particular that of determining the most pressing health needs at the present moment even while being ready to change those goals when the circumstances change. A century ago it seemed self-evidently valuable to go after those infectious diseases that randomly killed children and young adults in large numbers. A reduction in mortality was appropriate as the highest goal when most people died before reaching old age. But that aim has been virtually achieved, and different priorities in setting goals are gradually becoming appropriate in most developed countries.

On the matter of de facto biases, a major complaint is that health promotion and disease prevention have systematically been given a place of low priority both in the care of patients and in setting research priorities. The chief culprit has been a bias in favor of cure, which has too often been seen as the highest goal of medicine in most circumstances. It is a bias that has led to a disproportionate amount of money being spent on biomedical rather than behavioral research, on the one hand, and to an emphasis in clinical practice on treatment rather than on patient education, on the other. An obviously important aim of setting proximate, context-dependent goals for medicine would be to counteract outdated goals and open the way for new priorities. The recent effort to give palliative care new force and sophistication is an example of this possibility.

Politics and Priority-Setting

While it might seem obvious that the setting and prioritizing of goals would be a wise move as part of setting health policy, some subtle and not-so-subtle pressures mitigate against doing so. The least noxious of those pressures arises from the play of politics and pluralism. It is better, many believe, to leave deep and possibly divisive matters safely buried away. Pragmatic concerns frequently engender resistance not only to the setting of formal goals but also to any concrete attempt to prioritize them. For many, particularly legislators, it is the give-and-take of politics, full of bargaining and compromise, that appears an attractive, less theoretical way to fashion policy. The setting of priorities means, moreover, that there will be winners and losers—but it is important for the legislators that this reality be obscured to take the sting out of the losses and to act as if the winners are not taking something from the losers.

Admittedly, I speculate here, but that seems necessary in the face of an international pattern of great interest. Despite considerable public and legislative interest in recent years, only in the state of Oregon has a priority-setting policy actually been put into effect; otherwise, it has remained just talk, provocative enough, but still just talk (Ham, 1997). At the same time, while there has of late been a greater interest in a population-based public health approach to setting policy, it is rare to see this approach coupled with any proposal to give an individual-based, biomedical approach a lesser place. It is, in a word, uncommon for reform recommendations that call for a greater emphasis on a fresh health-care strategy to be coupled with an equally strong emphasis on cutting back more established approaches. Reform is not looked upon as a zero-sum game, even though it often must be.

If the political willingness to call for a more precise definition of goals and a prioritizing of them is rare, still other threats exist to a serious discussion of goals. A setting of goals is clearly easier in small, relatively homogeneous societies than in those that are large and pluralistic, and it is considerably more possible when there is a centralized governmental control of policy—that is, in a closed system. Indeed, in a society such as the United States, where there is a mixed public and private health care system with no central authority, the explicit setting of goals is nearly impossible except at the most local level. I say "nearly," for it is possible, on occasion, to achieve a political consensus on policy and to thereby set some new directions, as happened in 1965 with the passage of Medicare and Medicaid. In that case, the aim was to provide coverage to the elderly and the poor. As such, this aim did not involve changing any traditional goals of medicine. Instead, it formally introduced into American health policy the goal of special care for the poor and the old.

It has not, however, been possible to significantly push health policy much beyond the 1965 level. While there are many reasons this has not happened, I stress three in particular: (*1*) the important and growing role of the market, which plays to individual preference and works against strong and universal goals and policies of any kind; (*2*) the unabated drive for constant biomedical progress and technological innovation, which turns any and all research interests into goals; and (*3*) the concomitant increase in health care costs that the combination of progress and market forces brings about, which are typically responded to with managerial and economic techniques, not a reconsideration of goals.

While those developments logically speaking, might seem ideal circumstances in which to press forward the question of goals, in practice they make it difficult even to open such a discussion. Consequently, the fitful drive for universal health care has stalled once again. If that drive can be stimulated again, an articulation of the goals of health care will become imperative: aims and priorities will have to be set, limits fashioned, and the relationship of health to other public goods reexamined.

The Goals of Public Health

Together with medicine, public health is the other principal ingredient of health care. Are the goals of public health different from those of medicine (Institute of Medicine, 1988)? The answer is yes, even though overlap occurs. The characteristic mark of public health is its interest in population, not individual, health. While a population perspective is hardly indifferent to the health of individuals, its focus is on overall trends of mortality and morbidity and their causes. Epidemiology is the key discipline for the measurement of those trends, while a number of other disciplines work to assess the causes and outcomes of health-related activities. Traditionally, public health has focused its efforts on disease and infection surveillance, food safety and sanitary conditions, and, more recently, health promotion and disease prevention.

While health promotion and disease prevention have always had a place in medicine, it is nonetheless true that most of medicine's goals and its common practice focus on dealing with those who are sick or injured. Public health does not attempt to find cures for disease, though it often works with those who do. Public health has no equivalent to the caring function of medicine, which includes providing assistance and palliation to those whose sicknesses or disabilities cannot be cured. Public health has no place in the recent efforts to improve palliative care and end-of-life treatment.

Yet by looking to the health of populations instead of care at the bedside or in the doctor's office, public health is a necessary and invaluable partner in health care. Its goals complement those of medicine. No less importantly, if public health does its work well, it can help society reduce its burden of sick care. For example, an effective immunization program or an antismoking campaign can make a great, and often greater, contribution to the goal of health than can the provision of good medical care. The fresh emphasis on health promotion and disease prevention in primary care medicine, helped along by managed care, shows that this perception, while hardly new, is finally beginning to take hold. By asking the question of what health and social practices will make the greatest statistical improvements in mortality and morbidity rates rather than in individual benefits, a population perspective focuses a wide-area lens on health, and that is invaluable. The combination of the medical lens, focused on the individual, and the wide-area lens, focused on populations, constitutes the realm of health care.

SETTING THE PROXIMATE GOALS OF HEALTH CARE

I have suggested that while there can be universal and timeless goals of health care—if only because the body and the mind have needs that cut across all cultures and eras—health policy requires the setting of proximate goals. This means giving a more specific meaning to the general goals, specifying some subgoals, and setting priorities among them. I will put to one side the important political question of the procedures by which those proximate goals should be set, other than to say they should be accomplished by democratic procedures by a populace well informed about the health needs of the community. I will instead propose some ways in which the setting of goals can and should be tied intimately to ethics, reducing the possibility of a sharp gap between the ethics of ends and the ethics of means. I offer three policy directions toward that end bearing on the needs of subgroups in the population, on the enhancement of population health, and on the promotion of equitable health care.

Goals That Are Responsive to the Needs of Population Subgroups

For the purposes of policy, it is valuable to understand the full population of a society as made up of various subgroups, each of which will have some overlapping but also some different health-care needs. A basic respect for persons and a sensitivity to the variability in health needs of different population groups connects health-care goals and ethical demands. The most useful way to classify the subgroups is three-fold: by virtue of age, by virtue of economic status, and by virtue of racial, ethnic, sex, or other important social characteristics. To show how this might be done, I will paint only with the boldest strokes.

Age should make a vital difference in the understanding and prioritization of the four goals of medicine sketched above. Health promotion and disease prevention should have the highest priority with children, and here the role of public health measures and socioeconomic conditions is crucial. The point is to get children off to the best start possible, which will serve not only their childhood welfare but their welfare for rest of their lives as well. The cure of disease becomes comparatively more important in adulthood, when it is important to keep workers and parents alive and well-functioning for their own sake as well as for the well-working of their society. With the elderly, cure as a high-priority goal should give way to an increased emphasis on the relief of pain and suffering, rehabilitation, and palliative care in the face of chronic, ultimately fatal disease. Of course, it does not matter (for the aim of my argument) whether the reader agrees with my particular choice of goals for each age group; the point is to establish subgoals for each group based on a combination of health needs and social considerations.

The economic characteristics and disparities of different social groups is another obvious criterion for the establishment of subgoals. Money matters. It is not so much that poor children necessarily have health needs radically different from those found among more affluent children (low birth weight, for instance, will be found in both groups), but that their needs are more demanding and widespread. While health promotion is equally important for both groups, a stronger curative emphasis may be needed to compensate for poor socioeconomic conditions afflicting some groups. A similar kind of analysis may be appropriate in responding to racial, ethnic, and sex differences, shifting priorities to take account of different needs.

In each of these cases—age, economic status, and racial/ethnic/sex differences—the aim is to fashion goals that avoid setting inappropriate goals for different groups; that shape the goals to meet the special needs and social situations of different groups; and that seek to avoid, in the setting of goals, an exacerbation of existing health problems.

Goals That Enhance Population Health

The bias of American health care has been toward individual health. That bias is compatible both with the Hippocratic tradition, which puts individual patient welfare as its highest goal, and with American individualism, which is uncomfortable with most value systems that stress the common good. But ethics ought to encompass the welfare and vitality of entire communities as well, if only because the general welfare of a community influences the general welfare of each of its individual members. An excessive individualism fails to take account of the social life of communities and the interdependence of individuals. It has long been known that it is not high technology, cure-oriented medicine that best promotes population health. Instead, public health measures and socioeconomic improvement accounted for most of the reduction of mortality over the past century. That knowledge should lead to an obvious conclusion: goals and priorities oriented to population health should, in general, have the highest place in health care, in research, and in health policy. Yet this has not happened and may never happen. Measures that improve population health will not improve the health of everyone. Many people will get sick anyway, and for that reason ordinary medicine devoted to the cure of the sick and the relief of suffering will always play an important role. There is probably a basic, not fully resolvable tension here: population-oriented strategies have the compelling logic of likely success and overall health improvement in their favor, yet individual-oriented medicine, aimed at dealing with people who are sick, responds best to people's greatest fear, which is what will happen to them when health runs out, as it always does sooner or later.

As mortality declines for younger groups, it makes sense to shift the main goals of health care from their present de facto priorities, which are now heavily oriented toward cure. It is not that cure is irrelevant any longer; far from it. However, a persistent priority of cure leads to a medical perfectionism with diminishing health and economic benefits. By contrast, a shift in goals toward, first, improving the quality of health of the young and reducing their morbidity and disability burdens and, second, greater health promotion and disease prevention would aim to have people reach old age in the best possible physical and mental state. The viability of the idea of a compression of mortality depends on strategies that also have the advantage of benefits prior to old age.

Goals That Facilitate Equitable Health Care

There is widespread agreement that health care should be equitable, even if there is considerable disagreement about the best political and economic means of achieving that aim. Yet remarkably little notice has been taken of what is, I believe, a fundamental condition for future health-care equity: that the kind and quality of available health care be economically affordable. The current pursuit of unlimited medical progress, regardless of its potential cost, is in direct conflict with that condition. It has led to ever-increasing health-care costs and ever-higher aspirations for good health.

I offer as a primary example of this threat to equity the rising costs of pharmaceuticals. They are proving to be one of the main contributors to rising health-care costs. That rise is exacerbated by direct advertisements to consumers, by the development of expensive drugs that have only marginal health benefits, and by the argument on the part of pharmaceutical manufacturers that high costs are necessary to provide money to continue high-quality research. The inevitable result, it should now be obvious, is a steady growth in the number of uninsured individuals (traceable, in great part, to rising insurance costs), a steady rise in co-payments for drugs, and the inability of many people to pay for prescribed drugs. The trail to this result leads back, I am convinced, to the high priority given to individual health care and, consequently, the lower place given to health promotion and disease prevention. The research money invested in neonatal intensive care units, for instance, would be better spent (as has long been argued) to improve prenatal care to mothers. The money invested in expensive heart surgery for the elderly might better be invested in programs for the young designed to reduce heart disease, and so on.

My approach to the goals of health care has been dominated of late by the idea of developing sustainable medicine and health care (Callahan, 1999). By "sustainable" I mean health care that is economically affordable in the long run and equitably available to all. Our current health care is neither. It is gradually becoming unaffordable, as biomedical progress develops ever more costly treatments, and inequitable, in that rationing is imposed, but imposed on the poor and near-poor, not on those able to buy health care out of their own pockets. When the de facto ideal is unlimited progress and cure is the highest goal, then an ethic of equity is rendered almost impossible. Infinite aspirations cannot be met with finite resources, and the problem is present not only in the United States: The same forces are putting great pressures on the Canadian and western European universal health-care systems to reduce their benefits and to privatize parts of their systems.

The ultimate cause behind these pressures is not, as is commonly assumed, inefficiency (though there is still plenty of that), but instead a set of health-care goals that invites non-sustainability. They are, most notably, the goal of constant, unlimited, and open-ended progress combined with a focus on individual health benefits. Health policy reforms that look only to the mechanisms of policy are bound to fail without a parallel, overlapping reform of the goals of health care. And those goals must be reoriented in the direction of methods to help hold down costs, moderate desires for constant progress, and focus on population rather than individual health.

If sustainable health care were to become a high-priority policy goal, then it might be necessary to qualify the stress I have placed on determining goal priorities by determining the most urgent health care needs for any given historical moment. There are, in fact, two goals that would seem to command a high priority in almost every circumstance—health promotion and disease prevention programs for children and the relief of pain and suffering. The former seems to be required in order to start people out in life with the best possible health prospects, which will have long-term and life-long benefits, and the latter because medicine and health care will always fail at some point to provide cure or relief from illness. It is typically pain and suffering, the palpable symptoms of physical or psychological problems, that bring people to health care; it is the relief of those symptoms that has a prima facie claim upon resources. As with all matters of health care and health policy, then, balance must be sought, and the setting of priorities in the goals of health care will have to balance the claims of the moment against the long-term need for sustainability and the equity that would come with it.

There is obviously plenty of work to be done here and room for many arguments, but I will be satisfied if I have established the cogency of my main convictions. The most important is that it is no longer sensible to distinguish between the ends and means of health care. If equitable access is an aim of health policy, as it should be, it can only be brought about by devising goals of health care that make such access possible or (more minimally) that do not put obstacles in its way. If the improvement of the health of the population as a whole is the principal policy aim, as it should be, then it is a mistake to allow individual benefit to remain the test of successful policy and for the provision of high-technology, acute care medicine to remain as the highest de facto goal. If, finally, there is to be any hope of weathering the long-range health policy problem of aging societies, then it will be necessary to devise goals of health care for the elderly that are different from those of younger age groups; and then to put in place policies for the young that will help bring them into old age in good health.

REFERENCES

Callahan D (1999) *False Hopes: Overcoming the Obstacles to a Sustainable, Affordable Medicine*. New Brunswick, NJ: Rutgers University Press.

Daniels N, Kennedy BP, and Kawachi I (1999) Why justice is good for our health: The social determinants of health inequalities. *Daedalus* 128:4.

Evans RG, Barer ML, and Marmor TR (eds) (1994) *Why Are Some People Healthy and Others Not? : The Determinants of Health of Populations*. New York: Aldine DeGruyter.

Ham C (1997) Priority setting in health care: learning from international experience. *Health Policy* 42:49–66.

Hanson MJ and Callahan D (eds) (1999) *The Goals of Medicine: The Forgotten Issues in Health Care Reform*. Washington, D.C.: Georgetown University Press.

The Hastings Center (1996) The goals of medicine: setting new priorities. *Hastings Center Report* Supplement:S1–28.

Institute of Medicine (1988) *The Future of Public Health*. Washington, D.C.: National Academy Press.

Nordenfeldt L (1999) On medicine and other means of health enhancement. In Hanson and Callahan (1999) (eds) *The Goals of Medicine: The Forgotten Issues in Health Care Reform*. Washington, DC: Georgetown University Press, pp. 69–81.

Parens E (1998) *Enhancing Human Traits: Ethical and Social Implications*. Washington, D.C.: Georgetown University Press.

Pellegrino E (1999) The goals and ends of medicine: how are they to be defined. In Hanson and Callahan, (1999) (eds) *The Goals of Medicine: The Forgotten Issues in Health Care Reform*. Washington, D.C.: Georgetown University Press, pp. 55–68.

2

Justice, health, and health policy[1]

NORMAN DANIELS, BRUCE P. KENNEDY, AND ICHIRO KAWACHI[2]

Much thinking about ethics and health policy focuses on issues of access to medical services and the special problems created when we must limit access to potentially beneficial services as a result of resource limitations. This narrow focus is the result of many things—the widely held belief that it is medical care, especially new medical technologies, that are primarily responsible for population health, the prominence of health expenditures in the budgets of developed economies, and the enormous demand for medical services created by the medical and health promotion industries. Our goal in this essay is to put other issues on the ethics and health policy agenda and to broaden the perspective of those thinking about health policy in light of increased understanding of the social determinants of health. We argue in what follows for a broad view of ethics and health policy.[3]

THE NEED FOR A BROAD VIEW

To bring ethics and health policy together, we need a broad view of what justice requires society to do in the promotion of health and the provision of health care. Such a broad view, of course, involves surveying the familiar terrain of medical care at the point of delivery. We must consider how effectively and efficiently the health sector promotes population health under reasonable resource constraints and how fairly it distributes the benefits and burdens of such care. A broad view of the requirements of justice also means looking upstream from the point of medical delivery to traditional public health measures. We must consider disease vectors and environmental hazards in the air and water as well as in work and living spaces; we must consider the adequacy of nutrition and shelter; and we must educate people about the risks of tobacco, alcohol, and unsafe sexual practices. These familiar risk factors pose a threat to the health of all, but their unequal distribution also raises specific issues of equity.

A broad view also requires that we look even further upstream to a less familiar set of factors, the social determinants of health. We have known for more than 150 years that an individual's chances of life and death are patterned according to social class: the more affluent and better educated people are, the longer and healthier their lives (Villerme, 1840, cited in Link et al, 1998). To these effects of class we may add the additional effects of race, or caste, and sex.

These patterns of inequality persist even when there is universal access to health care, a fact quite surprising to those who think financial access to medical services is the primary determinant of health status. In fact, recent cross-national evidence suggests that the greater the degree of socioeconomic inequality that exists within a society, the steeper the gradient of health inequality. As a result, middle income groups in a more unequal society will have worse health than comparable or even poorer groups in a society with greater equality. Of course, we cannot infer causation from correlation, but plausible hypotheses exist about pathways that link social inequalities to health. Even if more work remains to be done to clarify the exact mechanisms, it is not unreasonable to talk here about the social "determinants" of health (Marmot, 1999). Justice requires that we ask whether these social determinants of health are fairly distributed, and where they are not, that we take steps to address these sources of health inequality.

Our purpose in this chapter is to stimulate further deliberation about the implications of this broad view for justice and health policy. First we describe the findings from the recent literature on social determinants. Then we suggest one way to broaden an account of justice and health care so that it encompasses this broader picture. Specifically, we describe Rawls's theory of justice as fairness (Rawls, 1971), earlier extended by one of us to address issues of health-care delivery (Daniels, 1981, 1985), and show how it actually—and with some surprise—includes this broader view. Our contention is that, quite unintentionally, Rawls's (extended) theory provides a defensible account of how to distribute the social determinants of health fairly. If we are right, this unexpected application to a novel problem demonstrates a fruitful generalizability of the theory, analogous to the extension in scope of a non-moral theory, and permits us to think more systematically across the disciplines of public health, medicine, and political philosophy.

Athough unintended, this surprising result is not just serendipity. Justice as fairness was formulated to specify terms of social cooperation that free and equal citizens can accept as fair. Its principles of justice assure people equal basic liberties, including the value of political participation, guarantee a robust form of equal opportunity, and impose significant constraints on inequalities. Together, these principles aim at meeting the "needs of free and equal citizens," a form of egalitarianism Rawls calls "democratic equality" (Rawls, 1971; Daniels, 2002). A crucial component of democratic equality is providing all with the social bases of self-respect and a conviction that prospects in life are fair. As the empirical literature we review demonstrates, institutions conforming to these principles of justice together focus on several crucial pathways through which many researchers believe institutional inequality works to produce health inequality. Consequently, securing fair terms of cooperation that are good for our social and political well-being helps to secure conditions good for our physical and mental health, as well. Later, we point to a convergence between Rawls's view that we must provide for our capabilities as free and equal citizens and Amartya Sen's focus on "positive liberty" (Sen, 1980, 1992, 1999).

Justice, together with this view of the influence of the social determinants, thus requires that we broaden our policy agenda. Of course, detailed determinations of what policies to pursue require more information than theories of justice can provide, but the theory at least helps us define the full scope of our policy agenda. This theory does not answer all our questions about justice, health inequality, and health policy, since there are some crucial points on which it is silent, but it does provide considerable guidance on central issues.(In any case, the theory must be supplemented with democratic, deliberative procedures in order to address a variety of resource allocation problems. See Daniels and Sabin, 1997.)

SOCIAL DETERMINANTS OF HEALTH: SOME BASIC FINDINGS

We highlight five central findings in the literature on the social determinants of health, each of which has implications for an account of justice and health inequalities. First, the income/health gradients we observe are not the result of some fixed or determinate laws of economic development but are influenced by policy choices. Second, the income/health gradients are not just the result of the deprivation of the poorest groups. Rather, a gradient in health operates across the whole socioeconomic spectrum within societies.

Third, the slope, or steepness, of the income/health gradient is affected by the degree of inequality in a society. Fourth, relative income or socioeconomic status is as important as, and may be more important than, the absolute level of income in determining health status, at least once societies have passed a certain threshold. Fifth, identifiable social and psychosocial pathways exist through which inequality produces its effects on health (with little support for "health selection," the claim that health status determines economic position) (Marmot, 1999, 1994). These causal pathways are amenable to specific policy choices that should be guided by considerations of justice.

Cross-National Evidence on Health Inequalities

The pervasive finding that prosperity is related to health, whether measured at the level of nations or individuals, might lead one to the conclusion that these "income/health gradients" are inevitable. They might seem to reflect the natural ordering of societies along some fixed, idealized teleology of economic development. At the individual level, the gradient might appear to be the result of the natural selection of the most "fit" members within a society who are thus better able to garner socioeconomic advantage.

Despite the appeal and power of these ideas, they run counter to the confirmation. Figure 2–1 shows the relationship between the wealth and health of nations as measured by per capita gross domestic product (GDPpc)

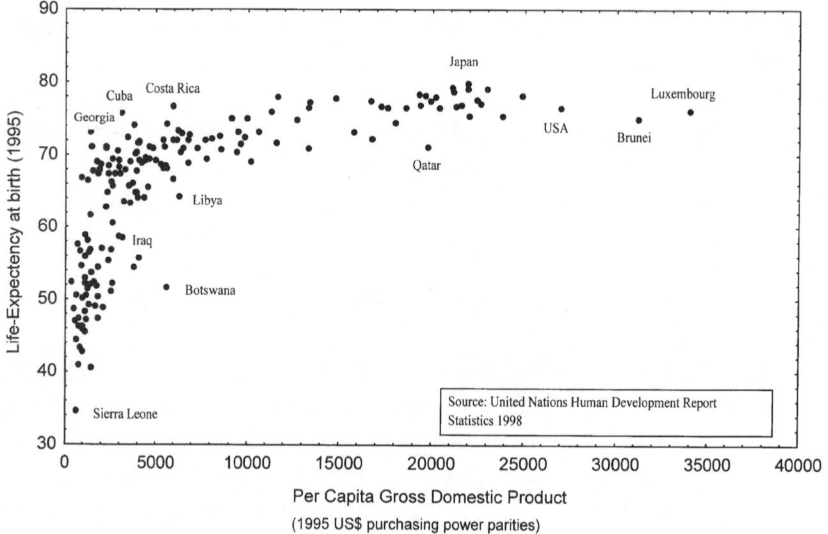

FIGURE 2–1. Relationship between national wealth and life expectancy.

and life expectancy. A clear association exists between GDPpc and life-expectancy, but only up to a point. The relationship levels off beyond about $8,000-$10,000 GDPpc, with virtually no further gains in life expectancy.

This leveling effect is most apparent among the advanced industrial economies (Fig. 2–2), which largely account for the upper tail of the curve in Figure 2–1. The lack of relationship between wealth and health is true within individual countries as well.

Closer inspection of these two figures points up some startling discrepancies. Though Cuba and Iraq are equally poor (GDPpcs about $3100), life-expectancy in Cuba exceeds that in Iraq by 17.2 years. The difference between the GDPpc for Costa Rica and the United States, for example, is enormous (about $21,000), yet Costa Rica's life-expectancy exceeds that of the United State's (76.6 vs. 76.4). In fact, despite being the richest nation on the globe, the United States performs rather poorly on health indicators.

Taken together, these observations support the notion that the relationship between economic development and health is not fixed and that the health achievement of nations is mediated by processes other than wealth. To account for the cross-national variations in health, it is apparent that other factors such as culture, social organization, and government policies are

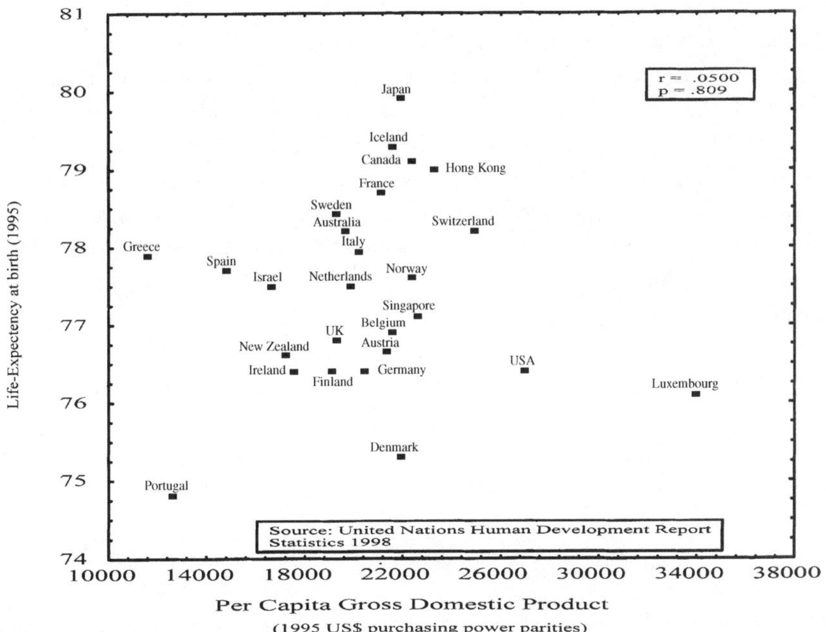

FIGURE 2–2. Relationship between national wealth and life expectancy among advanced industrialized countries.

significantly involved in the determination of population health and that variations in these factors may go some distance in explaining the differences in health outcomes among nations.

If we are right that the health of nations does not reflect some inevitable natural order, but that it reflects policy choices—or features of society that are amenable to change via policies—then we must ask which of these policies are just ones.

Individual Socioeconomic Status (SES) and Health

At the individual level, numerous studies have documented what has come to be known as the "socioeconomic gradient." On this gradient, each increment up the socioeconomic hierarchy is associated with improved health outcomes, as measured by life expectancy or mortality rates, over the rung below (Black et al, 1988; Davey-Smith et al, 1990; Pappas et al, 1993; Adler et al, 1994). It is important to observe that this relationship is not simply a contrast between the health of the rich and the poor but is observed across all levels of SES.

What is particularly notable about the SES gradient is that it does not appear to be explained by differences in access to health care. Steep gradients have been observed even among groups of individuals, such as British civil servants, with adequate access to health care, housing, and transport (Davey-Smith et al, 1990; Marmot et al, 1998).

Importantly, the steepness of the gradient varies substantially across societies. Some societies show a relatively shallow gradient in life expectancy or mortality across SES groups. Others, with comparable or even higher levels of economic development, show much steeper gradients in mortality rates across the socioeconomic hierarchy. The determining factor in the steepness of the gradient appears to be the extent of income inequality in a society. Thus, middle income groups in a country with high income inequality may have lower health status than comparable or even poorer groups in a society with less income inequality. We find the same pattern within the United States when we examine state and metropolitan area variations in inequality and health outcomes (Kennedy et al, 1998a; Lynch et al, 1998). These results lead to the question: How much socioeconomic inequality should a society tolerate in order to avoid health inequalities?

Relative Income and Health

The apparent connection between the distribution of income in a society and the level of health achievement of its members is a relatively recent finding (Wilkinson, 1992, 1994). Simply stated, it is not just the size of the economic pie, but how the pie is shared, that matters for population health. It is not the absolute deprivation associated with low economic development (lack of access to the basic material conditions necessary for health such as clean water, adequate nutrition and housing, and general sanitary living conditions) that explains health differences among developed nations, but the degree of relative deprivation within them. Relative deprivation refers not to a lack of the "goods" that are basic to survival, but rather to a lack of sources of self-respect that are deemed essential for full participation in society.

Numerous studies have provided support for the relative income hypothesis, demonstrating that income inequality is strongly associated with population mortality and life-expectancy both between and within nations (Wilkinson, 1992, 1996). This finding helps to explain the anomalies highlighted in Figures 2–1 and 2–2. Much of the variation in life-expectancy for the rich countries in the upper tail of Figure 2–1 is explained by income distribution, where countries with more equal income distributions, such as Sweden and Japan, have higher life-expectancies than do countries such as the United States, regardless of GDPpc. Furthermore, countries with much lower GDPpc, such as Costa Rica, appear to be able to obtain their remarkably high life-expectancy through a more equitable distribution of income.

Within the United States, income inequality accounts for about 25% of the between-state variance in age-adjusted mortality rates independent of state median income (Kennedy et al, 1996; Kaplan et al, 1996). Moreover, the size of this relationship is not trivial. A recent study across U.S. metropolitan areas, rather than states, found that areas with high income inequality had an excess of death compared to areas of low inequality that was equivalent in magnitude to all deaths due to heart disease (Lynch et al, 1998).

While most of the evidence so far has been accumulated from cross-sectional data, time trend data support similar conclusions. Widening income differentials in the United States and the United Kingdom appear to be related to a slowing down of life-expectancy improvements. In many of the poorest areas of the United Kingdom, mortality for younger age cohorts have actually increased during the same period that income inequality widened (Wilkenson, 1996). In the United States, states with the highest income inequality showed slower rates of life-expectancy improvement compared to states with more equitable income distributions between 1980 and 1990 (Kawachi et al, 1999; Kaplan et al, 1996).

As noted in the previous section, income distribution appears to affect the health of populations by shifting the slope of the curve relating individual income to health. This can be clearly seen in Figure 2–3, where the prevalence of self-reported fair/poor health is higher for almost every income group (and the gradient steeper) for those living in the highest income in-

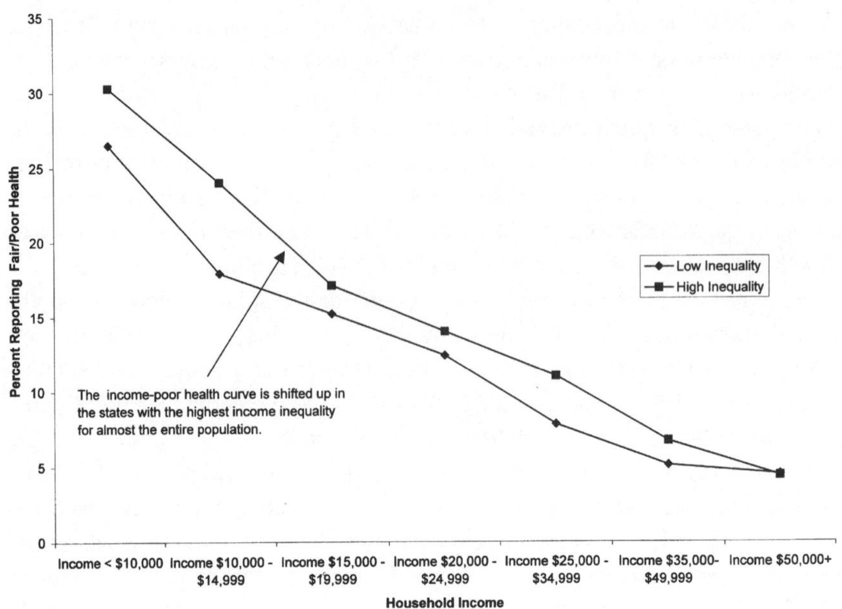

FIGURE 2–3. Self-rated health and individual household income.

equality states (Kennedy et al, 1998a). Nearly identical patterns have been found for individual mortality rates (Lochner, 1999).

Pathways Linking Social Inequalities to Health Inequalities

Our final contention is that there are plausible and identifiable pathways through which social inequalities produce inequalities in health. Some of these occur at the societal level, where income inequality patterns the distribution of social goods, such as public education, that affect the access to life opportunities that are in turn strong determinants of health.

The evidence for these associations, while fairly new, is quite striking. In the United States the most inegalitarian states with respect to income distribution invest less in public education, have larger uninsured populations, and spend less on social safety nets (Kaplan et al, 1996; Kawachi and Kennedy, 1997). Differences in human capital investment are particularly striking. These are demonstrated for educational spending and, more importantly, for outcomes, where, even when controlling for median income, income inequality explains about 40% of the between-state variation in the percentage of children in the 4th grade who are below the basic reading level. Similarly, strong associations are seen for the percentage of high school drop-out rates. It is quite evident from these data that educational opportunities for children in high income inequality states are quite different from those in states with more egalitarian distributions. Furthermore, these early effects not only have an immediate impact on health, increasing the likelihood of premature death during childhood and adolescence (as evidenced by the much higher death rates for infants and children in the high inequality states), but also have lasting effects that show up later in life as part of the SES gradient in health (Bartley et al, 1997; Barker, 1998; Davey-Smith et al, 1998).

Differential investment in human capital is also a strong predictor of health across nations. Indeed, one of the strongest predictors of life-expectancy among developing countries is adult literacy, particularly the disparity between male and female adult literacy, which explains much of the variation in health achievement among these countries after accounting for GDPpc. For example, among the 125 developing countries with GDPpcs less than $10,000, the difference between male and female literacy accounts for 40% of the variance in life-expectancy after factoring out the effect of GDPpc. The fact that sex disparities in access to basic education drives the level of health achievement further emphasizes the role of broader social inequalities in patterning health inequalities. Indeed, in the United States, differences between the states in women's status—measured in terms of their economic autonomy and political participation—are more strongly correlated with higher female mortality rates (Kawachi et al, 1999; Wilkinson, et al, 1999).

These societal mechanisms—for example, income inequality leading to educational inequality leading to health inequality—are tightly linked to the political processes that influence government policy. For example, income inequality appears to affect health by undermining civil society. Income inequality erodes social cohesion, as measured by higher levels of social mistrust and reduced participation in civic organizations (Kawachi and Kennedy, 1997; Kawachi et al, 1997). Lack of social cohesion leads to lower participation in political activity, such as voting, serving in local government, and volunteering for political campaigns. Lower participation, in turn, undermines the responsiveness of government institutions in addressing the needs of the worst-off in society. This is demonstrated by the human capital investment data presented earlier, but it is also reflected by the lack of investment in human security. States with the highest income inequality, and thus lowest levels of social capital and political participation, are far less generous in the provision of social safety nets (Kawachi and Kennedy, 1999).

The social science and public health literature sharpens our understanding of the causes of health inequalities, but it contains no systematic way to evaluate the overall fairness of those inequalities and and the socioeconomic inequalities that produce them. The philosophical literature has produced theories aimed at evaluating socioeconomic inequalities, but it has tended to ignore health inequalities and their causes. To produce an integrated view, we need the resources of a more general theory of justice.

JUSTICE AS FAIRNESS EXTENDED

We can better see the need for appealing to a theory of justce if we briefly examine what happens when we try to proceed without one. Consider, for example, the intuitively promising analysis, prominent in the international literature on health policy, that a health inequality between social groups is an inequity when it is avoidable, unnecessary, and unfair (Whitehead, 1992; Dahlgren and Whitehead, 1991; Braveman, 1999). If we can agree on what is avoidable, unnecessary, and unfair, and this analysis is correct, then we can agree on which inequalities are inequitable.

The poor in many countries lack access to clean water, sanitation, adequate shelter, basic education, vaccinations, and prenatal and maternal care. As a result of some or all of these factors, infant mortality differences exist between them and richer groups. Since social policies could supply the missing determinants of infant health—other poor countries have pursued development in a way that provides these factors—then the inequalities are avoidable.

Are these inequalities also unfair? Most of us would immediately think they are, perhaps because we believe that policies that create and sustain poverty are unjust, and we also believe that social policies that compound poverty with lack of access to the determinants of health are doubly unfair. Of course, libertarians would disagree. They would insist that what is merely unfortunate is not unfair; on their view, we have no obligation of justice, as opposed to charity, to provide the poor with what they are missing. Many of us might be inclined to reject the libertarian view as itself unjust because of this dramatic conflict with our beliefs about poverty and our social obligations to meet people's basic needs.

The problem becomes more complicated, however, when we remember one of the basic findings from the literature on social determinants: We cannot eliminate health inequalities simply by eliminating poverty. Health inequalities persist even in societies that provide the poor with access to all of the determinants of health noted above, and they persist as a gradient of health throughout the social hierarchy, not just between the very poorest groups and those above them.

At this point, many of us would have to reexamine what we believe about the justice of the remaining socioeconomic inequalities. Unless we believe that *all* socioeconomic inequalities (or at least all inequalities we did not choose) are unjust—and very few embrace such a radical egalitarian view—then we must consider more carefully the problem created by the health gradient and the fact that it is made steeper under more unequal social arrangements. Our judgements about fairness, to which we, rightly or wrongly, felt confident in appealing when rejecting the libertarian position, give us less guidance in thinking about the broader issue of the social determinants of health inequalities. Indeed, we may even believe that some degree of socioeconomic inequality is unavoidable or even necessary and therefore not unjust.

One reason we develop general ethical theories, including theories of justice, is to provide a framework within which to resolve important disputes about conflicting moral beliefs or intuitions of the sort we have just raised. For example, in *A Theory of Justice* Rawls sought to leverage our relatively broad liberal agreement on principles and judgments guaranteeing certain equal basic liberties into an agreement on a principle limiting socioeconomic inequalities, a matter on which liberals have considerable disagreement (Cohen J, 1989). His strategy was to show that a social contract that was designed to be fair to free and equal people ("justice as [procedural] fairness") would not only justify the choice of those equal basic liberties but would also justify the choice of principles guaranteeing equal opportunity and limiting inequalities to those that work to make the worst-off groups fare as well as possible.

Our contention is that Rawls's account, though developed to answer this general question about social justice, turns out to provide principles for the just distribution of the social determinants of health, unexpectedly adding to its scope and power as a theory. The extra power of the theory is a surprise, since Rawls deliberately avoided talking about disease or health in his original account. To simplify the construction of his theory, Rawls assumed his contractors were to be fully functional over a normal life span, that is, no one becomes ill or dies prematurely.

This idealization itself provides a clue about how to extend this theory to the real world of illness and premature death. The goal of public health and medicine is to keep people as close as possible to the idealization of normal functioning under reasonable resource constraints. (Resources are necessarily limited since maintaining health cannot be our only social good or goal.) Because maintaining normal functioning makes a limited but significant contribution to protecting the range of opportunities open to individuals, it is plausible to see the principle guaranteeing fair equality of opportunity as the appropriate principle to govern the distribution of health care, broadly construed to include primary and secondary preventive health care as well as medical services (Daniels, 1985; Rawls, 1993). This way of extending Rawls's theory also suggests that health status should be incorporated through its effects on opportunity into the index of primary goods (to be explained shortly), which is used to evaluate the lifetime prospects of contractors and citizens.

This extension of Rawls's theory thus gives us a perspective on two components of the broad view on which we remarked earlier. The account implies that we have social obligations to promote population health fairly through a system with universal access and that resource allocation should further be guided by concerns about the impact of disease and disability on the range of opportunities open to individuals, so that some priority must be given to preventing, curing, or compensating for the worst impairments of normal functioning (Daniels, 1985; Daniels et al, 1996). The account also forces us to look upstream toward traditional public health measures and the distribution of risk factors (Daniels, 1985). We note, as well, that the fair equality of opportunity account guides our thinking about disabilities, for it gives us a natural way to understand the requirement to provide reasonable accommodation in the workplace for people with disabilities (Daniels, 1996).

What about looking even farther upstream, adopting the very broad view noted earlier? What is particularly appealing about examining the social determinants of health inequalities from the perspective of Rawls's theory is that the theory is at once egalitarian in orientation and yet justifies certain inequalities that might contribute to health inequalities. In addition, Daniels's extension of Rawls links the protection of health to the protection of equality of opportunity, again setting up the potential for internal conflict. To see whether this combination of features simply leads to contradictions in the theory or to insight into the problem, we must examine the issue in more detail.

How does Rawls justify socioeconomic inequalities? Why wouldn't free and equal contractors simply insist on strictly egalitarian distributions of all social goods, just as they insist on equal basic liberties and equal opportunity?

Rawls's answer is that it is irrational for contractors to insist on equality if doing so would make them worse off. Specifically, he argues that contractors would choose his "difference principle," which permits inequalities provided they work to make the worst off groups in society as well off as possible. (A discussion of Rawls's argument for the difference principle and the extensive critical literature it has generated is beyond the scope of this chapter. It is important, however, to distinguish Rawls's own social contract argument from the many informal and intuitive reformulations of it. See Barry, 1989; Cohen GA, 1992, 1995; Cohen J, 1989; Daniels, 2002.) The argument for the difference principle appears to suggest that relative inequality is less important than is absolute well-being, a suggestion that is in tension with other aspects of Rawls's view. Thus, he also insists that inequalities allowed by the difference principle should not undermine the value of political liberty and the requirements of fair equality of opportunity. The priority given these other principles over the difference principle thus limits the inference that Rawls has no concern about relative inequality. Specifically, as we shall see, these principles work together to constrain inequality and to preserve the social bases of self-respect for all.

Two points will help avoid misunderstanding of the difference principle and its justification. First, it is not a mere "trickle-down" principle, but one that requires maximal flow in the direction of helping the worst-off groups. The worst-off, and then the next-worst-off, and so on (Rawls calls this "chain connectedness" [Rawls, 1971]) must be made as well-off as possible, not merely just somewhat better-off, as a trickle-down principle implies. The difference principle is thus much more demanding than a principle that would permit any degree of inequality provided there was some "trickle" of benefits to the worst-off. Indeed, it is more egalitarian than alternative principles that merely assure the worse-off a "decent" or "adequate" minimum. Part of the rationale for the more demanding principle is that it would produce less strain of commitment, less sense of being unfairly left out, at least for those who are worst-off, than would principles that allow more inequality (Cohen J, 1989). Indeed, from what we have learned about the social determinants of health, the more demanding difference principle would also produce less health inequality than any proposed alternative principles that allow inequalities. By flattening the health gradient, it also benefits middle income groups, not simply the poorest. In this regard, its benefits are important beyond the level where we have helped the worst-off to achieve "sufficiency." This point provides a reply to those who suggest that the difference principle has no appeal once the worst-off are sufficiently provided for (Gutmann and Thompson, 1995).

Second, when contractors evaluate how well-off the principles they choose will make them, they are to judge their well-being by an index of "primary social goods" (Rawls, 1971, 1993). The primary social goods, which Rawls thinks of as the "needs of citizens," include liberty, powers, opportunities, income, and wealth, and the social bases of self-respect. (These objective measures of well-being should be contrasted with measures of happiness or desire satisfaction that are familiar from utilitarian and welfare economic perspectives.) In his exposition of the difference principle, Rawls illustrates how it will work by asking us to consider only the simpler case of income inequalities. In doing so, he assumes that the level of income will correlate with the level of other social goods on the index.

This simplification should not mislead us, for, in crucial cases, the correlation may not obtain. For example, let us suppose that having "democratic" control over one's workplace is crucial to self-realization and the promotion of self-esteem (Cohen J, unpbl). Suppose further that hierarchical workplaces are more efficient than democratic ones, so that a system with hierarchical workplaces would have resources to redistribute that meant higher incomes for worst-off workers than democratic workplaces would permit. Then the difference principle does not clearly tell us whether the hierarchical workplace contains allowable inequalities since the worst-off are better-off in some ways but worse-off in others. Without knowing the weighting of items in the index, we cannot use it to say clearly what inequalities are permitted. When we are evaluating which income inequalities are allowable by asking which ones work to make the worst-off groups as well-off as possible, we must, in any case, judge how well-off groups are by reference to the *whole* index of primary goods and not simply the resulting income.

This point is of particular importance in the current discussion. Daniels's extension of Rawls treats health status as a determinant of the opportunity range open to individuals. Since opportunity is included in the index, the effects of health inequalities are thereby included in the index.

Unfortunately, Rawls says very little about how items in the index are to be weighted. This is one of the crucial points on which the theory says less than we might have wished. Therefore, we have little guidance about how these primary goods are to be traded off against one another in its construction. This silence pertains not only to the use of the index in the contract situation, but also to its use by a legislature trying to apply the principles of justice in a context where many specific features of a society are known. We return to this point shortly.

We can now say more directly why justice, as described by Rawls's principles, is good for our health. To understand this claim, let us start with the ideal case, a society governed by Rawls's principles of justice that seeks to achieve "democratic equality" (Daniels, 2002). Consider what it requires with regard to the distribution of the social determinants of health. In such a society, all are guaranteed equal basic liberties, including the liberty of political participation. In addition, there are institutional safeguards aimed at assuring all, richer and poorer alike, the worth or value of political participation rights. Without such assurance, basic capabilities of citizens cannot develop. The recognition that all citizens have these capabilities protected is critical to preserving self-esteem, on Rawls's view. In requiring institutional support for political participation rights, Rawls rejects the claim that freedom of speech of the rich is unfairly restricted by limiting their personal expenditures on their own campaigns, a limitation the Supreme Court ruled unconstitutional in *Buckley vs Valeo* (Rawls, 1993). After all, the limitation does not unduly burden the rich compared to others. Since there is evidence that political participation is itself a social determinant of health (see above), the Rawlsian ideal assures institutional protections that counter the usual effects of socioeconomic inequalities on participation and thus on health.

The Rawlsian ideal of democratic equality also involves conformity with a principle guaranteeing fair equality of opportunity. Not only are discriminatory barriers prohibited by the principle, but it requires robust measures aimed at mitigating the effects of socioeconomic inequalities and other social contingencies on opportunity. In addition to equitable public education, such measures would include the provision of developmentally appropriate day care and early childhood interventions intended to promote the development of capabilities independently of the advantages of family background. Such measures match or go beyond the best models of such interventions we see in European efforts at day care and early childhood education. We also note that the strategic importance of education for protecting equal opportunity has implications for all levels of education, including access to graduate and professional education.

We have already noted some implications for the design of the medical and public health systems. Because the principle aims at promoting normal functioning for all as a way of protecting opportunity for all, it at once aims at improving population health and the reduction of health inequalities. Obviously, this focus requires provision of universal access to comprehensive health care, including public health, primary health care, and medical and social support services.

To act justly in health policy, we must have knowledge about the causal pathways through which socioeconomic (and other) inequalities work to produce differential health outcomes. Suppose we learn, for example, that structural and organizational features of the workplace that induce stress and a loss of control tend to promote health inequalities. We should then view modifying those features of workplace organization in order to mitigate their negative effects on health as a public health requirement of the equal opportunity approach. It is thus on a par with the requirement that we reduce exposures to toxins in the workplace (Daniels, 1985).

Finally, in the ideal Rawlsian society, the difference principle places significant restrictions on allowable inequalities in income and wealth. G. A. Cohen (1992) argued that a strict interpretation of the difference principle would allow few incentive-based inequalities. (For a more permissive view, see Daniels, 2002.) The inequalities allowed by this principle (in conjunction with the principles assuring equal opportunity and the value of political participation) are probably more constrained than those we observe in even the most industrialized societies. If so, then the inequalities that conform to the difference principle would produce a flatter gradient of health inequality than we currently observe in even the more extensive welfare systems of northern Europe.

In short, Rawls's principles of justice regulate the distribution of the key social determinants of health, including the social bases of self-respect. There is nothing about the theory or Daniels's extension of it that should make us focus narrowly on medical services. Properly understood, justice as fairness tells us what justice requires in the distribution of all socially controllable determinants of health.

We still face a theoretical issue of some interest, however. Even if the Rawlsian distribution of the determinants of health flattens health gradients further than what we observe in the most egalitarian, developed countries, we must still expect a residue of health inequalities. In part, this may happen because we may not have adequate knowledge of all the relevant causal pathways or interventions that are effective in modifying them. The theoretical issue is whether the theory requires us to reduce *further* those otherwise justifiable inequalities because of the inequalities in health status they create.

We should not further reduce those socioeconomic inequalities if doing so reduces productivity to the extent that we can no longer support the institutional measures we already employ to promote health and reduce health inequalities. Our commitment to reducing health inequality should not require steps that threaten to make health worse off for those with less-than-equal health status. So the theoretical issue reduces to this: Would it ever be reasonable and rational for contractors to accept a trade-off in which some health inequality is allowed in order to produce some nonhealth benefits for those with the worst health prospects?

We know that, in real life, people routinely trade health risks for other benefits. They do so when they commute longer distances for a better job or take a ski vacation. Some such trades raise questions of fairness. For example, when is hazard pay a benefit workers gain only because their opportunities are unfairly restricted, and when is it an appropriate exercise of their autonomy (Daniels, 1985)? Many such trades are ones we think it unjustifiably paternalistic to restrict; others we see as unfair.

Rawlsian contractors, however, cannot make such trades on the basis of any specific knowledge of their own values. They cannot decide that their enjoyment of skiing makes it worth the risks to their knees or necks. To make the contract fair to all participants and to achieve impartiality, Rawls imposes a thick "veil of ignorance" that blinds them to all knowledge about themselves, including their specific views of the good life. Instead, they must judge their well-being by reference to an index of primary social goods (noted earlier) that includes a weighted measure of rights, opportunities, powers, income and wealth, and the social bases of self-respect.

When Kenneth Arrow (1973) first reviewed Rawls's theory, he argued that this index was inadequate because it failed to tell us how to compare the ill rich with the well poor; Sen (1980, 1992) argued that the index is insensitive to the way in which disease, disability, or other individual variations would create inequalities in the capabilities of people who had the same primary social goods. By extending Rawls's theory to include health care through the equal opportunity account, some of Arrow's (and Sen's) criticism is undercut (Daniels, 1990). But our theoretical question about residual health inequalities reminds us that the theory says too little about the construction of the index to provide us with a clear answer.

One of Rawls's central arguments for singling out a principle protecting equal basic liberties and giving it (lexical) priority over his other principles of justice is his claim that, once people achieve some threshold level of material well-being, they would not trade away the fundamental importance of liberty for other goods (Rawls, 1971). Making such a trade might deny them the liberty to pursue their most cherished ideals, including their religious beliefs, whatever they turn out to be. Can we make the same argument about trading health for other goods?

There is some plausibility to the claim that rational people should refrain from similar trades of health for other goods. Loss of health may preclude us from pursuing what we most value in life. We do, after all, see people willing to trade almost anything to regain health once they lose it.

If we take this argument seriously, we might conclude that Rawls should give opportunity, including the effects of health status, a heavier weighting in the construction of the index than income alone. (Rawls [1971] suggests that, since fair equality of opportunity is given priority over the difference principle, we can assume that, within the index, opportunity has a heavier weighting.) Such a weighting would mean that absolute increases in income that might otherwise have justified increasing relative income inequality, according to the difference principle, now fail to justify those inequalities because of the negative effects on opportunity. For although in this scheme income of the worst-off would increase, they would not be better-off according to the whole (weighted) index of primary social goods, and so the greater inequality would not be permitted. Rawls's simplifying assumption about income correlating with other goods fails in this case (as it did in the hypothetical example about workplace democracy cited earlier).

Nevertheless, there is also strong reason to think the priority given to health and thus opportunity is not as clear-cut as the previous argument implies, especially where the trade is between a *risk* to health and other goods that people highly value. Refusing to allow any (ex ante) trades of health risks for other goods, even when the background conditions on choice are otherwise fair, may seem unjustifiably paternalistic, perhaps in a way that refusals to allow trades of basic liberties is not.

We propose a pragmatic route around this problem, one that has a precedent elsewhere in Rawls. Fair equality of opportunity, Rawls admits, is only approximated, even in an ideally just system, because we can only mitigate, not eliminate, the effects of family and other social contingencies (Rawls, 1971; Fishkin, 1983). For example, only if we were willing to violate widely respected parental liberties could we intrude into family life and "rescue" children from parental values that arguably interfere with equal opportunity. Similarly, though we give a general priority to equal opportunity over the difference principle, we cannot achieve complete equality in health any more than we can achieve completely equal opportunity. Even ideal theory does not produce perfect justice. Justice is always rough around the edges. Specifically, if we had good reason to think that "democratic equality" had flattened inequalities in accord with the principles of justice, then we might be inclined to think we had done as much as was reasonable to make health inequalities fair to all. The residual inequalities that emerge with conformance to the principles are not a "compromise" with what justice ideally requires, they are acceptable as just.

So far, we have been considering whether the theoretical question can be resolved from the perspective of individual contractors. Instead, suppose the decision about such a trade-off is to be made through the legislature in a society that conforms to Rawls's principles. Because those principles require effective political participation across all socioeconomic groups, we can suppose that groups most directly affected by any trade-off decision have a voice in the decision. Since there is a residual health gradient, groups affected by the trade-off include not only the worst-off, but those in the middle as well. A democratic process that involved deliberation about the tradeoff and its effects might be the best we could do to provide a resolution of the unanswered theoretical question (Daniels and Sabin, 1997).

In contrast, where the fair value of political participation is not adequately assured—and we doubt it is so assured in even our most democratic societies—we have much less confidence in the fairness of a democratic decision about how to trade health against other goods. It is much more likely under actual conditions that those who benefit most from the inequalities, that is, those who are better-off, also wield disproportionate political power and influence decisions about trade-offs to serve their interests. It may still be that the use of a democratic process in nonideal conditions is the fairest resolution we can practically achieve, but it nevertheless falls well short of what an ideally just democratic process involves.

We have focused on Rawlsian theory because it provides, however fortuitously, a developed account of how to distribute the social determinants of health. Some other competing theories of justice, including some recent proposals about "equal opportunity for welfare or advantage" (Arneson, 1988; Cohen GA, 1989) offer no similarly developed framework for distributing the key social determinants of health. On the other hand, Sen's most developed account (1999) of the importance of an egalitarian distribution of "capabilities" actually resembles the Rawls/Daniels account of equal opportunity and normal functioning more than it seems to at first glance (Daniels,

1990, 2002; Buchanan et al, 2000). Anderson (1999) has imaginatively focused the discussion of capabilities on those needed if citizens are to have "democratic equality." The result is a striking convergence with Rawls's view of democratic equality, though Rawls's ability to talk about the fair distribution of social determinants of health follows directly from his principles, whereas Anderson must appeal intuitively to an account of the capabilities needed by citizens.

POLICY IMPLICATIONS FOR A JUST DISTRIBUTION OF THE SOCIAL DETERMINANTS OF HEALTH

The Rawlsian account of justice as fairness provides a robust account of what is fair and unfair in the distribution of the social determinants of health. The theory provides a more systematic way to think about which health inequalities are inequities. Compared to that ideal, most health inequalities that we now observe worldwide among socioeconomic and racial or ethnic groups are "inequities" that should be remedied. Even some countries with the shallowest health gradients, such as Sweden and England, have viewed their own health inequalities as unacceptable and initiated policy measures to mitigate them. A National Public Health Commission in Sweden, for example, has targeted restrictions on socioeconomic inequality as a means for improving population health and reducing health inequalities (Ostlin and Diderichsen, 2000). Clearly, the broader World Health Organization efforts in this direction are, probably without exception, also aimed at true inequities.

A central policy implication of our discussion is that reform efforts to improve health inequalities must be intersectoral and not just focused on the traditional health sector. Health is produced not just by having access to medical prevention and treatment, but, to a measurably greater extent, by the cumulative experience of social conditions across the life course. In other words, by the time a 60-year-old patient presents to the emergency room with a heart attack to receive medical treatment, that encounter represents the result of bodily insults that accumulated over a lifetime. Medical care is, figuratively speaking, "the ambulance waiting at the bottom of the cliff." Much of the contemporary discussion about increasing access to medical care as a means of reducing health inequalities misses this point. An emphasis on intersectoral reform will recognize the primacy of social conditions, such as access to basic education, levels of material deprivation, a healthy workplace environment, and equality of political participation in determining the health achievement of societies (Lavis and Stoddart, 1994).

Before saying more about intersectoral reform, we want to head off one mistaken or exaggerated inference that may be drawn from our view, namely that we should ignore medical services and health sector reform because other steps have a bigger payoff. Even if we had a highly just distribution of the social determinants of health and of public health measures, people would still become ill and need medical services. The fair design of a health system arguably should give some extra weight to meeting actual medical needs.

We might think of those who are ill and who have known needs as "identified victims," whereas we might think of those whose lives would be spared illness by robust public health measures and a fair distribution of social determinants as "statistical victims." Several theoretical perspectives, both utilitarian and nonutilitarian, imply that we should consider all these lives impartially, judging statistical lives saved to be just as valuable or important as identified victims. Utilitarian approaches, for example, would then push us immediately to maximize net benefit by allocating resources from saving identified lives to saving statistical ones.

Other reasonable considerations, however, temper our inclination to reallocate in such an impartial way from identified to statistical victims. Many of us give some extra moral weight to the urgent needs of those already ill. Others, through their roles as medical providers, may legitimately believe that the good they can control through their delivery of medical care has a greater claim on them than the good that would be brought about by more indirect measures beyond their control. More generally, many of us will be connected as family members and friends to the identified victims and will feel that we have "agent-relative" obligations to assist them that supersede the obligations we have to more distant, statistical victims.

It is impossible to dismiss the relevance of these other considerations. (We cannot here address this deep issue within moral theory.) Consequently, we do not draw the inference that impartiality or rationality considerations might seem to support, namely, that we should immediately reallocate resources away from medical services to public health measures or a fairer distribution of social determinants in accordance with some algorithm based on the relative benefit, neutrally calculated, between statistical and identified lives. This is not, however, to imply that no reallocations are justifiable. No doubt some are in light of what we have argued (Lavis and Stoddart, 1994).

What sorts of social policies should governments pursue in order to reduce health inequalities? Certainly, the menu of options should include equalizing access to medical care, as we emphasized earlier, but it should also include a broader set of policies aimed at equalizing individual life opportunities, such as investment in basic education, affordable housing, income security, and other forms of antipoverty policy. Though the connection between these broad social policies and health may seem somewhat remote, and they are rarely linked to issues of health in our public policy discussions, growing evidence suggests that they should be so linked. The kinds of policies suggested by a social determinants perspective encompass a much broader range of instruments than would ordinarily be considered for improving the health of the population. We discuss three such examples of social policies that hold promise of abating socioeconomic disparities in health: investment in early childhood development, improving the quality of the work environment, and reduction in income inequality.

The Case for Early Life Intervention

Growing evidence points to the importance of early childhood environment in influencing the behavior, learning, and health of individuals later in the life course. Providing equal opportunities within a Rawlsian framework translates into interventions as early in life as possible. Several studies have demonstrated the benefits of early supportive environments for children. In the Perry High/Scope Project (Schweinhart et al, 1993), children in poor economic circumstances were provided a high-quality early childhood development program between the ages of 3 and 5. Compared to the control group, those in the intervention group completed more schooling by age 27; were more likely to be employed, own a home, and be married with children; experienced fewer criminal problems and teenage pregnancies; and were far less likely to have mental health problems.

Compensatory education and nutrition in the early years of life (as exemplified by the Head Start and WIC [Women, Infants, and Children] Programs) have been similarly shown to yield important gains for the most disadvantaged groups. As part of the War on Poverty, the U.S. government introduced two small compensatory education programs, Head Start for preschoolers and Chapter 1 for elementary school children. Evaluations of these programs indicate that children who enroll in them learn more than those who do not. In turn, educational achievement is a powerful predictor of health in later life, partly because education provides access to employment and income and partly because education has a direct influence on health behavior in adulthood, including diet, smoking, and physical activity (Acheson et al, 1998).

A similarly persuasive case can be made for nutritional supplementation in low-income women and children. An analysis of the National Maternal and Infant Health Survey (Moss and Carver, 1998) found that participation of low-income pregnant women in the WIC program was associated with about a 40% reduction in the risk of subsequent infant death. A mother's nutritional state affects her infant's chance of death not just in the first year of life, but also throughout the life course. Thus, a woman's prepregnant weight is one of the strongest predictors of her child's birth weight, and, in turn, low birth weight has been shown to be linked with increased risks of coronary heart disease, hypertension, and diabetes in later life. It follows that investing in policies to reduce early adverse influences may produce benefits not only in the present, but also in the long run for future generations.

The Case for Improving the Quality of the Work Environment

We alluded earlier to the finding that the health status of workers is closely linked to the quality of their work environment, specifically to the amount of control and autonomy available to workers on their jobs. Low-control work environments—such as monotonous machine-paced work (e.g., factory assembly lines) and jobs involving little opportunity for learning and utilization of new skills (e.g., supermarket cashiers)—tend to be concentrated among low-income occupations. The work of Marmot and colleagues (Marmot et al, 1997) has shown that social disparities in health partly arise as a consequence of the way labor markets sort individuals into positions of unequal authority and control. Exposure to low-control, high-demand job conditions is not only more common in lower-status occupations, but they also place such workers at increased risks of hypertension, cardiovascular disease, mental illness, musculoskeletal disease, sickness absence, and physical disability (Karasek and Torell, 1990).

A growing number of international case studies have concluded that it is possible to improve the level of control in workplaces by several means: by increasing the variety of tasks in the production process, by encouraging workforce participation in the production process, and by allowing more flexible work arrangements, such as altering the patterns of shift work to make them less disruptive of workers' lives (Acheson et al, 1998). In some cases it may even be possible to redesign the workplace and to enhance worker autonomy without affecting productivity (since sickness absence may diminish as a consequence of a healthier workplace).

The Case for Income Redistribution

Many policies suggested by the social determinants perspective tend to fall under the category of antipoverty policy. However, research on the social determinants of health warns us that antipoverty policies do not go far enough in reducing unjust health disparities. Though none would disagree about putting priority on reducing the plight of the worst-off, the fact is that health inequalities occur as a gradient; the poor have worse health than the near-poor, but, in turn, the near-poor fare worse than the lower-middle class, the lower middle class does worse than the upper-middle class, and so on up the economic ladder. Addressing the social gradient in health requires action above and beyond the elimination of poverty.

To address comprehensively the problem of health inequalities, governments must begin to address the issue of economic inequalities per se. As we mentioned earlier, growing international and within-country evidence suggests that the extent of socioeconomic disparities—that is, the size of the gap in incomes and assets between the top and bottom of society—is itself an important determinant of the health achievement of society, independent of the average standard of living (Kawachi et al, 1999). Most importantly, economic disparities seem to influence the degree of equality in political participation (in the form of voting, campaign donations, contacting elected officials, and other forms of political activity): the more unequal the distribution of incomes and assets, the more skewed the patterns of political participation and, consequently, the greater the degree of political exclusion of disadvantaged groups (Kawachi and Kennedy, 1997; Kawachi and Kennedy, 1999).

Inequalities in political participation in turn determine the kinds of policies passed by national and local governments. For example, Hill and colleagues (Hill et al, 1995) carried out a pooled time series analysis for the fifty U.S. states from 1978 to 1990 to examine the relationship between the degree of mobilization of lower class voters at election time and the generosity of welfare benefits provided by state governments. Even after adjusting for other factors that might predict state welfare policy—such as the degree of public liberalism in the state, the federal government's welfare cost-matching rate for individual states, the state unemployment rate and median income, and the state tax effort—robust relationships were found between the extent of political participation by lower-class voters and the degree of generosity of state welfare payments. In other words, *who participates* matters for political outcomes, and the resulting policies have an important impact on the opportunities for the poor to lead healthy lives.

For both the foregoing reasons—that it yields a higher level of health achievement as well as greater political participation—the reduction of income disparity ought to be a priority of governments concerned about addressing social inequalities in health. Although beyond the scope of the this chapter, a number of levers do exist by which governments could address the problem of income inequality, ranging from the radical (a commitment to sustained full employment, collective wage bargaining, and progressive taxation) to the incremental (expansion of the earned income tax credit, increased child care credit, and raising the minimum wage) (Kawachi, Kennedy, Wilkinson, 1999).

IMPLICATIONS FOR INTERNATIONAL DEVELOPMENT THEORY

Our discussion has implications for international development theory as well as for economic choices confronted by industrialized countries. To the extent that income distribution matters for population health status, it is not obvious that giving strict priority to economic growth is the optimal strategy for maximizing social welfare. Raising everyone's income will improve the health status of the poor (the trickle-down approach), but not as much as will paying attention to the *distribution* of the social product. Within the developing world, a comparison of the province of Kerala in India with more unequal countries like Brazil and South Africa illustrates this point. Despite having only one-third to a quarter of the income of Brazil or South Africa (and thereby having a higher prevalence of poverty in the absolute sense), the citizens of Kerala nonetheless live longer, most likely as a result of the higher priority the government of Kerala accords to a fair distribution of economic gains (Sen, 1998).

The real issue for developing countries is what *kind* of economic growth is salutary. Hence Dreze and Sen (1989) and Sen (1999) distinguish between two types of successes in the rapid reduction of mortality, which they term "growth mediated" and "support-led" processes. The former works mainly *through* fast economic growth, exemplified by mortality reductions in countries like South Korea and Hong Kong. Their successes depended on the growth process being wide-based and participatory (for example, full employment policies) and on the gains from economic growth being used to expand relevant social services in the public sector, particularly health care and education. Their experience stands in stark contrast to the example of countries like Brazil, which have similarly achieved rapid economic growth but have lagged behind in health improvements.

In contrast to growth-mediated processes, "support-led" processes operate not through fast economic growth but through governments giving high priority to the provision of social services that reduce mortality and enhance the quality of life. Examples of such countries include China, Costa Rica, and the Indian state of Kerala, already mentioned above.

A similar choice between policies emphasizing growth versus more equality applies to developed nations as well. Application of the Rawlsian difference principle suggests that a society like the United States has much room to move toward a more equitable (perhaps a more European) distribution of its national income without suffering a loss in productivity or growth. Simultaneously, it would benefit from a gain in the health status of its citizens. That health benefit would be greatest in the bottom 60% to 80% of the socioeconomic scale, and it would occur without any loss in health for those who are best-off.

A REMARK ON RACE AND CLASS

Our survey of the social determinants literature has focused on measures of class, but our discussion would be remiss if we did not comment on the importance of race in the social determinants of health. It is important to bring both class and race into policy focus, since the literature sometimes makes it seem as if we should attend to one or the other, but not both, as if they are in competition with each other and attending to one means ignoring the other (for an excellent review, see House and Williams, 2000). Historically, racism has been used to widen class divisions, for example by splitting union movements and potential political alliances. Understanding this history suggests it is difficult to address problems of class without also opposing overt and institutional forms of racism. In addition, there are residual and clear effects of race even when socioeconomic status is held constant. Understanding the lingering, intergenerational effects of racism will help us understand better the mechanisms through which social determinants of health work on both races and classes. Focusing on race alone will result in addressing only part of the social gradient in health, which does not respect racial boundaries (i.e., the majority of the poor and nonpoor are white). We must therefore give priority to the worst-off (poor blacks), but not stop at the dividing line of race (which has too often been used to justify a limited, and ultimately politically unsustainable, vision of social justice).

A theory of justice, such as Rawls's (or Sen's) requires us to pay attention to both race and class and to think broadly about addressing both in constructing a policy agenda. Some of our specific suggestions above—the emphasis on early childhood interventions, for example—have the effect of addressing both race and class issues. A key task for further policy analysis is to focus on strategies and tactics that similarly unite people concerned about either race or class.

A broad view of justice and health policy gives us strong reason to expand what is on our traditional policy agenda. The suggestions we have made are aimed at the modest goal of expanding the policy domain, not resolving just how resource allocations should be made among all the options we should consider. Further work in ethics and health policy must tackle the specific issues raised by such decisions about priorities.

NOTES

1. This essay is substantially based on our "Why Justice is Good for Our Health: The Social Determinants of Health Inequalities," *Daedalus* 128:4 (Fall 1999): 215–51. We gratefully acknowledge permission to use this material here.

2. Norman Daniels, Bruce P. Kennedy, and Ichiro Kawachi are recipients of Robert Wood Johnson Foundation investigator awards in health policy research.

3. A brief aside about terminology: Throughout, we view disease and disability as departures from (species typical) normal functioning and view health and normal functioning as equivalent (Daniels, 1985).

REFERENCES

Acheson D et al (1998) *Report of the Independent Inquiry into Inequalities in Health.* London: Stationary Office.

Adler NE, Boyce T, Chesney MA, Cohen S, Folkman S, Kahn RL, Syme SL (1994) Socioeconomic status and health: The challenge of the gradient. *American Psychologist* 49:15–24.

Anderson E (1999) What is the point of equality? *Ethics* 109:287–337.

Arneson RJ (1988) Equality and equal opportunity for welfare. *Philosophical Studies* 54: 79–95.

Arrow K (1973) Some ordinalist-utilitarian notes on Rawls's theory of justice. *Journal of Philosophy* 70:9:251.

Barker D (1998) *Mothers, Babies and Health in Later Life.* Edinburgh: Churchhill Livingstone.

Barry B (1989) *Theories of Justice.* London: Harvester Wheatsheaf.

Bartley M, Blane D, Montgomery S (1997) Socioeconomic determinants of health: Health and the life course: Why safety nets matter. *British Medical Journal* 314:1194.

Black D, Morris JN, Smith C, Townsend P, Whitehead M (1988) *Inequalities in Health: The Black Report; The Health Divide.* London: Penguin Group.

Braveman P (1999) *Monitoring Equity in Health: A Policy-Oriented Approach in Low- and Middle-Income Countries* Geneva: World Health Organization.

Buchanan A, Brock D, Daniels N, Wikler D (2000) *From Chance to Choice: Genetics and the Just Society.* New York: Cambridge University Press.

Cohen GA (1989) On the currency of egalitarian justice. *Ethics* 99:906–44.

Cohen GA (1992) Incentives, inequality, and community. In: Petersen GB (ed) *The Tanner Lectures on Human Values, Volume Thirteen.* Salt Lake City: University of Utah Press.

Cohen GA (1995) The Pareto argument for inequality. *Social Philosophy and Policy* 12: 160–85.

Cohen J (1989) Democratic equality. *Ethics* 99:727–51.

Cohen J (unpbl ms) The Pareto Argument.

Dahlgren G and Whitehead M (1991) *Policies and Strategies to Promote Social Equity in Health.* Stockholm: Institute of Future Studies.

Daniels N (1981) Health-care needs and distributive justice. *Philosophy and Public Affairs* 10:146–79.

Daniels N (1985) *Just Health Care.* New York: Cambridge University Press.

Daniels N (1990) Equality of what: welfare, resources, or capabilities? *Philosophy and Phenomenological Research* 50 (Supplement): 273–96.

Daniels N (1996) Mental disabilities, equal opportunity and the ADA. In: Bonnie RJ and Monahan J (eds) *Mental Disorder, Work Disability, and the Law.* Chicago: University of Chicago Press.

Daniels N (2002) Democratic Equality: Rawls' Complex Egalitarianism. In: Freeman S (ed) *Companion to Rawls* Oxford: Blackwell (in press).

Daniels N, Light D, Caplan R (1996) *Benchmarks of Fairness for Health Care Reform.* New York: Oxford University Press.

Daniels N and Sabin JE (1997) Limits to health care: Fair procedures, democratic deliberation, and the legitimacy problem for insurers. *Philosophy and Public Affairs* 26: 303–50.

Davey-Smith G, Shipley MJ, Rose G (1990) Magnitude and causes of socioeconomic differentials in mortality: Further evidence from the Whitehall Study. *Journal of Epidemiology and Community Health* 44:265–270.

Davey-Smith G, Hart C, Blane D, Hole D (1998) Adverse socioeconomic conditions in childhood and cause specific adult mortality: A prospective observational study. *British Medical Journal* 316:1631–5.

Dreze J and Sen AK (1989) *Hunger and Public Action.* Oxford: Clarendon Press.

Fishkin J (1983) *Justice, Equal Opportunity, and the Family.* New Haven, CT: Yale University Press.

Gutmann A and Thompson D (1995) *Democratic Disagreement.* Cambridge, MA: Harvard University Press.

Hill KQ, Leighley JE, Hinton-Andersson A (1995) Lower-class mobilization and policy linkage in the U.S. states. *American Journal of Political Science* 39:75–86.

House J and Williams D (2000) Understanding and reducing socioeconomic and racial/ethnic disparities in health. Unpublished ms presented at the IOM/CBSS Conference on Capitalizing on Social Science and Behavioral Research to Improve the Public's Health, February 2–3, 2000.

Kaplan GA, Pamuk ER, Lynch JW, Cohen RD, Balfour JL (1996) Inequality in income and mortality in the United States: Analysis of mortality and potential pathways. *British Medical Journal* 312:999–1003.

Karasek R and Theorell T (1990) *Health Work.* New York: Basic Books.

Kawachi I and Kennedy BP (1997) Health and social cohesion: Why care about income inequality? *British Medical Journal* 314:1037–40.

Kawachi I and Kennedy BP (1999) Income inequality and health: Pathways and mechanisms. *Health Services Research* 34:215–27.

Kawachi I, Kennedy BP, Lochner K, Prothrow-Stith D (1997) Social capital, income inequality and mortality. *American Journal of Public Health* 87:1491–8.

Kawachi I, Kennedy BP, Prothrow-Stith D, Gupta V (1999) Women's status and the health of women: A view from the states. *Social Science and Medicine* 48:21–32.

Kawachi I, Kennedy BP, Wilkinson R (eds) (1999) *Income Inequality and Health: A Reader.* New York: The New Press.

Kennedy BP, Kawachi I, Glass R, Prothrow-Stith D (1998a) Income distribution, socioeconomic status, and self-rated health: A US multi-level analysis. *British Medical Journal* 317:917–21.

Kennedy BP, Kawachi I, Prothrow-Stith D (1996) Income distribution and mortality: Test of the Robin Hood Index in the United States. *British Medical Journal* 312:1004–8. Published erratum appears in *British Medical Journal* 312:1194.

Kennedy BP, Kawachi I, Prothrow-Stith D, Gupta V (1998) Income inequality, social capital and firearm-related violent crime. *Social Science and Medicine* 47:7–17.

Lavis JN and Stoddart GL (1994) Can we have too much health care? *Daedalus* 123: 43–60.

Link BG, Northridge ME, Phelan JC, Ganz ML (1998) Social epidemiology and the fundamental cause concept: On the structuring of effective cancer screens by socio-economic status. *Milbank Quarterly* 76:375–402.

Lochner K (1999) *State Income Inequality and Individual Mortality Risk: A Prospective Multilevel Study*. Harvard University PhD dissertation.

Lynch JW, Kaplan GA, Pamuk ER, Cohen RD, Balfour JL, Yen IH (1998) Income inequality and mortality in metropolitan areas of the United States. *American Journal of Public Health* 88:1074–80.

Marmot MG (1994) Social differentials in health within and between populations. *Daedalus* 123:197–216

Marmot MG (1999) Social causes of social inequalities in health. Harvard Center for Population and Development Studies, Working Paper Series 99.01, January 1999.

Marmot MG, Bosma H, Hemingway H, Brunner E, Stansfield S (1997) Contributions of job control and other risk factors to social variations in coronary heart disease incidence. *Lancet* 350:235–9.

Marmot MG, Fuhrer R, Ettner SL, Marks NF, Bumpass LL, Ryff CD (1998) Contribution of psychosocial factors to socioeconomic differences in health. *Milbank Quarterly* 76:403–48.

Moss NE and Carver K (1998) The effect of WIC and Medicaid on infant mortality in the United States. *American Journal of Public Health* 88:1354–61.

Ostlin P and Diderichsen F (2000) Equity-oriented national strategy for public health in Sweden. WHO Regional Office for Europe, European Centre for Health Policy, Brussels.

Pappas G, Queen S, Hadden W, and Fisher G (1993) The increasing disparity in mortality between socioeconomic groups in the United States, 1960 and 1986. *New England Journal of Medicine* 329:103–9

Putnam RD (1993) *Making Democracy Work. Civic Traditions in Modern Italy*. Princeton, NJ: Princeton University Press.

Rawls J (1971) *A Theory of Justice*. Cambridge, MA: Harvard University Press.

Rawls J (1993) *Political Liberalism*. New York: Columbia University Press.

Schweinhart LJ, Barnes HV, Weikart DP (1993) *Significant Benefits: The High/Scope Project Perry Preschool Study Through Age 27*. Ypsilanti, MI: The High/Scope Press.

Sen AK (1980) Equality of what? In McMurrin S (ed) *Tanner Lectures on Human Values*, Vol 1. Cambridge: Cambridge University Press.

Sen AK (1992) *Inequality Reexamined*. Cambridge, MA: Harvard University Press.

Sen AK (1998) Mortality as an indicator of economic success and failure. *The Economic Journal* 108–25.

Sen AK. (1999) *Development as Freedom*. New York: Alfred A. Knopf.

Villerme L. (1840) *Tableau d'Etat Physique et Moral des Ouvriers*, Vol 2. Paris: Renourard.

Whitehead M. (1992) The concepts and principles of equity and health. *International Journal of Health Services* 22:429–45.

Wilkinson RG. (1992) Income distribution and life expectancy. *British Medical Journal* 304: 165–8.

Wilkinson RG. (1994) The epidemiological transition: From material scarcity to social disadvantage? *Daedalus* 123:61–77.

Wilkinson RG. (1996) *Unhealthy Societies: The Afflictions of Inequality*. London: Routledge.

Wilkinson RG, Kawachi I, Kennedy B. (1998) Mortality, the social environment, crime and violence. *Sociology of Health and Illness* 20:578–97.

Wilkinson RG, Kennedy BP, Kawachi I. (1999) Women's status and men's health in a culture of inequality. *Sociology of Health and Illness* (in press).

II

Connecting ethics and health policy

3

What ethics can contribute to health policy

LARRY R. CHURCHILL

Why bring ethics to health policy? Of course, in one sense it is already there. There are ethical assumptions and implications for all health policies and ethical aspects to every process of policy making. For example, issues of who receives the burdens and benefits under various policies are irreducibly moral issues, and Eli Ginsberg's essay in this volume describes some of these issues for U.S. policy in the last century. Likewise, policy-making rules and procedures can be fair or morally arbitrary, and the essay by Amy Gutmann and Dennis Thompson presents a deliberative model they believe satisfies the requirements for fairness. These ethical dimensions are so pervasive that it is hard to imagine a health policy or policy-making procedure without them. But while these ethical dimensions are easy to identify, they are rarely given systematic scrutiny. Aside from a handful of scholars working on issues of justice in allocation or on the social goals and priorities in health care, policy questions are not a routine part of the work of most bioethicists.

What accounts for this lack of engagement? Many inhibiting factors exist, but two deserve special mention. The first is the pervasive American commitment to individualism (Tocqueville, 1990; Reisman, 1954; Slater, 1970; Bellah, et al, 1985). To date, American bioethics has largely mirrored this commitment. As such, it has been preoccupied with issues of individual autonomy, that is, with how to protect and extend personal freedoms. Reflecting both a political and a cultural commitment to the individual as the key unit of moral analysis, bioethicists tend to analyze policy questions for their effect on persons as independent entities rather than as members of society, and to focus on discrete, individualized goods rather than public and social goods. Moreover, even among those who have made health policy issues the major emphasis of their work, a focus on individuals is apparent. For example, the prevailing arguments for a right to health care are frequently interpreted not as expressions of social solidarity or advocacy for population health, but as supportive of a personal entitlement the absence of which thwarts individual opportunities and thereby creates problems of fairness (Daniels, 1985).

A second inhibiting factor is the American cultural aversion to rationing health services, which is an aversion not only to rationing itself but also a disinclination to recognize that health resources are finite. Of course, in the final analysis, every society must allocate and ration health services, since the health needs of populations always exceed the supply of available resources. Most Western democracies have chosen to ration according to national health policies and to strive for some degree of equity in access for all citizens. The United States also rations health care, but not according to national health policies. Instead, we ration by price, allowing market forces to determine who receives care and subsequently creating special programs for some groups who are undesirable to private insurers, such as the elderly and impoverished children.

But there is a pervasive distaste for calling these market-driven practices "rationing." Indeed, the disdain for rationing has been so strong that the term has often been used to castigate one's opponents in health policy debates, as occurred repeatedly during the 1993–1994 demise of the Clinton health reform proposal. Only in Oregon has it been possible to openly discuss finite resources and policy-making processes that explicitly include rationing, and even this conversation was heavily criticized by those outside Oregon (Kitzhaber, 1990).

This deep cultural aversion has had a quelling effect on exchanges between ethicists and shapers of health policy. More specifically, policy makers may be understandably reticent to join forces with bioethicists since some of the first issues bioethicists are likely to raise are those that are the most contentious. Indeed, when a group of bioethicists was assembled in the early 1990s to help draft the values statement that would accompany the Clinton health plan, they were specifically instructed to draft principles that did not include the term *rationing*.

I mention these inhibiting factors briefly because they are two of the largest barriers to any lasting engagement between health policy and ethics, and also because I believe it is possible to overcome them. While individualism and the antipathy for candid conversions about rationing are inhibiting, they are not prohibitive. A fruitful engagement between ethics and health policy is both possible and highly desirable. The chief barrier to this engagement is, quite simply, a lack of understanding of the benefits it will reap. Exploring these benefits is my chief objective in this essay.

WHAT ETHICS CAN CONTRIBUTE TO HEALTH POLICY

Ethics in its broadest sense concerns how we live and the choices we make. More precisely, ethics is the field that seeks to understand which values are worthy of our embrace, and why. Finding this out is an endeavor in which both theory and practice are important. Indeed, some of the missteps and slippage in ethics come from an improper balance between the two. On the one hand, ethical problem solving without the benefit of theoretical reflection is like digging a garden with one's bare hands rather than using the appropriate tools. Theories are tools and can be used with greater or lesser skill, and skill only comes with practice. On the other hand, theoretical reflection that is untested by involvement in the concrete particulars of life is like reading about gardens without ever planting and tending one. Accordingly, the flourishing of ethics, both for individuals and for societies, depends upon this dialectic between careful theoretical deliberation and practical experience. There is no substitute for either.

Ethics is too often thought to be the province of experts—an esoteric field in which the major texts are in Greek or German and in which even the translations are abstruse and the reasoning beyond the keen of ordinary people. While I believe there is real benefit to studying Aristotle and Kant, I am convinced that the insights of these moral theorists can be made accessible to anyone and, more importantly, that the essential theoretical maneuvers and practical skills of ethics are already available to much of the population, although not often used. It is these commonplace but important aspects of ethical reflection and deliberation that I will emphasize here. In other words, whatever the reasons that ethics has not been a major part of health policy, it is *not* because ethics as a field requires highly specialized knowledge or recondite theories. The things that are valuable about ethics for health policy and for other fields are things that all of us can do, given the will to undertake them.

The Humanizing Function of Ethical Dialogue

So far as I can tell, we humans are the only members of the animal kingdom—perhaps the only living things, period—that do ethics. It seems clear that other primates, and perhaps many other forms of life, are capable of moral behavior and exercise it routinely. My dog, for example, can be taught to be ashamed of himself as well as to exhibit loyalty; porpoises and other aquatic dwellers seem capable of helping behaviors and perhaps even altruism. But none of these nonhuman animals seems to be able to reflect systematically and critically on their moral behaviors or to creatively oscillate between the theoretical and the practical, which is the essence of ethics. The core capacity for ethics is not simply a matter of doing good, but knowing *why* what one is doing can be called "good," having self-consciously chosen it from among the alternatives. It would be hubris to insist that only our species can possibly do this, so I couch my thesis with the requisite agnosticism. Still, as I will explain, there is a great deal to be learned about ethics from studying the moral behavior of primates.

Ethics is not only a distinctively, if not uniquely, human capacity, it is a humanizing activity. Here I mean something very elementary. In order to have an ethical discussion with someone, I must seriously and respectfully entertain values, both my interlocutor's and my own. Values are simply not accessible unless they are approached in this way. Ethical conversations require accrediting others with respect and regard; an exchange in ethics begins with the assumption that others have values that are as important to them as mine are to me. This simple act of accrediting is itself a humanizing activity, for it means that I am willing to set aside, at least for the moment, differences in power and status in order to consider matters afresh. Ethical conversations, in order to be productive, must suspend hierarchy and minimize power differences. This suspension of status to enable attention to values is not easy and is perhaps why ethical conversations between parents and children and between supervisors and employees are so rare.

Engaging in ethical deliberation means listening—paying attention—and this calls into play our innate empathic capacity. David Hume, Adam Smith, and others philosophers of the Scottish Enlightenment were the most systematic and sophisticated students of this capacity, which they termed "sympathy" or "fellow feeling" (Hume, 1978; Smith, 1976). The education and refinement of this universal capacity for sympathy through reasoned reflection was for them the core of ethics. Thus, as Hume and Smith saw it, ethics could be said to be humanizing because it called for the higher development of a basic capacity we seem to share with other life forms. Attaining this higher development necessarily requires respectful engagement with other persons as sentient and reflective beings like ourselves whose values hold for them the same primal place that mine hold for me.

In his essay in this volume Kingdon expresses a concern that infusing policy deliberations with ethics could tend to harden discussion and make coalition building and consensus more difficult. My conception of ethics is just the opposite. While discussion of moral values can take ideological turns and lead to ossification, the true spirit of ethical inquiry involves exploration and openness to differences undertaken in the spirit of moral agnosticism—the assumption that I do not possess the final truth on most issues. Such a demeanor is the very opposite of moralizing or proselytizing for one's position; rather, it involves seeking to find the best policy through a careful examination of the ethical implications of all the options. I do not claim that this is simple. Yet when it is present, the assumption that all engaged parties have a morally equivalent voice can make consensus and coalition building easier rather than more difficult.

Ethical engagement is humanizing in another obvious way. Because it involves the mutual flow of empathy and respectful regard for differences that lets values emerge in an exchange, it is also a mode of interacting that is vastly less harmful to the participants than the other modes of handling disagreements, such as shouting matches, holding grudges, filing suits, or shooting people.

If ethics is considered a mode of conflict resolution, perhaps there is much to learn from studying the moral behavior of other primates. The primatologist Frans de Waal, wary of quasi-Darwinian theories that make aggression the bedrock explanation for primate behavior, has spent the last 25 years investigating how relationships are repaired and normalized following outbreaks of aggression. Most reconciliatory rituals, he discovered, take minutes or hours, whereas humans sometimes hold grudges and seek revenge over decades or even across generations. Waal concludes his book *Peacemaking Among Primates* by saying that "forgiveness is not . . . a mysterious and sublime idea that we owe to a few millennia of Judeo-Christianity. . . . The fact that monkeys, apes and humans all engage in reconciliatory behavior means it is probably over thirty million years old. . . ." (Waal, 1989).

The findings of Waal signal both the immense antiquity of reconciling behaviors and also their profound importance for human well-being. Consistent with my approach above, it would be accurate to say that while only humans engage in ethics, understood in the deep sense of reflective weighing to guide actions and find justifications, the higher primates are clearly capable of moral activity that is respectful and constructive. I find it helpful to think of ethical discussion and deliberation as a higher form of the conciliatory physical gestures of our primate relatives such as hand-holding, food sharing, and grooming. In other words, our ethical practices are simply a sophisticated verbal and cognitive extension of attitudes of respectful interaction with evolutionary roots extending back several million years. Ethics, as 21st-century peoples know it, is the most recent flowering of this ancient rootage.

Moreover, ethical deliberation, as one of the modes of recognition and reconciliation, can have a positive effect on human bonding even when it fails as a mechanism of problem solving or consensus. Ethics has intrinsic and not just instrumental value, so the benefit of ethical deliberation and discussion can be significant even when consensus is not possible or an "answer" is not reached. Health policy questions inevitably concern questions of conflict, of social choices in which issues of distributing burdens and benefits arise and for which no technological fixes exist. Respectful accommodation is thus almost always necessary. As such, health policy questions represent an area in which ethics, if properly understood, might play a substantial role.

But what role? Even readers who have followed me thus far and see the civilizing capacity of ethics as compared to other ways of approaching contentious issues are likely to feel dissatisfied, for I have not yet identified any specific benefits obtainable from the application of the tools of ethics to health policy issues. What, more precisely, can we hope to gain by a more routine engagement of ethics with health policy? I will discuss two salutary effects, although others could be mentioned. As we shall see, ethics can, first, lead to a broader and more stable basis for health policy initiatives. Second, ethics can help us step back and identify, clarify, and assess the aims and purposes of health policy.

Broadening the Moral Basis for Health Policies

Discussions of moral values are occasionally marred by moralizing, by dichotomous categorizations into "good" and "bad," and by villainization of those whose opinions differ from ours. Because of this, it is sometimes assumed that bringing ethics into a discussion is harmful to consensus building. But, as I argued earlier, just because ethics is sometimes done poorly does not mean that it cannot be done well. And when done well, it stretches our powers of empathy and lays the basis for a more attentive and respectful exchange. When this occurs, ethics can be a powerful aid to consensus building, revealing unexpected common ground and providing a broader and more stable foundation of support for policy initiatives.

For example, the past few years have seen a variety of initiatives aimed at covering more children for basic health services. In some cases these initiatives are conceived as preliminary steps in attaining the goal of universal care for children, which is itself conceived as a step toward universal care for all citizens. An ethics approach to these policy initiatives would, of course, inquire into the values they seek to embody and probe the various moral rationales for such policies. Such probing requires going beyond the moral rationales provided by the sponsors of these children's health initiatives and asking about the potential interests of those who are uncommitted and potentially opposed to them. In other words, ethics always involves asking what policy looks like from different vantage points, with the values of multiple perspectives in mind.

To illustrate, most of the rationales given in support of expanded health care for children address the needs of the children themselves and focus on the declining coverage of children through employer-based insurance, the increasing number of children who grow up in poverty, and, in general, the "crisis" in children's health (Hughes, 1999; Miller, 1998; Kopelman and Palumbo, 1997). This is a natural focal point for those advocating children's health programs. Ethics can broaden and strengthen this advocacy. More specifically, one role of ethics in this context is to imagine what parents of insured children—and even those who are not parents and will never be parents—might think of these initiatives, including what possible ethical reasons they might have to support such a policy. Seeking to explore multiple rationales for children's health initiatives, one might argue in the following ways (Churchill, 2001).

(*1*) All parents have a stake in avoiding intrafamilial struggles about whose health care needs will be met. Consider the following dynamic. Employers in the heavily commercial managed care environment have a diminishing willingness and/or ability to offer policies to cover the spouses and children of workers, and this means tragic choices and sacrifices for low-income workers or for any family whose coverage is unstable. For example, as a North Carolina state employee, the premium for my individual health insurance is paid completely by the state. It costs me nothing, and the costs I do incur are modest co-payments and deductibles at the time services are rendered. To ensure coverage for my family, I pay a monthly premium of $365, for which I receive a federal tax subsidy, reducing the actual payroll deduction to roughly $240. The housekeeper who cleans my office also receives fully funded coverage for herself, and she has the same opportunity to purchase coverage for her spouse and children. Yet, since her salary is roughly one-sixth of mine, this becomes for her a far more difficult calculation, and the cost of providing for her children the same coverage she enjoys becomes a strategic survival choice among food, clothing, transportation, and other fundamental goods. Many housekeepers have no insurance for their children, whereas it is virtually unheard of for faculty to choose not to cover their children.

It could be argued that this example illustrates the unfairness of a system that charges everyone the same amount to fund services, rather than dividing costs proportionally. My chief point, however, is the resulting unfairness within a family unit of having some members of a household covered while others are not, especially when those not covered are one's children. Most parents consider obligations to their children their primary obligations. A policy of broader coverage for children should be supported, then, because it would assure that no matter what a person's employment status now or in the future, one's children would not suffer. Such a policy would relieve parents of the agonizing choice between health needs and other needs. It would also obviate choices about which child's needs to meet, for example, who to take to the doctor or dentist when one child requires treatment for her asthma and another child suffers chronic infections from impacted teeth. No parent should have to make such choices.

It might be thought that this argument will appeal only to low-income, working-class parents. I think it applies to all parents, since few of us can be confident that, over the two decades required to raise a child, we can be assured of adequate health coverage for him or her. Even tenured professors, who tend to think of their jobs as relatively secure, must worry about pre-existing condition clauses, changes in health plans and eligibility rules, and other cost-reduction schemes that will jeopardize the ability to care adequately for children. This reasoning might encourage parents to be concerned with other people's children as well, given that a system that covers all children may well be a system they will someday need to use. It should be noted that both self-interest as well as benevolence inform this motivation, illustrating how both self-regarding and other-regarding motivations have ethical weight and can eventuate in the same policy.

(*2*) But why should adults who no longer have children or who have never been parents and never plan to become parents be concerned about the health needs of children? Of course, they may simply be caring and generous people, but other considerations exist that an empathetic imagination can uncover. For example, any working adult should be concerned with the health of future workers and the ways the current health status of children affect the chances that those children will become productive, tax-paying citizens. Every child who has diminished opportunities from ill health is a drain upon the common resources from which each of us hopes to draw in retirement. Unless one's head has been completely buried in the sand over the past decade, she will understand that the soundness of both the health-care and income provisions of the Social Security system depend upon future workers. That is, no one has a secure individual account in the U.S. Treasury awaiting her retirement. Each has only the willingness of future generations to carry on a tradition of medical and social care for the elderly, nothing more. Thus each has a powerful interest in supporting a system that enhances the life opportunities of the young and maximizes their future productivity.

A self-interested adult might also be deeply invested in how younger generations think and feel about the system of intergenerational subsidies that will support her retirement income and medical care. Persons who twenty years hence will be asked to shoulder a substantial financial burden to care for the growing number of elderly will have a greater willingness to do so, I surmise, if they themselves have been cared for in their youth. While health services are only a part of that care, they are a significant part. In terms of how they think of a health-care system, young adults who have grown up in a society in which income and social class are not admission tickets to health providers may approach their tax burden with a sense of solidarity with other citizens, rather than seeing themselves as pitted against others in competition for scarce resources. Given that my own health-care needs will increase with age, anything that can be done to strengthen the sense of community among different age groups is likely to benefit me, and benefit me more the older I become.

These are, to be sure, only sketches of arguments, and they form only a small part of the larger effort to probe diverse perspectives for common causes. I cite them not to defend them as persuasive, but as illustrations of the kind of thinking that ethics can bring to health policy. By probing the various rationales of those who are uncommitted and potentially opposed to such policies, ethics can sometimes find new bases for agreement. However, even when ethics does not work, trying to think from the perspectives of others can provide the basis for future conversations in which consensus building may be more successful.

Grounding Health Policy in Ethical Goals and Purposes

Ethics can serve the very important function of clarifying and examining the larger goals and purposes of health policies, aspects of which are often left tacit and unexamined. The goals and purposes of health policies can be said to be "ethical" in the sense that they necessarily involve the ranking of some goods over others and the distribution of benefits and burdens in some way. Yet just what that ranking of goods and distribution of benefits and burdens should be is not always evident until a crisis occurs.

A 1999 U. S. Supreme Court ruling illustrates how crises in health care serve to display the values embedded in health policies. The ruling in question concerned Illinois resident Cynthia Herdrich, who went to her HMO for a pain in her side. A diagnostic test that might have detected her problem was delayed, and subsequently Herdrich's appendix burst, requiring emergency surgery. Herdrich and her attorneys claimed that the delay in properly diagnosing her problem was due to the cost-cutting practices of her HMO and that its zeal for profit-driven efficiency made her physicians negligent in her care. This case was one in a long line of horror stories from angry patients who believed their care was compromised in order to increase corporate profits or to fill the pockets of physicians who are paid bonuses to keep costs down. The Supreme Court unanimously ruled that Herdrich could not use existing federal law to sue her HMO, and, moreover, in the words of Justice Souter, "inducement to ration care goes to the very point of any HMO scheme . . . and rationing necessarily raises some risks while reducing others" (*Pegram v. Herdrich*, 2000).

I am not arguing that rationing can be avoided, nor would I contend that Justice Souter was wrong to emphasize that HMOs necessarily ration services. Indeed, he showed a refreshing degree of candor. Rather, the problem is the way the Court's decision seems to focus so narrowly on what HMOs are and are not permitted to do, a focus that is perhaps legally appropriate but morally troubling. Such a narrow focus separates the responsibility for cost containment from accountability for health outcomes. Justice Souter's phrasing shows that what is needed is not so much a different decision from the Court, but a different kind of accountability from HMOs. This enhanced accountability for HMOs and for managed care more generally is not within the purview of the judicial system. Instead, it is the policy initiatives from the legislative and executive branches that are responsive to the public interest. What Justice Souter's remarks make clear is the need for larger purposes and goals within which specific policies and practices can be framed and interpreted. What is at stake is not what HMOs are, but what they ought to be.

In these and similar situations the role of ethical analysis lies in asking if the outcome of *Pegram v. Herdrich* is what we want not just from HMOs but from the health care policies that permit and encourage HMOs to function in this way. Are the larger goals or purposes of health policy being achieved by a system that permits delays and inattention to the extent that patients suffer avoidable harm, such as a ruptured appendix? We should note that this question cannot be answered by consulting the ERISA law and clarifying the role of the federal judiciary, which is what the Supreme Court (appropriately) did in the Herdrich case. Nor can it be answered by asking about the financial or managerial soundness of Herdrich's HMO, which is what state insurance commissioners are charged to do. These sorts of inquiries are merely particulars in the service of some larger agenda yet to be specified and give us little sense of the overall purposes and goals of health policy. Rather the ethical interrogation of larger aims and justifications strives to be clear about precisely what any given health policy seeks through its various programs and subjects these goals to critical scrutiny.

It is part of the genius of market-dominated health care that this question of the larger aims and justifications of policy is rendered very difficult to address since the workings of the market in the U.S. environment are made to seem natural and obvious and therefore not in need of moral justification (Churchill, 1987). It takes a crisis, or a sense of being harmed and wronged, as in the Herdrich situation, to uncover these goals and purposes. When we do uncover them they may be quite different from what we had assumed.

One important role for ethics in policy matters is, then, fundamentally, the identification of the ends sought in policies, the examination of the values embodied in these ends, and the assessment of the extent to which these ends are in keeping with social values. Of course, it is always possible to argue that the U.S. health-care system has no social purposes or goals as such, or at least no goals that can be isolated for moral scrutiny. While doctors have their particular goals in delivering care and patients in receiving it, and HMOs have goals in organizing and marketing it, and so on, there is no larger set of social goals being pursued. Indeed, just as there are no social goals for the automobile industry, it could be argued, there are no social goals for the health-care industry. Of course, there are regulations on automobiles for purposes of safety, such as laws mandating seat belts, shatter-resistant glass, and restrictions on the amount of pollution from automobile exhaust systems, yet there are no social goals or purposes concerning the importance of driving or car ownership. In a similar fashion, the dominance of market forces could be taken to mean that health policies are like automobile policies, that is, their function is to regulate (minimally) the actors on matters at the outer boundaries of public safety and fair business dealings. Such minimalist tinkering does not express any positive or important social goal; it only ensures a modicum of safety and fair play for the individual participants. This is precisely what is exemplified in the ruling of Justice Souter, who in effect said that Herdrich got just what she should have expected, while completely ignoring any sense of larger purpose for HMOs in providing good health care or exercising fiduciary obligations toward Herdrich and other patients.

To express this somewhat differently, it could be argued that ethical analysis of health policies is not needed because health policy aims are both known and routinely accomplished. They are accomplished through the satisfaction of the millions of actors, agencies, and organizations as they negotiate and bargain for health services, making whatever deals they can in an environment minimally affected by government interference. From this perspective, health policy has no purpose beyond the separate purposes of the individual actors, and the only appropriate role of specific health policies, rules, and regulations is to make the bargaining process among providers and consumers at all levels devoid of fraud and abuse.

The idea that well-functioning markets are the true goal of health care policy has always enjoyed a following in the United States, and it has gained more popularity since the failure of the Clinton reform proposals in 1994.

Of course, a countervailing argument can be made based on the long-standing popular support for health programs for special populations that cannot compete in the market, such as the elderly, the chronically ill, and children. But, despite the support for these programs, consensus on their overall social aims and their fit into a larger social agenda is elusive. Are we, through these programs, seeking better health status for individuals? Or is the goal to maximize health benefits from limited resources for the affected population? Or is the goal medical progress, as the burgeoning NIH budget and the increasing conflation of clinical research with therapeutic standards would suggest? Is the aim security from impoverishment from medical bills? Is it fair equality of opportunity, as Norman Daniels has argued (Daniels, 1985)? Of course, different health policies, such as Medicare, Medicaid, the Veterans Administration health programs, the Indian Health Service, the Childrens Health Insurance Programs, and so on, were devised at different times in our national history. Each affects different constituencies and has appropriately divergent aims. To this extent, each program should be judged on its own merits, yet it is also important to ask about the social values that underwrite these separate programs and whether there are purposes and goals that underwrite health policies for the nation in some more generic sense. Is there anything of which these separate programs are a part? Lack of clarity about this larger question inevitably leads to the inability to judge whether these separate programs are playing their parts well or poorly (Reinhardt, 1997). As Victor Fuchs puts it, "If you don't know where you're going, any road will get you there" (Fuchs, 1995, p. 186). Thus ungrounded, it is no surprise to find that these programs are altered and sometimes fundamentally changed with changes of the federal executive or legislative branch.

I have argued in another volume that the two large civic purposes of any modern health-care system should be security and solidarity (Churchill, 1994). Security here refers to the freedom of persons to live both without fear that their basic health needs will go unattended and without fear they will become impoverished when seeking or receiving care. Solidarity refers to the sense of community that emerges from acknowledgment of shared benefits and burdens. Both these aims are endorsed by the vast majority of modern industrial democracies, but they have yet to be embraced by the United States. My aim here is not to argue for these two purposes but to point to the role of ethical reflection in bringing to the foreground a particular kind of thinking that interrogates purposes, that probes for clarity about both particular program goals and larger social goals, and in this way seeks to ground and stabilize health policy. Such grounding is a sine qua non for evaluating health policies and establishing accountability for their effects. Dan Callahan's chapter in this volume is a good example of the kind of contribution ethics can make to health policy in clarifying and critically examining purposes and goals, yet it is only a beginning for what must become an on-going conversation.

CONCLUSION

This essay highlights some of the contributions that systematic ethical reflection can bring to health policy. I have not discussed the benefits that would accrue to the field of ethics from this dialogue, although I believe they would be substantial. In a 1982 essay Stephen Toulmin claimed that engagement with medicine had "saved the life of ethics" by bringing it down from its abstract metaethical preoccupations and into contact with practical problems, thus giving ethics a "seriousness and human relevance" that it had lacked (Toulmin, 1982). I believe something similar can be said for the emerging engagement of ethics with health policy. The formal training of most academic ethicists emphasizes theoretical justifications and general norms and thus provides poor preparation for delving into the murky details and the predominantly pragmatic concerns of health policy. While health policy may not save the life of ethics, it may help to correct its individualistic bias, sharpen awareness of the irreducibly social and political character of ethical issues, and enliven the more arid, theoretical approaches to which most ethicists are predisposed.

While I hope and believe that ethics as a field will benefit from a more sustained engagement with health policy, I have also stressed an approach in this essay that deemphasizes the technical skills of ethicists and illustrates the sort of ethical contribution to health policy matters that might be made by any reflective person. Graduate training in ethics or some closely aligned discipline can, of course, be very useful. Yet connecting ethics to health policy requires both less (no advanced degrees in philosophy are needed) and more (getting one's hands—or one's theories—dirty). The most important resources to call upon are a willingness to suspend moral certainty long enough to make human contact with those who differ, a demeanor of respectful empathy, and a critical focus on the values involved. These are resources rarely mastered in graduate programs, but they are often attained in the warp and woof of the conversations, debates, and compromises that go into policy formation.

It may be that our lack of interest in the ethics of health policy has given us the health-care system we deserve. When ethical reflection becomes a more routine part of health policy studies, we will be in a position to decide if this is the health care system we want.

REFERENCES

Bellah R, Madsen R, Sullivan W, Swidler A, Tipton S (1985) *Habits of the Heart: Individualism and Commitment in American Life*. Berkeley, CA: University of California Press.

Churchill L (1987) *Rationing Health Care in America: Perceptions and Principles of Justice*. Notre Dame, IN: University of Notre Dame Press.

Churchill L (1994) *Self-Interest and Universal Health Care: Why Well-Insured Americans Should Support Coverage for Everyone*. Cambridge, MA: Harvard University Press.

Churchill L (2001) Universal health care for children: Why every self-interested person should support it. *Journal of Medicine and Philosophy* 26:179–191.

Daniels N (1985) *Just Health Care*. Cambridge: Cambridge University Press.

Danis M, Mutran E, Garrett J, Stearns S, Slifkin R, Hanson L, Williams J, Churchill L (1996) A prospective study of the impact of patient preferences on life-sustaining treatment and hospital costs. *Critical Care Medicine* 24:1811–17.

Fuchs V (1995) What every philosopher should know about health economics. *Proceedings of the American Philosophical Society* 140:186–95.

Hughes D, Johnson K, Rosenblum S (1999) Children's access to health care. In: Lille-Blanton M, Martinez R, Lyons B, Rowland D (eds) *Access to Health Care: Promises and Prospects for Low-Income Americans*. Washington, D.C.: The Kaiser Commission on Medicaid and the Uninsured.

Hume D (1978) *A Treatise of Human Nature, Book III*, 2d ed, edited by Nidditch P. Oxford: Clarendon Press.

Kitzhaber J (1990) *The Oregon Basic Health Services Act*. Oregon State Senate, 2–5.

Kopelman L, Palumbo M (1999) The U.S. health care system: Ineffective and unfair to children. *American Journal of Law, Medicine and Ethics* 23:2.

Miller C (1998) A snapshot of children's health. In: Mouradian W (ed) *Children Our Future*. Seattle, WA: Washington State Department of Health.

Pegram v. Herdrich (2000) U.S. Supreme Court. No. 98–1849. June 12, 2000.

Reinhardt U (1997) Wanted: A clearly articulated social ethics for American health care. *Journal of the American Medical Association* 278:1446.

Reisman D (1954) *Individualism Reconsidered*. Garden City, NY: Doubleday Anchor.

Slater P (1970) *The Pursuit of Loneliness: American Culture at the Breaking Point*. Boston, MA: Beacon Press.

Smith A (1976) *The Theory of Moral Sentiments*, Raphael D, Macfie A (eds). Indianapolis, IN: Liberty Classics.

Tocqueville A (1990) *Democracy in America, Vol. I & II*. New York: Random House.

Toulmin S (1982) How medicine saved the life of ethics. *Perspectives in Biology and Medicine* 25:736–750.

Waal F (1989) *Peacemaking Among Primates*. Cambridge, MA: Harvard University Press.

4

Health-care policy in the United States in the 20th century

ELI GINZBERG

I begin with some summary observations about the role that ethics has played in helping to shape health-care policy in the United States in the 20th century. The fact that the United States consists of fifty states occupying an area of about three million square miles with a population of around 270 million with substantial variations in culture, politics, and family wealth and taxable revenue has contributed to substantial variations in private insurance and public services. These variations include large-scale disparities in both the geographic distribution of health care resources and the costs and quality of medical care. These disparities invite inquiry into the dynamic between ethics and health policy. I will be concerned here with the absence of national health insurance in the United States, an absence that serves to contrast this country with all other advanced nations, each of which has implemented universal coverage.

Part of the explanation for the failure to provide basic health insurance coverage for all the country's people is the population's deep-seated unease about extending the scale and scope of the powers of the federal government. Most service programs are viewed as the primary responsibility of state governments, which have found it impossible to cover the high costs of health insurance coverage for all of their residents, but as the conclusion of this chapter suggests, what has long been established practice may soon be changed.

Although President Theodore Roosevelt, running on the Bull Moose ticket for the presidency in 1912, included support for national health insurance in his platform, the subject was conspicuously absent from the New Deal agenda of President Franklin Roosevelt in the mid-1930s. It did not reappear on the national agenda until the early post–World War II years, when Harry Truman was in the White House.

Yet Truman's efforts were ultimately unsuccessful. Once the War Labor Board had responded favorably to the request of the trade unions early in World War II (1942) to permit them to negotiate with employers for private health insurance benefits, most labor leaders focused their future efforts on securing and expanding private health insurance coverage for their members (Dunlop JT). Truman's efforts for the enactment of national health insurance coverage died aborning.

For all practical purposes, national health insurance did not reemerge on the national agenda until the Clinton health reform proposals made their appearance in 1993–1994. These died in Congressional committee in September 1994. At the century's end, the United States is alone among the advanced nations in having no national health insurance coverage for its population.

Of course, one must note that during the course of the 20th century, as well as earlier, state governments provided long-term care for selected groups of patients, particularly for those suffering from mental illness and tuberculosis. Also, the predominantly not-for-profit community and teaching hospitals provided considerable amounts of free clinic and in-patient care to the poor and near-poor, and many members of the medical profession provided care to considerable numbers of patients who could not meet their full charges or were unable to pay toward their care at all. Further, most acute care hospitals resorted to cross-subsidies, overcharging the patients with private rooms to enable them to admit and treat larger numbers of poor patients. After World War II the federal and state governments started to make selected funding available for hospital construction and operations, biomedical research, and the expansion of education and training of medical, nursing, and other health professional students, with much expanded federal and state funding following the passage of Medicare and Medicaid in 1965.

In 1999 the United States spent about $1.2 trillion, close to 14% of its gross domestic product (GDP), on national health expenditures (Smith, 1998). As a percentage of the GDP, the United States spends approximately 40% more than its two closest rivals in this area, Canada and France. Federal actuaries forecast that the country will pierce the $2 trillion level for expenditures on health by 2008, amounting to more than 16% of its estimated GDP in that year (Smith, 1998). Clearly, the steep upward trend in U.S. health care expenditures suggests that the nation has been responsive to a diversity of ethical issues even as it continues to avoid providing essential health insurance coverage as a governmental right to all of its citizens.

Considering these broad generalizations about the relations between ethics and health policy as markers of U.S. developments during the 20th century, we are better positioned to look more closely at the key policy transformations that occurred in the financing and delivery of health-care services to the American people. I will examine these transformations in three key periods: (*1*) from the Flexner Report (1910) to the end of World War II, (*2*) during the two decades from the end of World War II to the passage of Medicare and Medicaid (1965), and (*3*) the twenty year period leading to managed care, roughly 1965–1985. In this last period I will emphasize the "disconnect" between dollars and services, which is one of the chief sources of ethical problems in American health policy. I will conclude with a brief look at what the future is likely to hold.

THE PRE–WORLD WAR I PERIOD

The first and, according to many, defining event of 20th-century U.S. medical reform was the publication of Abraham Flexner's report *Bulletin Number Four* in 1910 by the Carnegie Foundation for the Advancement of Teaching. This publication recommended the closure of nearly 80% of the nation's medical schools then in operation. It also contained the model and the methodology for assuring that the surviving and new medical schools would be able to respond to the potential challenge of science-based medicine. With strong support from the American Medical Association (AMA) and the deans of the nation's leading medical schools, Flexner's report set the stage for health policy reform at least up to World War II and led to the continuing dominance of the AMA up to the passage of Medicare and Medicaid in 1965.

What was critically important about these many decades of the AMA's dominance? The AMA played a leading role in reducing the number and improving the quality of U.S. medical schools, though many more schools survived than Flexner had initially proposed. From the standpoint of ethics, it is significant that neither the AMA nor its allies—the medical school deans—considered it important to provide opportunities for men and women of all backgrounds to be admitted to mainline U.S. medical schools.

The second important observation regarding the period of AMA domination was the organization's insistence that fee-for-service should govern the patient–physician payment relationship, with the understanding that physicians would treat the poor as charity cases. There is little question that many physicians provided considerable amounts of care at no charge or at reduced charges when they saw and treated patients in their offices or in their homes. They also contributed a considerable amount of time and effort to taking care of the poor, meeting the needs of community and teaching hospitals, and instructing medical students and residents.

Despite the predominance of the AMA in setting the goals of medical education and practice, the mid 1920s saw the beginnings of a restiveness among many interested physicians, academics, businessmen, and other concerned parties that led to the establishment of the Committee on the Costs of Medical Care (CCMC). The CCMC was chaired by Ray Lyman Wilbur, a past president of the AMA, president of Stanford University, and Hoover's Secretary of the Interior. The committee released its final report in 1932, at the very height of the Great Depression, with major disagreements among its 50+ members. The vast majority of the committee favored group practice and group payment for medical care but opposed compulsory health insurance.

The AMA, while not in principle opposed to the idea of private health insurance coverage, spelled out ten principles, or conditions, it required of private health plans (Starr, 1982). In a sense, it was protecting its turf from what it considered a possible precursor to compulsory health insurance. When he was shaping his New Deal reforms for Congressional action, President Roosevelt decided that it was better to avoid submitting a health insurance proposal rather than risk his entire reform program.

WORLD WAR II AND ITS EFFECTS

A complete assessment of the impact of World War II (WWII) on the U.S. health-care system remains to be written, but, as a minor contributor to that unwritten book, I will briefly note some of my impressions during the three years I served as the Chief Logistical Advisor to the Surgeon General of the Army. The army and the navy absorbed 40% of the physician supply and put them into uniform to take care of the 15 million soldiers and sailors who served in uniform, together with millions of their dependents in the United States who presented at military hospitals far away from civilian centers. These individuals constituted one-fifth of the total population at the time, and many had their first encounter with a well-functioning clinic and hospital system during the war, which helps explain the pressures on Congress at war's end to make more federal dollars available to the health care sector. Congress did so in 1946, when it passed the Hill-Burton Act, which helped smaller-sized communities build or upgrade their hospitals and thereby attract and retain practitioners who would care for the local populations.

The federal government also made considerable funding available via the GI Bill of 1944 to facilitate the return to school of honorably discharged servicemen and officers. In the case of many physicians, the GI Bill helped them obtain their board certification as specialists, which, in turn, accelerated the trend toward specialization (Ginzberg, 1999).

The immediate post-WWII years were ripe for a much enlarged federal funding effort in biomedical research. The successful development of the atomic bomb, the arrival of the penicillin era, and the high optimism portrayed in books such as Vannevar Bush's *Science: The Endless Frontier* set the stage for the extraordinary investment in the development of high-tech medicine from 1950 through the end of the century.

Possibly the most striking change of all, precipitated by the U.S. engagement in WWII, was the explosive growth of employer health and hospital benefits provided to workers and their dependents. Encouraged by the U.S. Treasury, which enabled employers and their high-earning employees to enjoy a tax subsidy, large numbers of workers and their dependents were provided benefits by their employers. This subsidy has grown with the costs of health insurance, and in 1999 it was estimated at more than $100 billion a year. With hindsight on our side, we can say that the country more or less stumbled into private health insurance coverage for the majority of the nation's working population.

The much improved economy that followed WWII did much to permit the nation's leading hospitals to upgrade their facilities. Among other factors, this upgrading became possible because of the increasing percentage of the workforce that was covered by hospital, and later by hospital and physician insurance policies. Still, the 10- to 15- year-period following WWII was one of relative stability and quiet in terms of health policy innovation. The AMA, although challenged by new positions within the profession and the public, remained the dominant force in U.S. health policy.

The stability characterizing the period immediately following World War II was upset somewhat by the challenges faced during the second Eisenhower administration (1957–1961). For simplicity's sake, these challenges are here restricted to the efforts to deal with the retired population that no longer had health insurance, the struggle facing Congress about whether to make funding available to increase the physician supply, the reform of the immigration statute, with its subsequent impact on the inflow of International Medical Graduates, and some important issues relating to discrimination against women and African Americans. As we shall see, each of these issues led to major policy changes during the 1960s.

The Elderly

In the late 1950s and early 1960s, Congress responded to the growing numbers of retirees aged 65 or more who could no longer gain broad access to mainline health and hospital care services. This response provided new funding for state commissioners of welfare to help underwrite the hospital care of the elderly. But the elderly balked at having anything to do with the welfare system. Most of them had had no prior contacts with welfare and did not want to start having them late in life. What they wanted was the insurance coverage that they finally got with Medicare in 1965, despite the all-out opposition to this program on the part of the AMA, a defeat from which the AMA never recovered.

Physician Supply

The AMA was challenged, together with the mainline medical community, for opposing federal support for the education of more physicians. After holding the line successfully against Congressional action, the AMA finally withdrew its opposition in 1963 in order to focus all its energies on the defeat of Medicare, with which Congress and the country was then struggling. The federal government began a modest—and later a much broadened—effort over 13 years to expand not only the physician supply but also the supply of other health professionals, from nurses to veterinarians.

International Medical Graduates (IMGs)

In 1965 the United States revised its immigration and naturalization statutes and paved the way for the large-scale relocation of IMGs to this country. Today IMGs account for about one quarter of all practicing physicians (Iglehart, 1996).

Minorities and Women

President Kennedy's assassination in November 1963 gave the Democratic Party in Congress the opportunity to submit a strengthened Civil Rights Act. I am proud to relate that I helped to persuade Senator Joseph Clark and his staff to try to move the much strengthened bill past the Southern chair of the House Rules Committee by suggesting that the bill address sexual, as well as racial, equality. Clark took this advice and the bill sailed through, opening the way to a doubling of the number of African Americans admitted and graduating from U.S. medical schools. The number of women physicians increased from around 8% in the late 1960s to 37% of the current resident force (JAMA, 1998).

MEDICARE, MEDICAID, AND THE COMING OF MANAGED CARE

With the advantage of a long-term perspective, one can recognize that the passage of Medicare (less so in the case of Medicaid) radically transformed the national outlays for health care, making the federal government the single largest provider. Medicare and Medicaid raised the federal share of expenses for health care from about 10%–11% in 1965 to around 40% today (Smith, 1998). This increase is important from an ethical standpoint because the piecemeal and incremental approaches that programs such as Medicaid embody have made it politically possible for the United States to avoid facing up to providing health insurance to the entire population. Indeed, the 50%–80% contribution that the federal government pays for Medicaid set the stage for additional benefits for the poor, the near-poor, and the elderly via nursing home care, as well as for joint coverage for low-income Medicare beneficiaries after 1989 and, among other additions, for the introduction of home health benefits.

The Great Society initiatives also had a profound impact on the nation's leading academic health centers (AHCs), permitting them to take off and "do their own thing" with little concern about future funding, staffing, or other constraints. By considering all patients to be "teaching patients," the AHCs no longer were under pressure to admit considerable numbers of charity patients in order to meet their teaching responsibilities. With multiple billions of graduate medical education funds, the AHCs could—and did—expand their training of future specialists and use many senior residents and fellows to supplement their research staffs.

Because Medicare reimbursed hospitals on a cost-plus basis (up to the mid-1980s), it created a market for the ever-larger numbers of well-trained specialists the AHCs were turning out. And, what is more, the cost-plus system of reimbursement enabled many suburban hospitals to upgrade themselves into good tertiary care institutions by appointing increasing numbers of the newly certified specialists to their staffs.

THE GREAT "DISCONNECT" BETWEEN DOLLARS AND HEALTH CARE SERVICES

In seeking to buoy the spirits of the AMA leadership after their failure to block the enactment of Medicare, President Johnson assured them that nothing would change in the relations of patients to their physicians except that, henceforth, the government (and employers) would pay the bills. A few months after replacing Johnson in the White House, President Nixon told the nation of his deep concern about prospective health care expenditures being so seriously out of control that he feared not only for the future viability of the health-care system but, in fact, for the future stability of the economy as a whole. Nobody except the president and a few of his close advisers took note of his warning. In point of fact, Johnson's optimistic forecast about the government picking up most of the bills was confirmed by later events. By the mid-1980s, various large employers and profit-seeking entrepreneurs were moving to correct the long-standing and growing "disconnect" between dollars and services.

More specifically, by the early 1980s, in locales such as southern California, the Twin Cities, and eastern Pennsylvania, profit-seeking entrepreneurs saw the opportunity, with assistance from the stock market and venture capitalists, to step between hospitals with increasingly empty beds and physicians who had free time in their appointment books. These entrepreneurs offered to each of the two major providers (hospitals and physicians) larger referrals for significant reductions in their customary prices. The entrepreneurs were also able and willing to offer the companies that provided health care coverage to their workers some of the cost reductions that they extracted from providers, especially if the companies cooperated and encouraged or mandated that their employees shift over to some type of managed care plan.

Nonetheless, except for these few locations, the era of "disconnect" between dollars and health services continued throughout most of the 1980s. Between 1980 and 1989, national health expenditures (NHE) increased from just under $250 billion to around $650 billion (Smith, 1998). It was not until the early to mid-1990s, when most corporate employees had been moved to some type of managed care plan, that employers were able to enjoy a major retardation in what had earlier been double digit increases in their annual premium rate, yet medical inflation spiked once again in 1998, headed substantially higher in 1999, and will likely continue to increase.

For all these increasing expenditures, concern continues about the substantial differences in health access and in quality of life and longevity among subgroups of the population, particularly between whites and African Americans. Even after making adjustments for income and education, a significant gap remains of around four to five years with respect to the average age of death between whites and blacks. Nonetheless, we must not forget that after four decades of the National Health Service in the United Kingdom significant differentials continue to exist as to the year of death for members of the "upper classes" compared to those at the bottom of the occupational scale. Accordingly, we may conclude that longevity and years of healthy life are determined by much more than ready access to the health-care system.

More specifically, the research findings suggest that ready access to medical care of good quality may account for about 20%–25% of the differences that have been noted among the years of healthy life enjoyed by groups at the upper end of the educational–income ladder compared to those at the lower end. Another 20%–25% of the explanation for the differential between those with longer and shorter lifespans awaits more research and definitive analysis of environmental factors.

Despite the fact that these disparities are understudied, we can surmise from the findings just mentioned that about half the explanation for enjoying a longer and healthier life span reflects the differences in the health behavior patterns followed by those who live longer compared to those who die earlier. What one eats, how much one drinks, whether one smokes, how long one sleeps, whether one exercises regularly, whether one engages in unsafe sex, and a great number of additional risky behavior patterns appear to be critical variables. The question here is whether people should be held financially accountable, and to what degree, for behaviors like these? The answer is a difficult one, but one that has to be faced.

There are at least three questions of ethics that arise from the efforts of the 1980s and 1990s to reduce or eliminate the "disconnect" between dollars and medical services. First, the nation's annual health-care spending increased between the beginning of the 1980s and the end of the 1990s (1998) by about $1 trillion. In light of this tremendous increase, the question that warrants more attention than it has received is this: What did the country get by way of improved medical care and health status for such a large increase in annual outlays? Second, how can one account for the fact that despite such an enlarged annual outlay the two key parties in health care, patients seeking care and physicians rendering care, suffered a serious loss of trust and confidence in the health-care marketplace? Finally, how is it that the prosperous 1990s saw a steady increase of about 1 million uninsured persons per year, so that at the end of 1998, the total number of uninsured individuals approximated 44 million, with an estimated additional 30 million possessing inadequate coverage? In short, about one of every four Americans lacks any or essential coverage at a time when national health expenditures are in the $1.2 trillion range (Thorpe, 1997).

Put differently, how much spending on health care is enough, and who should get it? Thus far in America, we have increased the amount of dollars that go into health care with little debate about the clinical distribution of these moneys. We have instead approached different groups of the population incrementally and dealt with each one separately. This is a practice that continues even today. But change may be coming.

THE FUTURE

The major challenge that the American people confront in the health policy arena does not concern whether Congress grants Medicare beneficiaries a significant drug benefit, though this is clearly a matter of considerable concern to many lower-income elderly people. It does not even concern whether Congress will pass a patients' bill of rights, which will affect a great number of people. Rather, the challenge concerns whether the American public gains a clearer understanding of who is paying for what in the current multiple-payer health-care system.

Two widespread contradictory beliefs are held by large segments of the American public. We are a people who, from the outset, believed that it was the right of every American to pursue and accumulate increasing wealth by any and all legal means. Further, we believe that the wealthy are entitled to spend their money on any legal good or service without interference from government. But these deeply held and respected beliefs about wealth accumulation and spending conflict with the contradictory belief that all Americans insured against health risks are entitled to enjoy the same range and quality of health-care services, regardless of socioeconomic status. What, then, is to be done to resolve the disjunction between two central points in U.S. ideology and reality?

A first step in the resolution of this basic dilemma is to engage the American people in a realistic discussion of who is paying at the present time for the health care of most insured persons below the age of 65. Most employees see their employer group health insurance policy as a "fringe benefit" they receive from their employer. Most economists see it as an exchange for a lower wage.

Second, most current and potential Medicare beneficiaries believe that they have paid sufficient taxes into the federal tax system to cover their current and prospective Medicare benefits, yet the fact is that many, perhaps most, beneficiaries are receiving benefits far in excess of their earlier Medicare tax payments, even taking into account the parallel tax payments of their employer.

Further, many of the below-65 workforce with employer health-care benefits are unsettled by the fact that the scale and scope of their benefits have been reduced and that their co-payments have increased, emphasizing that, in their view, it is the employer's responsibility to keep providing them with the same benefits without asking them for larger co-payments. Finally, the bulk of the tax-paying public is not aware of the fact that the taxes they pay to federal and state governments cover about 50% of all current NHEs, or about $650 billion once one allows for the $100 billion plus tax subsidy that the federal government provides to employers and employees with group health insurance coverage.

In light of the foregoing misunderstandings and confusions about who pays for health care and the further fact that about one of four Americans is either not insured or inadequately insured against health-care risks, the time has come—in fact, some believe it is long overdue—for the federal government to take the lead and provide *essential* health-care coverage to all citizens and permanent immigrants. The government must also explain to the public that if they want more, better, quicker, more responsive, higher-quality care like that the affluent often seek and obtain, they will have to pay for it themselves, persuade their employer to cover the extras, or take out supplemental health insurance coverage. The current system needs immediate attention. The crucial steps are improved information for the public and new legislation providing essential universal coverage. There is also every reason for the government to inform the American public that it will increase its spending on essential health care services commensurate with increases in the nation's GDP, assuring citizens that they will continue to reap the benefits of future gains in medical research.

CONCLUSION

It appears that the time is long overdue in the United States for a stronger *connection between ethics and health policy*. But caution and fine balancing of interests is always required when ethics enters the debate. Questions concerning the amount and distribution of dollars for health care always carry with them ethical implications about who is supposed to receive what from the future disbursement of tax dollars and to what extent individuals and families must continue to look to their own income and wealth to provide ready access to desirable goods and services, such as more and better health care.

We have assiduously avoided opting for universal health insurance coverage despite the contrasting behavior of all other advanced nations. More and more Americans, from both the laity and health professions, are distressed by the fact that more than 44 million Americans lack health insurance, while another 30 million or so are poorly covered. The American public is surely closer to enacting essential health insurance coverage for all. Further, the political wisdom of continuing to adhere to a policy that views most extensions of governmental power to be a loss, no matter how inefficient and inequitable the competitive market may have proved itself to be, has to be questioned. On the grounds of political pragmatism, if not ethical imperatives, the time is fast approaching when the American people are likely to institute essential health insurance coverage for all. This will not solve *all* the problems of efficiency and equity in health care, but at least it will put us on the path to achieving these goals.

Acknowledgments

The author would like to acknowledge Mr. Panos Minogiannis for his assistance with this manuscript.

REFERENCES

Bush V (1960) *Science: The Endless Frontier*. Washington, DC: National Science Foundation, reprint.

Dunlop JT Appraisal of the wage stabilization policies. Washington, DC: U.S. Department of Labor, Bulletin No. 1009.

Flexner A (1910) A medical education in the United States and Canada: A report to the Carnegie Foundation for the Advancement of Teaching. Bulletin No. 4. Boston, MA: Updyke.

Ginzberg E (1999) The shift to specialism: The U.S. Army in World War II. *Academic Medicine* 74: 522–5.

Iglehart JK (1996) The quandary over graduates of foreign medical schools in the United States. *New England Journal of Medicine* 334: 1679–83.

Journal of the American Medical Association (*JAMA*) (1999) Appendix 11: Table 1: Resident Physicians, August 1, 1998. *JAMA* 282: 895.

Smith S et al (1998) The next ten years of health spending: What does the future hold? *Health Affairs* 17: 128–40.

Starr P (1982) *The Social Transformation of American Medicine*. New York: Basic Books.

Thorpe K (1997) The rising number of uninsured workers: An approaching crisis in health care financing. Paper prepared for the National Coalition on Health Care, Washington, DC.

5

Just deliberation about health care

AMY GUTMANN AND DENNIS THOMPSON

What standards should be used to assess the process of making decisions about health-care policy? These decisions are increasingly made not only in governmental institutions such as legislatures, courts, and presidential commissions but also in HMOs, hospitals, ethics committees, review boards, professional associations, and task forces. By focusing on a case study that involves decision makers in a for-profit HMO, we show how a political theory of deliberative democracy can be relevant to institutions that make important decisions concerning health care, even when those institutions are nongovernmental. We propose some generally applicable standards by which such decisions can be evaluated by both participants in the decision-making process and outside observers of that process.[1]

The guiding principle of deliberative democracy on which we base the standards is reciprocity: Citizens or their accountable representatives seek to give one another mutually acceptable reasons to justify the laws and policies they adopt. Their aim is to justify the policies in question to the people who are bound by them. Reciprocity sets four standards, or criteria, to assess the decision making about health care: The justifications that decision makers give should consist of reasons that are accessible, moral, respectful, and revisable. This chapter illustrates how these four standards of reciprocal reasoning are applicable to the making of public policy concerning health care.

In the leading case in a published text on ethical issues in managed care, readers are asked to consider whether DesertHealth, a for-profit HMO, should cover a new test called PUREPAP (Gervais et al, 1999).[2]

Approved by the FDA for assessing the efficacy of the standard Pap smear tests for cervical cancer, PUREPAP detects some of the cell abnormalities that the standard test misses. PUREPAP would benefit some individual patients but at some cost to others enrolled in the DesertHealth Plan.

The case is neither dramatic in its details nor earth-shaking in its consequences, but it is therefore all the more significant because it raises questions that are typical of the kind of issues that health care decision makers increasingly—and routinely—face. What benefits should health care plans provide and to whom? In deciding as a matter of policy what services to cover, HMO decision makers act more like public officials than private individuals, and they face many of the same challenges confronting government, even though their decisions directly affect only those enrolled in their plan. The pattern of economic and political trade-offs that must be made and the various interest groups that must be consulted create a microcosm of the larger political process. The case therefore can help uncover a set of standards that could be used quite generally in making health-care decisions by institutions that significantly affect the health care received by individuals, whether or not those institutions are governmental.

Political theories of democracy suggest standards for assessing how these often controversial decisions can be justifiably made. The most promising theories defend a central role for deliberation in dealing with controversies such as those that characterize the making of health-care policy. These theories of deliberative democracy offer the most promising perspective for judging health-care debates because they defend a kind of politics that is explicitly designed to respond morally to moral controversies, conflicts over what count as justifiable trade-offs among valued ends or between valued means and ends. These controversies have become increasingly common in health care. Many people now recognize that more medical care is not always better. Even when it is better, its costs cannot always be justified (in light of other ways of using the resources). Regardless of whether a certain kind of medical care is better on balance, it still may be desired and demanded by many people and opposed by health care organizations concerned about cost saving.

In a deliberative democracy, citizens or their accountable representatives seek to give one another mutually acceptable reasons to justify the laws and policies they adopt (Gutmann and Thompson, 1996). These reasons are not merely procedural ("because the majority favors health care") or purely substantive ("because health care is a human right"). They appeal to principles that citizens who are motivated to find fair terms of cooperation can reasonably accept. These principles are thus both substantive and procedural.

Both the content of the deliberators' reasoning and the conditions under which they are deliberating should manifest the aim of justifying the policies in question to the people who are bound by them. This aim may never be perfectly realized in practice, but the theory of deliberative democracy offers a useful standard by which to judge actual decision making as better or worse to the extent that the reasons for the decisions are mutually justified.

Reciprocity, the fundamental value of deliberative democracy, is both a moral principle and a mode of justification. In general terms, reciprocity means "making a proportionate return for the good received" (Becker, 1986). The "good received" is that others make their claims on terms that each can accept in principle. The "proportionate return" is that each makes claims on terms that can be accepted in principle by fellow citizens. Reciprocity is a characteristic of justice that has special force in a democracy, where people should be regarded and regard one another as free and equal members of a cooperative social system.

Reciprocity deals with disagreements in a way that expresses the equal status of citizens. Citizens are not merely objects of preference aggregation or of moral principles that others use to judge them (but that they cannot use to judge others). Citizens are active subjects who can accept or reject the reasons for mutually binding laws and policies, either directly in a public forum or indirectly through their accountable representatives. Reciprocity asks citizens and their representatives to try to justify their political views to one another and to treat with respect those who make a good faith effort to engage in this mutual enterprise, even when they cannot resolve their disagreements. When citizens morally disagree about public policy, reciprocity suggests that they should deliberate with one other, seeking moral agreement when they can and maintaining mutual respect when they cannot.

But deliberation that aims at mutual justification does not guarantee a just outcome. A well-designed deliberation that considers whether to fund PUREPAP may still yield the wrong answer. No decision-making process in the realm of policy making is perfect. Deliberative democracy explicitly recognizes this and therefore expresses a set of principles, not only a deliberative process. Those principles can help citizens and policy makers recognize the limitations as well as the strengths of deliberation in specific contexts. The principles suggest the possibility of justifying nondeliberative means when, for example, they are necessary in order to establish the socioeconomic conditions for a decent democracy and for more deliberative decision making.

The distribution of health care may offer an example of how nondeliberative means could, in principle, be defended by deliberative principles. Suppose that less affluent American citizens are unable either to insure themselves adequately for decent health care or to influence the political process sufficiently to overcome this inequity. This situation may be manifestly unjust by the principles of deliberative democracy. The claim of injustice would be based on reciprocity and might begin as follows: A cooperative social system under conditions of affluence cannot be justified to citizens who are denied the basic opportunities that decent health care affords (Gutmann and Thompson, 1996). If a nondeliberative process offers the only way to gain adequate health-care coverage for these citizens, then deliberation may justifiably be limited for the sake of furthering basic opportunity and better deliberation in the future. This argument proceeds according to the terms of deliberative democracy itself. Note, however, that the argument is hypothetical ("if" a nondeliberative process offers the only way . . . , then limitations on deliberation may be justified).

Deliberative processes are likely to work less well to the extent that the conditions under which they operate fail to treat people as free and equal citizens. When a political system is structured to give rich citizens far more political power than warranted by their numbers or their regard for justice, then deliberative processes will suffer. Poorer citizens will have less access to decision makers and less decision-making power than warranted. When, in addition, the government fails to secure an adequate level of basic opportunities, such as education, for all citizens, deliberative processes are likely to suffer as well.

Thus, the deliberation in DesertHealth and other HMOs and health organizations is often distorted by what might be called the burdens of injustice, the constraints that existing injustices place on what less-advantaged citizens can reasonably expect to accomplish, given their relative power. An example of a burden of injustice is that many patients today have no legal recourse against an HMO that denies them medical coverage for treatments that they, their own physician, and an independent panel of physicians all would deem medically necessary. Deliberation within one HMO is unlikely to rectify this situation for many reasons. A for-profit HMO operating in a competitive system would suffer a serious competitive disadvantage if it unilaterally extended patients' rights to include such legal recourse.

Suppose that DesertHealth refuses to cover a procedure simply because it cannot afford it, while other, better-endowed plans decide to cover it because they regard it as medically necessary. Suppose further that people who are poor through no fault of their own have access only to DesertHealth and similarly endowed plans. Under such circumstances, there is reason to question whether the basic distribution of resources for medical care in the society as a whole is just. If a deliberative process at DesertHealth concludes against coverage under these conditions, we should not blame deliberation itself. The problem is the scope of the decision: One HMO, no matter how deliberative, cannot solve the problem itself. (That is why cases limited to a single HMO cannot tell the whole story about social justice with respect to medical care.) Deliberation in a different forum may be necessary to address the problem. The best alternative to deliberation within HMOs may be publicly accountable deliberation in Congress, which has the power to set the legal parameters within which all HMOs must operate. Of course, deliberation at the Congressional level is also flawed because of the far greater power possessed by rich citizens and insurance companies in our politics. But the question remains as to whether any alternative nondeliberative method of decision making would be better in actual practice.

The imperfection of deliberation under nonideal conditions is no reason to favor nondeliberative means unless those means can be shown to be more valuable in themselves or to promise more mutually justifiable results. Neither is generally likely to be the case. Because deliberative processes put a premium on mutual justification, they are generally more valuable than are nondeliberative means, and they are also more likely to aid victims of social injustice than are power-based processes of decision making, such as interest-group bargaining. The participants in a deliberative process are expected to give not merely self-interested reasons for their positions, but reasons that satisfy a standard of mutual justification.

What kinds of reasons satisfy a standard of mutual justification, which reciprocity requires? We focus here on four core characteristics of reasons that make them reciprocal. These characteristics provide standards for judging the reasons given for decisions about health care and the institutions within which the decisions are made (Gutmann and Thompson, 1997). (The standards should be regarded as necessary conditions, which can be satisfied to varying degrees.)

ACCESSIBLE REASONS

First, the reasons that decision makers give should be accessible. The basic rationale for this requirement is clear: If you are trying to justify imposing your will on others, your reasons should be comprehensible to them. You would expect no less from them if they were imposing their will on you. The justification, if it is to be mutual, is irrelevant if those to whom it is addressed cannot understand its essential content. It would be unacceptable, for example, to appeal only to the authority of revelation, whether divine or secular. Revelation, by its very nature, is not accessible to many citizens. Simply citing a revelatory source therefore has no reciprocal value, but making an accessible argument that includes citing a revelatory source is not ruled out by this criteria. If someone says that God demands that fetal tissue not be used for research, and he also offers accessible reasons for not using fetal tissue—reasons that happen to be based on what God tells him—then it is those accessible reasons that satisfy the standard. The source of those reasons, even if inaccessible, is irrelevant to their mutual justification.

If the appeal to revealed authority is inaccessible, then why should a similar appeal to scientific authority and expertise not also be inaccessible? The conclusions and the essentials of the reasons that support scientific authority may be made publicly accessible and therefore satisfy this criterion. For example, it is perfectly legitimate for doctors to refuse to provide some kinds of treatment on the grounds that they are generally regarded, based on the best scientific evidence and evaluative standards, as ineffective, medically futile, or even excessively risky. These grounds often are not purely technical or medical, because they involve weighing of risks and benefits for the individual as well as others who might be affected, but their technical or medical aspects are critical to the justification, and they often may be difficult to explain to patients or even well-informed citizens who are not trained in medicine. Why, then, does the accessibility criterion not rule out such justifications?

Consider the justification for the decision that the benefit committee at DesertHealth is likely to make about PUREPAP. (Although the narrative of the case ends as the committee is about to make its decision, the arguments all point toward a definite conclusion.) The decision the committee is likely to reach is to decline to cover this new test on the grounds that it is not cost-effective. Here is part of the reasoning (as presented by the case writer):

> PUREPAP provides a computerized rescreening process that is about 7 percent more effective in detecting false-negatives than manual rescreening of negative Pap smears. In other words, if 10 percent false-negatives are detected under the current manual rescreening system, 10.7 percent would be detected using PUREPAP. For example, if manual rescreening detected 8 false-negatives out of a 100-slide pool, PUREPAP would detect 8.56. . . . The [annual] cost to [DesertHealth] would be $4.8 million. . . . The plan's underwriters estimate that PUREPAP would cost approximately $30,000 to detect one false-negative
>
> Gervais et al., 1999, 17–18

Ordinary patients, and even not so ordinary ones, may be excused if they do not fully follow this reasoning, but that does not necessarily make the justification inaccessible. The basic conclusion can be expressed in accessible terms by clarifying what the cost means (for example by showing what other treatments might be provided for $30,000) and what the benefit actually provides (by explaining that the test only identifies abnormal, not necessarily cancerous, cells, and that those that are cancerous are likely to be picked up in time by later tests because cervical cancer develops slowly). Behind these conclusions lie technical knowledge and some professional judgments that may not be unanimous, but this is true of many conclusions of experts that we reasonably accept in modern life.

We should not, of course, accept these conclusions uncritically. Accepting the justification for such conclusions presumes a certain amount of trust, but not blind trust. More specifically, the trust is not blind if two conditions hold. First, there is some independent basis for believing the experts are trustworthy (such as a past record of reliable judgments). Second, the experts can describe the basis for their conclusions in an understandable way. The justification then would be accessible in the way that reciprocity requires.

What kind of institutional arrangements would be likely to facilitate offering accessible justifications? Health-care decisions are best defended in forums that include representatives of the people whose health care is in the hands of the institution. The reasons are more likely to be accessible to people if accountable representatives are present when policies are being made and defended. (The consumer affairs committee in DesertHealth, which includes "consumer representatives" as well as members of the medical board, may go some way toward filling this role.) The representatives should be former or potential patients, and they should routinely be encouraged to ask critical questions and to challenge answers until the reasoning satisfies them.

In light of the generally greater power of health-care institutions than their consumer base, such institutions should also be required to give reasons for their policies to a patient tribune charged with acting more generally as an ombudsman would. Among other responsibilities, the patient tribune would make sure that the explanations the experts gave on behalf of the institution were comprehensible to the patient representatives. Representatives should have access to records of the past decisions and qualifications of the major decision makers. Detailed technical material supporting the justification of decisions like whether to cover PUREPAP should also be available for evaluation by independent experts. Individual patients or their representatives should be able to consult independent experts as a check on the reliability of the organization's experts, whose judgment about what constitutes reasonable and affordable health-care risk may be unintentionally skewed in some way that can be discovered only by considering technical details that are beyond what patients or their representatives are able to analyze on their own.

MORAL REASONS

Reciprocity demands more than accessible reasons. Self-interested reasons—or reasons that serve the interests of one's employer—are among the most conspicuously accessible. We understand only too well the argument that a policy of not covering some health-care services would increase the profits of a profit-making HMO. But reciprocity presumes a moral point of view. The reasons given must not only be accessible, they must also be moral. Thus, decision makers should justify policies by offering moral reasons.

What counts as a moral reason according to a deliberative perspective? The basic criterion of a moral reason, sometimes called generality, is one that deliberative democracy shares with many other moral and political theories. The criterion of generality is so widely accepted that it is often identified with the moral point of view (Baier, 1958; Rawls, 1971). Moral arguments apply to everyone who is similarly situated in morally relevant respects. Women who ask that DesertHealth reimburse them or their doctors for PUREPAP do not assert that only some women (or some doctors) should be reimbursed, but that all women so tested (or their doctors) should be. Similarly, the medical policy committee that recommends against reimbursing PUREPAP does so for reasons that are general in this sense, stressing "that most cervical cancer grows slowly over the course of ten to fifteen years, and . . . the implications of a false-negative are greatly overstated . . ." (Gervais et al., 1999, 18).

Generality is not a purely formal standard, as the controversy about covering PUREPAP shows. Generality always raises a substantive question: What are the morally relevant respects in which people are similarly situated? One possible moral response to arguments for and against recommending PUREPAP for all women who have PAP tests is to recommend (and therefore reimburse) PUREPAP only for women who are shown to be at particularly high risk for cervical cancer (Gervais et al., 1999, 24). Although this response picks out a more specific group to be rescreened and reimbursed by DesertHealth, it does so for morally relevant reasons and therefore satisfies the test of generality. A morally relevant characteristic—being at high risk for cancer—is being generally applied. As this example suggests, a reason that qualifies as moral by deliberative standards may be opposed by another moral reason. Moral reasoning therefore leaves room for reasonable disagreement because moral reasons may be multiple and may support opposing policy conclusions.

The requirement that reasons be moral distinguishes the deliberative approach from another common approach to public decision making. The other approach, prudence, is amoral. Prudential decision makers give reasons that are intended to show that a policy is the best that all parties to the decision, given their relative decision-making power, can expect to achieve. Prudential reasons and their outcomes reflect the balance of power of the decision makers. The morality of both the reasons and their results would be purely coincidental. Prudence aims not at justice (or a moral outcome), but rather at a modus vivendi, in which self-interested citizens deal with their disagreements through various forms of bargaining. Their reasoning aims at striking the best bargain for themselves, regardless of moral considerations.

The trouble with prudential reasoning as a criterion for public decision making is that some people have far greater bargaining power than others, and prudence authorizes them to use that power in a self-interested, or group-interested, way to gain still more benefits for themselves or their group. If the managers of DesertHealth get away with offering self-serving reasons to the detriment of their patients' well-being, they should be criticized, not commended for their successful bargaining strategy. The proponents of prudence cannot justify the outcomes of self-serving reasoning to those who are at a disadvantage when the bargaining begins. What can they say to a low-income patient who is denied health care that she needs and that would be provided if only the people in power were less powerful or less self-serving? They can suggest that she got the best deal she could in light of her relative bargaining power and their self-interested behavior. But this response gives her no moral reason to accept the decision as justified. At best, it tells her what she surely already knew: that she is the victim of an injustice because the people in power failed either to reason or to act morally.

Institutions should be designed to encourage more moral rather than more self-interested reasoning and action. Forums for deliberation that include representatives of less-advantaged citizens encourage decision makers to take a broader perspective on the matters that come before them. John Stuart Mill presented one of the most cogent accounts of such a deliberative process in democracy. Participating in public discussions, a citizen is "called upon . . . to weigh interests not his own; to be guided, in case of conflicting claims, by another rule than his private partialities; to apply, at every turn, principles and maxims which have for their reason of existence the common good . . ." (Mill, 1865, 68). Deliberation will not suddenly turn self-centered individualists into public-spirited citizens. Members of the benefits committee at DesertHealth are not automatically transformed from delegates of special interests into trustees of the public interest just as a result of talking to one another. Background conditions make a big difference and need to be considered in constituting such a committee or any deliberative forum. These conditions include the level of competence (how well-informed deliberators are), the distribution of resources (how equally situated they are), and the open-mindedness of deliberators (the range of arguments they are likely to take seriously). To urge more deliberation, we need only assume that most people are more likely to take a moral view in a deliberative process that puts a premium on moral reasoning than in a process in which assertions of political power are expected to prevail.

How can deliberative forums provide incentives for moral reasoning? These forums are likely to work best when they are designed to resemble as little as possible the processes of power politics and interest group bargaining. Members of the committees in health-care organizations like DesertHealth should not think of themselves as merely group-interested delegates, even if they inevitably and quite properly bring different perspectives to the meetings. They should not be chosen in a way that suggests that each represents the interests of a single constituent group whose interests the representative is therefore bound to articulate and promote. A forum that is so organized is likely to replicate the results of interest-group bargaining and eschew moral reasoning. Governmental institutions should also be designed to encourage deliberation on the merits of issues rather than engage only in interest group bargaining, which puts a premium exclusively on power at the complete expense of moral persuasion.

From this deliberative perspective, the committee structure of DesertHealth is not ideal. Separate bodies—the medical committee, the benefit committee, and the consumer affairs committee—that each concentrate on a different aspect of policy are likely to encourage a process of decision making that resembles interest group bargaining. Each committee is likely to advocate a position that reflects its own special perspective or particular interest. They arrive at policy conclusions with little exposure to the perspectives or interests of the individuals represented by the other committees. To some extent, this effect may be mitigated by the overlapping membership on the consumer affairs committee (which includes some people who are also members of the medical committee), but the consumer affairs committee is not the final decision-making body. To promote moral reasoning, the forum in which final decisions are made should include voices that represent as many relevant perspectives as is feasible. The challenge is to make sure that many perspectives are represented without encouraging the representatives to act as mere delegates.

RESPECTFUL REASONS

One of the virtues of a deliberative conception is that it recognizes that much moral disagreement will persist even among good-willed and intelligent people. Some of the moral disagreement that persists in politics is reasonable: Moral positions conflict, and there is no morally definitive perspective that, for public purposes, settles the disagreement. Health-care policy poses some of the most intractable of these issues. Should individuals be held responsible for health problems that are partly the product of their own choices? Should children who cannot give informed consent ever be subjects of experimental medical research? These questions have moral answers, some of which each of us is able to offer. From a public perspective, the problem is that our answers, more often than not, conflict, and some of the conflicts will be moral and reasonable.

In the face of disagreement of this kind, a deliberative conception specifies a third criterion of reasoning that strives for reciprocity: The reasons that decision makers give should be mutually respectful of those who are similarly striving for mutual respect. Mutual respect demands more than toleration or a benign attitude of indifference toward others. It requires a favorable attitude toward and constructive interaction with people with whom one reasonably disagrees when those persons are similarly willing and able to adopt such an attitude. In respecting one another as moral agents, participants in a deliberative process recognize the difference between morally respectable differences of opinion and merely tolerable ones. Differences that represent morally respectable conflicts are what we call *deliberative disagreements*, conflicts in which citizens seek a resolution that is mutually justifiable but continue to differ about moral principles or their practical implications.

Many disputes over how much emphasis to place on individual responsibility for certain health-care problems and how much of the cost of their health care consumers therefore should be required to bear through higher insurance premiums are examples of deliberative disagreements because conflicting sides can justify their views as reasonable within a reciprocal perspective. Consider, by contrast, a dispute in which some people defend de jure racial segregation or discrimination against non-Christians. This would be an example of a nondeliberative disagreement because one side can be rejected as unreasonable within a reciprocal perspective (Gutmann and Thompson, 1996). These positions reject the very premise of reciprocity, the idea that mutually binding laws and policies should be mutually justified to the people who will be bound by them. De jure racial segregation and discrimination against non-Christians cannot be justified to those who are severely disadvantaged by these policies.

The criterion of mutually respectful reasoning helps distinguish a reciprocal perspective from another kind of moral perspective, which bases itself on the criterion of impartiality. Reciprocity stands between prudence, which demands less from justifications, and impartiality, which demands more. Impartiality insists that reasons be impersonal. It requires citizens to suppress their own personal perspectives and partial projects when setting social policies and procedures. The prime example of an impartialist approach is utilitarianism. In practice, it favors expert decision making and implies that the medical professionals in DesertHealth should have the final say as long as their judgment is consistent with general professional opinion. The preferred impartialist method is neither bargaining nor deliberation, but demonstration, which aims as far as possible to establish the truth of a comprehensive moral view. In the face of moral disagreement, impartiality tells citizens and officials that they should affirm the view most consistent with the true morality as determined by impersonal justification. There is no further moral need for mutual respect or for actual political deliberation.

The trouble with impartiality is that it does not take moral disagreement seriously enough. More precisely, it fails to provide a satisfactory way to deal with the moral disagreements that inevitably remain on many issues when expert opinion on the technical and medical problems or the demonstration of a comprehensive moral philosophy such as utilitarianism are complete. In the face of a fundamental moral disagreement such as funding fetal tissue research, expensive organ transplants, or experimental diagnostic tests such as PUREPAP, the impartialist approach can only declare one side (or no side) correct. If one side is correct, it provides no reasons for recognizing moral value on the other side. It therefore offers no way, other than agreement, for the other side to respect the decision on moral grounds.

In a deliberative process characterized by mutual respect, participants recognize the moral merit in their opponents' claims (insofar as they have merit). Such a process can help clarify what is at stake in a moral disagreement by encouraging deliberators to sort out self-interested claims from public-spirited ones and to recognize those public-spirited claims that should have greater weight. Through a deliberative process, participants in a healthcare forum can isolate those conflicts that embody genuinely incompatible values on both sides. Conflicts that do not involve such deep disagreement can then easily be addressed and may turn out to be more resolvable than they at first appeared. Some may be the result of misunderstanding or lack of information, and some may be appropriately settled by bargaining, negotiation, and compromise. In this way, deliberation can use moral principles to put moral bargaining, negotiation, and compromise in their place.

In the face of deliberative disagreements, deliberative democracy recommends what we call an *economy of moral disagreement*. In justifying policies on moral grounds, citizens should seek the rationale that minimizes rejection of the position they oppose. By economizing on their disagreements in this way, citizens manifest mutual respect as they continue to disagree about morally important issues on which they need to reach collective decisions.

The economy of moral disagreement can be seen at work, for example, in two bodies that considered the issue of fetal tissue research, the Warnock Commission in England and the Fetal Tissue Research Commission in the United States. Both commissions sought to focus on those issues and justifications for positions that would help them reach some reasonable consensus rather than on those that were more likely to produce polarization. To the extent that they recognized and respected one another's conflicting values, commissioners helped realize the potential for mutual respect among citizens. Even when decision makers cannot responsibly avoid highly contentious issues, they can manifest mutual respect by seeking to help participants understand the perspectives of their opponents. The respectful quality of the reasoning that decision makers present—for example, how well they recognize the competing values at stake—has value in addition to that of the conclusion they reach.

An economy of disagreement is sometimes appropriate even when one side of the dispute seems mainly economic. In the dispute at DesertHealth, some patients and their doctors argued that any decision not to cover PUREPAP would be discriminatory. The money saved for all patients would be at the expense of the health of women. The decision would at least appear to be sacrificing lives of some women for improving the health care of men (and, of course, some other women). In the spirit of economizing on moral disagreement, the consumer affairs committee recommended that the plan spend the resources that would have been spent on PUREPAP instead on a program to promote regular Pap tests, which would not only be more cost-effective but also would be nondiscriminatory.

Suppose, for the sake of argument, that spending more on Pap smears would be more cost effective than funding PUREPAP, and suppose that the consumer affairs committee had not recommended that the money saved be used to fund more Pap smears so as thereby to help improve women's health. Or suppose the management of DesertHealth rejected the consumer affairs committee's recommendation with no comment. In either case advocates of funding PUREPAP could reasonably have thought that DesertHealth was putting profit-making above concern for women's health. Regardless of whether a decision not to fund PUREPAP was right, a defense of DesertHealth's decision—however accurate on the narrow merits—would have failed to appreciate the value of respectful reasoning and the correlative practice of economizing on moral disagreements. Mutually respectful reasoning may not always achieve the right results, but neither will bargaining or impartialist reasoning.

Although economizing on moral disagreement may reduce moral conflict, it does not eliminate disagreement. Indeed, in the process of clarifying and identifying moral differences, it may intensify the conflict. Some critics of mutual respect therefore may object that deliberative practices raise the moral stakes. Suppose DesertHealth rejected the recommendation of its consumer affairs committee and refused to spend the money saved on PUREPAP on improving women's health care. The internal conflict might have become greater than it would have been without any internal deliberative body. DesertHealth might have rued the day it instituted a consumer affairs committee. Critics are correct in suggesting that, in some contexts, the effort to economize on moral disagreements may turn what would otherwise be a simple bargaining situation into a conflict of moral principle and thereby encourage no-holds-barred opposition and political intransigence. Moral sensitivity sometimes makes necessary political compromises more difficult. But moral sensitivity often exists even without deliberative practices. When moral sensitivity exists (about the neglect of women's health care needs, for example), a bargaining situation may blow up in the face of the winners. Just as important, the absence of moral reasoning in bargaining situations makes unjustifiable outcomes and compromises more common.

What is even worse is a public philosophy that simply accepts unjustifiable outcomes and inequitable compromises because it assumes that self-interested bargaining is the best that politics in our society has to offer. If a disagreement about a change in eligibility for health care turns only on the question of costs, nothing is gained by invoking principles of justice and benevolence. But when a dispute raises serious moral issues—the avoidable deaths of less-affluent patients or the exclusion of certain groups, such as immigrants, for example—then it is not likely to be resolved more satisfactorily by avoiding arguments that are both moral and mutually respectful. Most disputes in health care raise serious moral issues and therefore put a social premium on parties' mutually seeking an economy of moral disagreement.

As they debate the future of health care in this country, members of Congress would be well advised to adopt, at least upon occasion, this practice. If Republican and Democratic senators, for example, could economize on their moral disagreements about patients' rights in managed care plans, citizens would be considerably better off than they are today. A moral compromise in this spirit would also signal that the parties were willing and able to put bipartisan concern for improving the welfare of Americans above partisan bickering.

REVISABLE REASONS

Like most case studies, the story about DesertHealth is presented as if the protagonists were making a one-time decision: Should they fund PUREPAP or not? This approach may be appropriate for pedagogical purposes, but it is a misleading guide for the practice of deliberation. A fundamental feature of deliberative reasoning is that its conclusions are morally revisable over time. If the benefit committee decides not to cover PUREPAP, DesertHealth officials should ensure that opportunities remain open to challenge and to reverse the decision in the future in light of new scientific information, fresh understandings of the moral values at stake, and other changes in the context within which the decision is made.

The revisable status of justifications is implied by the value of reciprocity. Decision makers owe justifications for the policies they seek to impose on other people. They therefore must take seriously the moral reasons offered by their opponents. If they take seriously their opponents' moral reasons, they must acknowledge the possibility that, at least for a certain range of views, their opponents may be shown to be correct in the future. This possibility has implications not only for the way citizens should treat their opponents, but also for the way they should regard their own views. It urges them to continue to test their own views, seeking forums in which their views can be challenged, and keeping open the possibility of their revision or even rejection. (The same obligation to justify policies that are imposed on other people supports the practice of the economy of moral disagreement described earlier.)

Deliberative forums that deal with moral disagreements put a premium on presenting justifications in a way that can stand the test of new moral insights, empirical evidence, and alternative interpretations of insights and evidence. Many other theories, of course, endorse something like this general outlook—for example, by adopting some form of fallibilism or, more simply, by expressing general approval of moral and intellectual open-mindedness—but the revisability that deliberative democracy recommends even for its own basic claims is integral to its substantive conception of justice. Deliberative democracy welcomes fundamental change in the content of the theory itself. This includes revisions, reinterpretations, and even rejections of its own principles. It also includes changes in the meaning and implications of a mutually justifiable deliberative process. All of these possibilities are consistent with—indeed they follow from—the fundamental idea of reciprocity: mutually justifying that which is mutually binding to the people who are most affected by the decision.

The purpose of revisability is not only to respect the moral status of the participants in the process, but also to improve the quality of the decisions they make. Revisability offers important protection against the mistakes that citizens, health-care professionals, and administrators all inevitably make. Ideally, all the participants recognize that their reasons and conclusions are revisable, but even when some or all of the participants do not recognize this before they deliberate, a well-constituted deliberative forum can foster revisability and its recognition. The give-and-take of moral argument in deliberative forums that reconsider existing laws and policies and propose new ones assumes revisability. Participants have an incentive to learn from one another, to recognize their individual and collective misapprehensions, and to develop new views and policies that can more successfully withstand others' critical scrutiny. When citizens bargain and negotiate, they may learn how better to get what they wanted to begin with, but when they deliberate, they can expand their knowledge, including their self-understanding of what is best for them and their collective understanding of what will best serve their fellow citizens.

The most important implication of the revisability criterion for health-care institutions is that decision-making bodies should be designed so that their conclusions are regarded as provisional and therefore revisable over time. Medical findings that are relevant to health-care decisions change rapidly and sometimes dramatically over time. The economic conditions of society that are relevant to the resources available to health-care institutions also vary. What counts as adequate health care changes with objective as well as subjective social conditions, and changes in one institution, such as government policy, are very relevant to other institutions, such as nonprofit and for-profit HMOs. At any given time, deliberative forums must, of course, reach conclusions, but the conclusions should always be open to challenge in a subsequent round of deliberation. Deliberation continues through stages as various health-care officials present their proposals, consumers respond, officials revise, consumers react, and the stages recur. This is what we call the reiteration of deliberation, which also recommends deliberative democracy and makes it more suitable to decision making under conditions of shifting uncertainties.

The potential strengths (and shortcomings) of this kind of deliberation can be seen in the process that the state of Oregon adopted in the early 1990s to set priorities for its publicly funded health care under Medicaid. The Oregon Health Services Commission's priorities list, based mainly on utilitarian cost–benefit calculations, provoked much justifiable criticism (for example, capping a tooth ranked much higher than an appendectomy). The commission then began an elaborate process of consultation, which included community meetings at which participants were "asked to think and express themselves in the first person plural . . . as members of a statewide community for whom health care has a shared value." Eventually, after still more deliberation, the commission presented a revised list, which was generally regarded as an improvement over the original plan.

Of course, the commission could not correct the most serious flaw in the scheme: because only poor people were eligible and the budget was very limited, some poor people would have to sacrifice for the sake of other poor people. Nevertheless, the process forced officials and citizens to confront a serious problem that they had previously evaded, and to confront it in a cooperative ("first person plural") spirit. As a result, even the basic unfairness in the policy was somewhat lessened in a way unexpected by the critics of the plan (and probably by its proponents as well). When the legislators finally saw what treatments on the list would have to be eliminated under the projected budget, they managed to find more resources and increased the total budget for health care for the poor. As a result, the state covered a greater percentage of the Medicaid-eligible population than it had done before.

Although some observers saw little connection between the earlier debate and the content of the revised list, the commission did correct most of the priorities that had been widely criticized. The year-long deliberations appeared to help citizens, legislators, and health care professionals come to a better understanding of their own values—those they shared and those they did not. The experience enabled citizens and their representatives to undertake, in a more reciprocal spirit, what is likely to be a long and difficult process of setting and adjusting priorities that could eventually affect the quality of health care of all residents of the state and even some in other states.

The distribution of health care is, of course, not the only issue that could benefit from such reiterated deliberation. When, if ever, is medical experimentation justified in the absence of informed consent? On what basis should organs for transplantation be allocated? Do physicians have a duty to treat AIDS patients? And, of course, should DesertHealth cover PUREPAP? The list of contestable questions could be expanded almost indefinitely simply by collecting the topics from the "Questions for Consideration" at the end of each case in *Ethical Challenges in Managed Care*, from which we took the DesertHealth case. Because moral disagreement in decisions about health care is not likely to diminish, the need for more and better deliberation is likely to grow.

If the values of deliberative democracy are to be more fully realized in the practices of health care forums, the justifications that the decision makers give should be more accessible, moral, respectful, and revisable. To the extent that the institutions for making these decisions are deliberation-friendly in these ways, the decisions that they produce will be more mutually justifiable, and the health care policies they represent will be more morally legitimate even if they are not always politically popular. By making the process in which citizens decide the future of their health care more deliberative, they stand a better chance of resolving some of their moral disagreements, and living with those that will inevitably persist, on mutually acceptable terms.

NOTES

1. Parts of this paper are based on material presented in Gutmann A and Thompson D (1996), (1997), (1999), and (2000).

2. The rescreening test PAPNET seems to be the model for PUREPAP in the case

study. *Medical Industry Today* (August 3, 1998) and *Biomedical Market Newsletter* (February 28, 1998) report on this test. *Biomedical Market Newsletter* report the results of a Centers for Disease Control CDC study released January 31, 1998 (Pt 2): "Given the high costs of using the automated system, the study suggests other ways to reduce cervical cancer death. These include implementing more effective screening programs, such as performing Pap smears on women who do not currently receive them."

REFERENCES

Baier K (1958) *The Moral Point of View*. Ithaca, NY: Cornell University Press.

Becker L C (1986) *Reciprocity*. London: Routledge and Kegan Paul.

Biomedical Market Newsletter (February 28, 1998).

Gervais K G et al (eds) (1999) *Ethical Challenges in Managed Care*. Washington, D.C.: Georgetown University Press.

Gutmann A and Thompson D (1996) *Democracy and Disagreement*. Cambridge, MA: Belknap Press of Harvard University Press.

Gutmann A and Thompson D (1997) Deliberating about bioethics. *Hasting Center Report* (May/June): 38–41

Gutmann A and Thompson D (1999) Democratic disagreement. In Macedo S (ed) *Deliberative Politics*. New York: Oxford University Press.

Gutmann A and Thompson D (2000) Why deliberative democracy is different. *Social Philosophy and Policy* 17: 161–80.

Medical Industry Today (August 3,1998).

Mill JS (1865) *Considerations on Representative Government*. London: Longmans, Green, and Roberts.

Rawls J (1971) *A Theory of Justice*. Cambridge, MA: Harvard University Press.

Weinstein MM (July 18, 1999) Beyond the bluster over health care. *The New York Times*, Sunday, "News of the Week in Review": 4.

III

Examining the ethics of how policy is made

6

The reality of public policy making

JOHN W. KINGDON

Many of us would like public policy making to be orderly. A tidy world, governed by transparent rules and rational decisions, would certainly make a scholar's life easier. In fact, any observer seeking to understand how this world works would be aided by more order. So would participants in the policy-making process. Lobbyists, for instance, might like a surer sense of the right levers to pull to manipulate this process.

Alas, for all of us, public policy making is extraordinarily messy. It does have a sort of structure, actually, which I outline here, but there is plenty of room for complexity, uncertainty, fluidity, and residual randomness.

This chapter presents what I think is a realistic picture of public policy making and then discusses some implications for those who might like to connect ethics and health policy. I begin with a description of the policy making process, concentrating particularly on processes of agenda setting and generation of alternatives. I then illustrate those processes by examining the experience of the Clinton administration in forming its proposal for national health insurance in the early 1990s. I consider next some constraints on the process, concentrating particularly on some features of American political culture. Finally, I discuss some implications for the relationship between ethics and health policy, highlighting especially some cautionary notes.

POLICY FORMATION

Final decisions are actually quite orderly, despite a surface appearance of chaos. On the floor of the U.S. House of Representatives, for example, decisions are governed by a previously determined set of parliamentary procedures. To the extent that there is disagreement over procedure, a rule is written to specify which amendments will be allowed and what the terms of debate will be. As I have discussed elsewhere (Kingdon, 1989), members' decisions are driven by a rather intelligible set of considerations that make it possible for scholars and other observers to understand what happens and why it happens. We know a lot about the importance of constituents, for example, about the place of interest groups and their effects, about the process by which members turn to their colleagues for cues on how to vote, and about the complex of political and ideological considerations that affect members' votes. We are able to reduce their decisions to equations and decision trees and succeed rather well in accounting for both individual and collective outcomes.

The processes leading up to final decisions, by contrast, seem much more free-form. In this section of the chapter, I dwell on those pre-decision processes, summarizing the argument in my book on the subject (Kingdon, 1995). While this account was based on research on the federal government, the principles apply to policy making more generally.

I begin with agenda setting. I define a governmental agenda as a list of subjects or problems to which governmental officials and those close to them are paying serious attention. So, an agenda setting process narrows the list of conceivable subjects within any given domain (e.g., health policy) to those that actually are the focus of attention. We want to understand why subjects rise and fall on that agenda. Within agenda subjects, quite a different process narrows the very large set of possible alternatives from which choices might be made to the set of alternatives that actually are considered. Agenda setting and the generation of alternatives are not the same as either final choices (e.g., a legislative enactment or a presidential decision) or the implementation of those choices.

Agenda setting exhibits a number of salient features. One is rapid change. We often think of public policy as changing slowly or incrementally, but policy agendas often change dramatically. Issues "hit" suddenly. There is a tremendous burst of activity, and government policy changes in major ways all at once. The New Deal, the Great Society, and the Reagan revolution in 1981 are all examples. After a period of intense change, the system adjusts to a new status quo, and a period of rest sets in, only to be followed by another spasm of activity. Baumgartner and Jones (1993) liken this pattern to punctuated equilibrium.

Other features of these processes include complexity, uncertainty, and fluidity. Neither scholars nor practitioners, even with the best knowledge and the best theory, can predict with great certainty what will happen and often find themselves surprised. The best we can do is to quote odds, sometimes quite reliably and sometimes less so. These systems may present an even greater challenge to analysts, because systems may not settle into equilibria at all. Development, adaptation, evolution, and what John Holland (1995) calls "perpetual novelty" characterize these processes.

To try to understand such complex and fluid processes, in my study of policy agendas (Kingdon, 1995) I use a revised version of the Cohen-March-Olsen (Cohen et al, 1972) "garbage can model" of "organized anarchies": large, multipurpose, fragmented entities like universities or the federal government. In their version, separate streams of problems, solutions, participants, and choice opportunities run through such organizations, each stream with a life of its own and largely unrelated to the others. People generate solutions whether or not they are solving problems, for instance, and then look for problems to which to hook their solutions. Advocates of urban mass transit, for example, have at various times portrayed public transportation as a solution to the problems of traffic congestion, air pollution, energy shortages, and even drunk driving, as each of these problems has heated up. Outcomes then depend heavily on how these rather separate streams are linked—which solutions get tied to which problems, which participants are present when decisions are made, and which problems and solutions are under consideration when a choice opportunity presents itself.

In my revised model, three streams—problems, proposals, and politics—flow through and around the federal government, each stream with a life of its own and largely unrelated to the others. First, policy makers and those close to them recognize and concentrate on certain problems rather than others at any given time. Second, policy proposals (alternatives) are generated and refined. Third, political events like changes of administration, party realignments, and interest group campaigns occur. These streams move along largely independently of one another. Proposals are generated whether or not policy makers are solving a problem, problems are recognized whether or not there is a solution, and political events move along according to their own dynamics.

Some policy change can be explained by the dynamics within each stream. A change of administration within the political stream, for instance, makes a big difference. But the greatest agenda change occurs at critical times of opportunity (open policy windows) when the three streams come together. A problem is recognized, policy alternatives are available that can be related to that problem, and the political conditions are right. Something is done when the window is open, or else the opportunity is lost, and advocates must wait for the next window to open. Lyndon Johnson realized that the election of 1964 and the tremendous influx of Democrats into the Congress opened a window for his Great Society proposals, for example, and he also knew that the window would close after two years. The Columbine High School shootings opened a window for advocates of many kinds (e.g., advocates for gun control, for harsher penalties for juvenile crime, for regulating the media, for more religious content in public institutions), a window that would stay open until memories of that horrible event faded.

I will now consider each of the three streams in turn and then discuss how they get joined.

Problem Recognition

Why do important people in and around government pay attention to some problems and not others at any particular point in time? Part of the answer is that they routinely monitor indicators of various conditions. Shifts in such indicators or performance contrary to expectations heighten attention. At other times, some focusing event, like a plane crash or a dramatic scientific discovery, draws attention to a particular problem.

But governmental attention does not always track on some objective indicator or even on focusing events. Government recognition of a problem also involves a process of interpretation that translates a condition into a problem. As a respondent in one of my studies said, "If you have only four fingers on one hand, that's not a problem; that's a situation." Problems are conditions that we feel we should do something to change. One way we come to the conclusion that we have a problem is when a condition conflicts with a prevailing value. Uneven access to health care is or is not a problem, for instance, depending on whether one thinks of health care as a right.

Another particularly fascinating way for conditions to become problems is through a struggle over framing. We treat conditions very differently depending on the category in which we place them. If transportation of disabled people in urban areas is viewed strictly as a transportation issue, for instance, then economical and effective approaches like dial-a-ride or subsidized taxi service are appropriate. But if transportation of the disabled is placed into a civil rights category, then retrofitting subways for elevators and providing bus lifts is called for to give disabled people the same access as everybody else. Framing this issue as one of transportation or as one of civil rights makes all the difference.

The Policy Stream of Proposals: A Policy Primeval Soup

Picture a community of specialists in health policy (or transportation, welfare, etc): researchers, congressional staffers, bureaucrats in planning and evaluation offices, academics, think tanks, analysts working for interest groups, and so on. Ideas float around in such communities. Specialists try out and revise their ideas by going to lunch, attending conferences, circulating papers, holding hearings, presenting testimony, writing reports, publishing articles, and drafting legislative proposals. Many, many ideas are considered at some point in the evolution of an issue.

The process by which proposals are selected from this very large set of ideas resembles biological natural selection. Much as molecules floated around in the "primeval soup" before life came into being, ideas float around in a "policy primeval soup" in these communities of specialists. Ideas, like molecules, bump into one another, combining and recombining in various ways. The policy primeval soup takes a long time to bubble around. Development of proposals must be done long before the opportunity for actual adoption presents itself because, at that point, it is too late to hone a proposal. In the process of policy evolution, some ideas fall away, others survive and prosper, and some are selected to become serious contenders for adoption.

The Political Stream

The third stream, the political stream, is composed of changes of administration, shifts in partisan or ideological balances in Congress, shifts in national mood, and interest group pressure. This stream is an important endogenous part of policy making, but it proceeds according to its own dynamics, such as elections, nominations, partisan politics, and interest group campaigns.

To illustrate the importance of this stream, a widespread perception that the national mood favors governmental activism at one point in time or favors smaller government at another time profoundly affects which items are possible and which are not. A change of administration or a shift in Congress changes governmental agendas. Likewise, social movements like civil rights, consumerism, environmental protection, and taxpayer revolts sweep across the land.

Joining the Streams

Advocates (policy entrepreneurs) continually push their pet proposals or push attention to particular problems and try to keep issues alive in good times and bad. But an open policy window presents them with a special opportunity. These entrepreneurs become particularly active when a problem floats by to which their proposals can be the solution or when a development in the political stream can be used to their advantage. At these critical points in time, entrepreneurs play a major part in joining the previously separate streams by hooking their solutions to problems or by ensuring that proposals from the policy stream are considered when the political conditions are right. Much like a window for a space shot, policy windows stay open only so long. Failure to seize an opportunity when it arises requires waiting for the next one to come along.

Generally, alternatives or policy proposals are generated in the policy stream, and agenda change comes from changes in the problems or politics streams. So windows sometimes open because problems become pressing or because the political stream changes. The election of the Reagan administration, for example, created many opportunities for the Heritage Foundation at the same time that it shut down any chance for comprehensive national health insurance. Sometimes, windows open predictably, as with the scheduled renewal of enabling legislation. Other windows open unpredictably, as with an airplane crash.

One of my respondents captured the whole process in an absolutely beautiful image. He showed how some of the process is governed by large events not under anybody's control, how advocates wait for their opportunities, how they must be prepared ahead of time, and how the joining of the streams is crucial. He said, "People who are trying to advocate change are like surfers waiting for the big wave. You get out there, you have to be ready to go, you have to be ready to paddle. If you're not ready to paddle when the big wave comes along, you're not going to ride it in."

AN ILLUSTRATION: THE CLINTON HEALTH PLAN

It is sometimes helpful to pin down theoretical abstractions to a particular case. The experience of the Clinton administration's health-care plan in 1993–1994 illustrates the operation of this model of policy formation quite well. Let us first consider the condition of the three streams in the early 1990s.

As to problems, there was a general agreement among health policy specialists, which extended well into the more general public, about the problems confronting the country in the health-care arena. First, the cost of health care had been rising sharply since the late 1960s, which produced severe constraints on federal and state government budgets, major conflicts over fringe benefits at bargaining tables across the country, and widespread concern about health care's share of the national economy. Second, gaps in health insurance coverage were also recognized as a serious problem. During the early 1990s the figure of 37 million Americans without health insurance (by late 1990s closer to 44 million) was widely discussed. The problem of gaps in coverage was exacerbated by the stubborn recession, as people lost their insurance when they lost or changed jobs. Some participants emphasized cost and others emphasized coverage, but there were sufficient problems recognized at the time to prompt government officials to pay attention to health care.

The political stream was not as clear. On the one hand, Senator Harris Wofford's 1991 Pennsylvania campaign ran television ads in which he said, "If criminals have the right to a lawyer, I think working Americans should have the right to a doctor." Events like Wofford's victory led many observers to the conclusion that the time was right for a major push for national health insurance. Bill Clinton took a page out of the Wofford campaign, making health-care reform a major theme of his 1992 campaign. Big business was also increasingly interested in reform, as the cost of their employees' health insurance put a major pinch on profits, complicated their bargaining with labor unions, and put them in a position of cross-subsidizing care for underinsured and uninsured Americans.

But politics was not all on the side of action. A generalized cynicism about government that had been spreading through the body politic since the mid-1960s made people suspicious of new initiatives. Taxpayer revolts further dampened expensive new federal programs. In addition, since most Americans did have health insurance, it was unclear to them how they would benefit from reform. Finally, the in-fighting among interest groups in this area was especially fierce. To see why this was so, consider that, at any time, advocates of national health insurance can count on the opposition of the insurance industry and, if a plan envisions employer mandates, on the opposition of small business. Physicians, hospitals, labor unions, and retired people all have well organized lobbies and well placed constituencies. In trying to build a proposal in that interest group environment, it is quite easy to step into quicksand and pay a hefty electoral price.

So in the late 1980s and early 1990s, there was a general recognition of the problems—cost and coverage—that needed attention. The problem stream, in other words, opened a window and produced a place on the governmental agenda. The direction of the political stream was less clear, however, with some aspects (e.g., the Wofford and Clinton campaigns and the interest of big business) in favor of action but other aspects (e.g., the generalized cynicism and the positions of the insurance industry and small business) opposed. On balance, the political stream probably at least tolerated some sort of action, leaving the window at least partly open.

In the early 1990s, however, the policy stream was in disarray. There were sharp, fundamental differences about which approach to take, even among vigorous advocates of reform. Some preferred single-payer national health insurance. Others, such as the "Jackson Hole" group, preferred "managed competition." The place of employer mandates was hotly disputed. Voucher plans and plans involving the extension of Medicare to the uninsured each had their advocates. For each approach, there were hybrids under consideration. I should emphasize that these were differences among advocates of change, not opponents, and no consensus had emerged in the policy community about which proposal to support.

The Clinton administration's proposal, as it turned out, did not forge that consensus. It came to be seen as an overly complicated, ambitious, and untested approach and was subjected to withering attacks from small business, insurance, and other opponents, from which it never recovered. Various politicians, including Senator George Mitchell, tried valiantly in 1994 to salvage some sort of initiative, but time ran out. If a policy window was open in 1993–1994, the election of 1994 slammed it shut.

The short version of these events is that the problems were widely recognized, the politics at least tolerated action, but the policy stream presented major difficulties. A policy window was open, but movement into position for enactment depended on a process of consensus building among advocates and specialists around a particular package. Such consensus is better built before the window opens, however, and the opportunity passed before agreement could be reached.

CONSTRAINTS, INCLUDING POLITICAL CULTURE

Even a system as fluid and unpredictable as the policy-making system I have described cannot produce just any result. Various factors constrain outcomes. Rules of procedure, for instance, including the constitution, statutes, prescribed jurisdictions, other legal requirements, and customary decision making modes, impose structures on participants. The budget imposes constraints, so that costly proposals are less likely to be considered in times of economic contraction and budget stringency than in more robust times.

Among the most important constraints is the content of the American political culture. Some approaches that are commonplace in other industrialized countries are out of bounds in the United States. Let us consider the limits on government, the roots of those limits in the American political culture, and the origins of that culture. (For a more complete treatment of this subject, including references to a very large literature, see Kingdon, 1999.)

Describing a Pattern of Limited Government

Compared to other industrialized countries, the United States can fairly be characterized as a system of more limited government. Combining federal, state, and local activity, government is less involved in most aspects of social and economic problems than is the case in other countries. With some exceptions, the state is less intrusive, our government programs are smaller and less far-reaching, our public sector is smaller relative to the private sector, and our taxes are lower. Government has grown over this century, to be sure, and aspects of a welfare state in America are not entirely absent. Still, compared to other industrialized countries, the United States has a less comprehensive welfare state and a smaller public sector. We are alone among industrialized countries, for example, in our lack of national health insurance.

This narrower reach of public policy is accompanied by limited institutions. The combination of separation of powers (division into legislative, executive, and judicial branches) and federalism (division of powers between national and state governments) constitutes an extraordinarily fragmented governmental system by comparison with other countries. The founders deliberately designed this fragmented system to limit the ability of any single branch or level of government to gain dominant power. In their effort to limit the possibilities of government tyranny, they also limited the capacity to mobilize government. They wanted these institutions to be unwieldy, prone to gridlock, and incapable of working smoothly. They succeeded.

Political parties, institutions that could mobilize majorities for action, are also weaker in the United States than they are in other industrialized countries. Individual candidates run and finance their own campaigns, and individual members of Congress and state legislatures are much more autonomous than are their counterparts in parliamentary systems. Again, this is no accident. The replacement of caucus nomination of parties' candidates with direct primary elections, for instance, took major powers from the hands of party leaders, thereby eroding party strength. So in terms of both our institutions and our public policies, government in the United States is more limited than is government in other industrialized countries.

American Political Culture

A proximate explanation for this pattern of limited government can be found in the content of American political thought. The United States has more limited government and less ambitious public policies than do other industrialized countries, in the first instance, because Americans have a different view of the proper authority, limits, and possibilities of government. What we might call the prevailing American ideology is different, in that it concentrates on limiting the power and reach of government.

Let me be clear that I do not mean that all Americans hold the same set of values or that there is a dominant, hegemonic ideology that drives out all other ideas. Far from it; there have been dramatic struggles over these ideas over the years that continue to the present day. By "prevailing," I simply mean that the location of the center of American politics is different from that found in other countries. Specifically, despite differing views, despite major increases in the size of the public sector over time, and despite the existence of a considerable edifice of social programs in the United States, the *center* of American politics still favors limited government *more than* the political centers in other industrialized countries do. Accordingly, I am simply drawing comparisons between countries, not making absolute statements about some sort of ideal or hegemonic American ideology.

There have been many attempts to distill the essence of American political thought into a set of themes, and authors' lists of themes differ. Let me concentrate here on two aspects of American political thought, individualism and equality.

Some historians and political philosophers have remarked that Americans, more than others, emphasize individual goals and individual advancement rather than community goals or the advancement of public or collective purposes. This individualism is closely connected to the much-noticed tendency of Americans to prize liberty and freedom. This emphasis on individual advancement and freedom implies a distrust of government, a concern about the potential for government tyranny, and therefore a need to limit government.

Other historians and political philosophers point to a more communitarian, republican strain in American political thought. This strain refers to a sense of community, in which people deliberate together to pursue the public good and place a high value on community. Quite a lot of disagreement exists in writings on American political thought about whether individualism or communitarianism dominates, when either might have dominated, whether and when individualism gained an ascendancy over early communitarianism, and so forth.

For the purposes of this chapter, however, both individualism and communitarianism came to similar views about limited government. On the face of it, individualists would want to limit government for reasons already discussed, but because many of the early communitarians were interested in the local autonomy of religious communities from central government authority, they also came to the conclusion that government should be limited. Both individualists and communitarians, in other words, were characterized by more suspicion of authority and more emphasis on limited government than one finds in the central thinking in other countries.

To turn to the second theme, observers from Tocqueville to the present remark that Americans prize equality. But in a distinctive approach, Americans seem to prize equality of *opportunity* rather than equality of result.

That is, Americans tolerate much larger differences between rich and poor (inequality of result) than one finds in most other industrialized countries, and do not consider those differences unjust. Americans think of this country as the land of opportunity, in which people are not simply born into their station in life but can change their economic, social, and geographical lot. In fact, instead of finding income disparities politically or morally repugnant, Americans tend to think that everyone can aspire to be rich one day, or at least that everyone's children can.

Indeed, in a fascinating twist, equality of opportunity is used to justify inequality of result. That is, if this is the land of opportunity, then unfortunate people are not poor because of forces beyond their control or because they are down on their luck, but because they did not take advantage of their opportunities and are responsible for their own condition. Of course, there is a very large literature that shows that people do not actually start their lives with equal opportunities, but we are dealing here with the world of political justification.

This emphasis on equality of opportunity rather than equality of result also reconciles the themes of individualism and equality. Individualism does imply that some people will get ahead faster than others, and if Americans prized equality of result, the two themes would conflict. But because Americans prize equality of opportunity, it is logical to believe that successful individuals are simply the ones who achieved, based on the same opportunities everybody else had rather than on inherited wealth or social class.

It is not hard to see the results of the dominant American political ideology, which starts with an impulse to limit government to a greater extent than one finds in other industrialized countries. The American founders deliberately built institutions—separation of powers, checks and balances, bicameral Congress, federalism, an independent judiciary—to ensure that no one faction could capture power and that mobilizing this cumbersome apparatus for action would be extremely difficult. In other countries strong political parties would coordinate actions and mobilize resources, but America set out to weaken parties. In terms of public policies, Americans do not tolerate taxes very well, the public sector as a percentage of gross domestic product is smaller than it is in other countries, and the United States has much less ambitious programs in health, welfare, housing, transportation, and many other areas.

Why Is American Political Culture As It Is?

Why did Americans, more than people in other countries, come to believe that there should be greater limits on government? The answer is complicated (see Kingdon, 1999), but a short version of the story begins with the first immigration of settlers from Europe. People who came to America were not typical of the people who stayed behind. They either came to escape religious or other discrimination or to better themselves economically. Either way, they carried with them a distinctive distrust of authority, including government authority, and they placed a priority on individual autonomy and advancement. Members of Protestant sects escaping from the Church of England and the close ties between the established church and the political regime, for example, brought with them a profound aversion to religious and governmental authority and a larger skepticism about authority and hierarchy in general. Those arriving to better themselves economically naturally placed their individual advancement and that of their families first. As such, they viewed taxes as confiscating what was theirs and placed a particular emphasis on equality of opportunity.

So the orientations of both these types of immigrants planted the seeds of the themes of individualism and equality of opportunity that are hallmarks of American political culture and fed their desire to limit government more than did those who stayed behind in the old countries. In short, because they came to these shores either to escape religious or political authority or to better themselves economically, the people who came to dominate American politics were more suspicious of government tyranny, less given to obey authorities, less tolerant of hierarchy, more inclined to see taxation as confiscating what was theirs rather than as a way to finance collective purposes, and less inclined to support ambitious government programs.

This distinctive orientation was combined with the pervasive localism of America. The country started with local communities. Each of the colonies was separate and each quite different from the others, so the institutions, such as a federal system, provided for only a minimal centralization. The political culture of limited government was enhanced by a particular suspicion of central government.

Subsequent events tended to reinforce this early emphasis on limited government. The American ideology of limited government, the tradition of localism, and the workings of the institutions perpetually reinforced one another. Ideology dictated continued limits on government, but because government institutions were limited, people also developed limited expectations about what government could or should accomplish, reinforcing these ideas. A cycle set in: Americans do not trust government, so they do not invest in it, so government does not work as well as it might, and the fears that government can never get anything right are thereby confirmed.

America also never developed the democratic socialist parties and movements of other industrialized countries. One reason for this difference is that, particularly after property qualifications for voting were eliminated, there was universal adult suffrage, at least for white males, from a very early date. So when workers came to unionize in response to the industrial revolution, they could concentrate single-mindedly on workplace issues and did not need to organize in both the political and economic spheres at once. In European countries, by contrast, workers were pressing for both the right to vote and the right to organize in the workplace at the same time, causing both unions and parties of the left to combine political and economic issues into one package wrapped in a general rhetoric of class consciousness. This feature of sequence, combined with the racial and ethnic divisions within the American working class, led to less working class solidarity and less pressure from the left than was true of other countries and to the absence of democratic socialism.

The Virtue of Pragmatism

The American approach of limited government compared to the style of government in other industrialized countries is rather firmly in place. But thoughtful observers often say that Americans, in addition to being driven by certain distinctive values and orientations, are also traditionally a practical, pragmatic people. We prize "know-how"; our biggest praise for a given approach is that it will "get the job done." In this pragmatic vein, we do not fully trust rigid ideologues; we regard them as a bit suspect or "extreme." An appeal to this pragmatism, under some circumstances, can modify the usual American impulse for limited government. Collective goods like environmental protection and national defense, for instance, will not be adequately provided by letting autonomous individuals go their own way. If people are persuaded that we cannot "get the job done" with the usual individualistic approach, then more collective approaches might well be adopted. But that persuasion process takes a long, long period of education and an uncommon persistence by people who are concerned about particular problems.

ETHICS AND HEALTH POLICY

My last task in this chapter is to reflect a bit on the relationship between ethics and health policy. The reality of policy making that I have discussed might contain a few hints concerning how ethics and health policy might be connected.

Let us first distinguish the domains of ethics and health policy. Most of us would think of the treatment of human subjects in research, whether to continue heroic treatment in terminally ill patients, or some aspects of fetal tissue research, for some examples, as involving ethical issues. Many people would generally regard whether to enact a system of single-payer national health insurance or how to regulate managed care companies, for instance, as important public policy issues. These issues involve central questions of who gets what from government and from medical care but often have not been regarded as ethical issues. One purpose of this volume, as I understand it, is to highlight the ways in which these policy issues and political fights involve ethical questions.

What is at stake here, it seems to me, is a process of framing issues. As I noted above with the example of transportation of disabled people in urban areas, the struggle over framing an issue is a critical process, one that often determines the outcome of a battle over a policy initiative. It made all the difference in the world, for instance, whether the Clinton health care proposal was framed as "big government" instead of "ensuring access to health care," and the struggle over how the issue would be framed was a huge part of the process. When the "big government" label took hold, advocates for the proposal were at a tremendous disadvantage, because that label resonates in the American political culture of limited government.

More generally, it makes a huge difference if access to health care is seen as a right, something to which every citizen in a humane society should be entitled, instead of being seen as something that is a good thing to have but not a right. Framing is everything, or if not everything, at least terribly important.

In this case, highlighting ethical dimensions in health policy discussions frames the issues quite differently from the ways in which they are conventionally framed. Consider the example of debates over national health insurance. The United States is the only industrialized country that does not have some version of national health insurance that covers virtually the entire population. Some 44 million Americans are uninsured, and the insurance for the remainder varies quite a lot in terms of its coverage, cost, and delivery mechanisms. If this incomplete coverage of the population is seen as an ethical issue, then the uneven access to health care is not simply unfortunate, sad, or inconvenient; it is wrong and immoral. That framing of the issue changes the debate significantly.

Notes of Caution

Here I introduce three notes of caution. First, some people are uneasy with the common practice of making public policy without a clear vision of goals and priorities. How can we make sensible policy choices, they reason, without an explicit definition of the ends we are trying to achieve?

Actually, clarifying goals often hinders action in the real world. Lindblom, in his classic article "The Science of Muddling Through" (1959), describes policy making as a process of incrementally trying out new initiatives in a kind of experimental way, learning from experience, and adjusting as we go. Beyond his description, he argues that a more comprehensive approach, in which one clarifies goals and chooses the alternatives to achieve those goals according to a comparison of benefits and costs, actually does not work well.

One reason for Lindblom's unease about clarifying goals involves the practical construction of coalitions. One person (e.g., a legislator) might be willing to join a coalition (e.g., in support of a particular bill) for one reason, and another for another reason. Given that situation, it is more productive to leave the goals fuzzy, so that various types of supporters can join for different and even incompatible reasons. Clarifying the goals ahead of time will only highlight those incompatibilities, complicating the process of building the coalition.

Transporting that logic to this case, it is quite possible that highlighting various ethical considerations in a debate over access to health insurance might prompt people who do not agree with those statements of the ethics of the situation to leave the coalition. Some of them, not all, but some, might have joined if the goal had been left vague.

Beyond that, there is a particular problem with ethical and moral discussions. They tend to harden positions and make compromises and coalition building more difficult. Opponents become not simply wrong about the facts, or myopic, but also tinged with immorality. Divergent points of view are not simply different, but also illegitimate. It may be better to conduct debates about health policy issues in a more pragmatic spirit, one that addresses issues while avoiding the adoption of positions that prove hard to alter. That approach has the additional advantage of appealing to the American pragmatism that I discussed above.

Now to the second note of caution: Too much discussion of ethics might strike some participants and observers as over-reaching, so it might be unsuccessful in any event. In the process of argumentation, various sides in a debate often introduce new rationales to justify their positions. In this case, advocates of national health insurance might well introduce a set of ethical considerations (e.g., "it's unjust to leave 44 million Americans uncovered"), complete with a developed literature on the ethical implications of failing to provide the entire population with access to health care. Their opponents would charge that old-fashioned tax-and-spend liberals are just bending the field of ethics around to provide yet another justification for their advocacy. This opposition would also rest on the American impulse to limit government, arguing that expansive government is itself unjust. At the least, an emphasis on ethical considerations in the debate might complicate the case for universal access; at most, it might backfire.

Discussions of health policy, of course, inevitably and appropriately involve issues of justice. The fact that 44 million Americans are without health insurance, for instance, does unavoidably raise questions about distributive justice. Does it violate our sense of just and fair outcomes that so many in the richest country on earth are uninsured? Many ethicists (e.g., Daniels, 1985) have considered the ethical dimensions of such health policy issues. Ethicists are increasingly turning their attention to such issues as access to health care, coverage of health insurance, and the regulation of managed care, often using their knowledge of theories of justice.

As with any discipline, however, it is important that the involvement of scholars in public policy debates be limited to the areas of their professional expertise. It is, of course, the right of all well-informed citizens to say what they think, but scholars' claim to a legitimate voice springs from their disciplinary knowledge. Ethics has its own expertise, but so do economics, medicine, law, sociology, anthropology, and political science. Any scholarly discipline loses some of its legitimate claim on policy makers' attention if its observations and positions stray too far from a grounding in its professional expertise. And without that grounding, pronouncements of ethicists or anybody else are little more than the venting of personal ideology.

Recognition of the comparative advantages and limits of various disciplines also argues for interdisciplinary approaches. For one thing, most important public policy issues involve empirical as well as philosophical questions. Returning to the uninsured, for instance, the fairness of uneven insurance coverage across a population involves not only theories of justice but also answers to a host of empirical questions that are not within the expertise of ethicists to answer. To what extent and in what ways does lack of health insurance actually affect access to health care? How much does access to health care actually affect health status? What should we make of the contribution of lifestyle choices (e.g., smoking, diet, seatbelt use) to mortality and morbidity, as well as the contribution of medical interventions? The importance of such questions argues for a collaboration between ethics and other disciplines, with each discipline bringing to the collaboration its own expertise.

My third caution is to point to the risk that an emphasis on ethics in health policy debates may dilute and damage the field of ethics itself. Ethicists do enjoy a certain credibility when confined to questions that are clearly ethical by general agreement. Providers, patients, and patients' families all need some ethical guidance with such questions as when to cease heroic treatments, for example, and whether to pursue certain fertility options. Their willingness to turn to ethicists in such circumstances depends on the ethicists' credibility. If ethics is bent to the purpose of ordinary policy advocacy, that credibility could be drawn into question in some quarters.

Ideas and Politics

None of the foregoing should diminish the importance of ideas in politics and policy formation. Indeed, I have become convinced that politics and policy making are not simply driven by such conventional political processes as reelection incentives, interest group pressure, campaign contributions, and marshalling votes and power. Instead, argumentation, persuasion, and marshalling evidence and information are also important. In other words, participants traffic in the world of ideas. There is a growing literature in political science and economics to which I have contributed (see Kingdon, 1993) on the importance of ideas in the political process.

One clue to the importance of ideas is the investment in time, money, and energy that people in and around government make in them. They hire analysts; they marshal arguments and collect evidence in support of those arguments; they reason and persuade. Even the most hard-bitten, self-interested lobbies have policy analysts and do not rely simply on appeal to their self-interest or their political muscle. If ideas were not important, savvy people like these, who know what is a productive use of their time, money, and other resources, would not invest so much in them. In addition to the "usual" process of mobilizing such assets as interest group pressure, reelection resources, and the positions of political parties, struggles over health policy involve, and should involve, debates over central ideas.

One relevant body of ideas is the considerable literature on justice. If I am right about the importance of equality of *opportunity* in American political thought as opposed to equality of result, then these arguments about justice might usefully be cast in terms of equality of opportunity. In what respects does inadequate access to health care or lack of health insurance limit a person's opportunities in the land of opportunity? Arguments about justice are likely to bear more fruit in American public policy debates if they are framed more in terms of opportunity than in terms of results. If we simply notice the result that some people lack health insurance, for example, we would have to argue that this inequality of result is somehow more unjust than the unequal distribution of fancy cars and huge houses. But if it can be plausibly argued that the lack of health insurance limits opportunities, then that argument ties more closely to themes in American political thought that are more widely accepted.

To turn to another idea, part of the debate over health policy involves a debate over compulsion. Other industrialized countries achieve universal health insurance coverage at lower cost than in the United States (see White, 1995) partly because of a degree of compulsion that Americans find hard to tolerate. They require all employers to furnish health insurance to employees, for instance; or they enroll all citizens in a government-sponsored insurance system, and pay for it with higher taxes. They achieve cost control by such devices as setting global budgets, negotiating fee schedules that will apply to all providers, rationing care, and other such practices. Patients may not be able to schedule elective procedures at their convenience and may have to wait in a queue.

These features of compulsion do not fit very well with the picture of the American political culture that I painted above, which stresses individual autonomy and limits on government. But the end result of a debate about compulsion might be a change in the way people in this country view the issues. It is worth pointing out, for example, that there is a lot of compulsion in the current American health-care system. Care is already rationed, for instance; it is just done by what someone called the "wallet biopsy" rather than by some criteria other than wealth. Employers also have been pushing their employees into managed care rather than fee-for-service care. The managed care companies, in turn, are quite strict about limiting access to specialists, shortening hospital stays, and implementing other cost-cutting measures. Debates surrounding a "patients' bill of rights" and other such initiatives reflect a recognition that nongovernmental systems result in undesirable compulsion. Indeed, national health insurance might result in less compulsion than currently exists. At any rate, Americans need to have a thorough debate about the topic of compulsion, which would be very much related to the view of limited government.

Americans also need a more thorough debate about costs. One of the curious features of the debates about "big government" or "returning people's money to them" is that taxes really are seen as family expenses that are quite different from other expenses. In the health-care arena, however, it is hard to see the practical differences between private health insurance premiums and taxes that might be collected to finance access to health-care through a government program. Indeed, ambiguity on that very point was at the center of the Congressional Budget Office's (CBO's) consideration of the Clinton health-care proposal. The issue was whether the premiums should be considered government revenue. When the CBO ruled that they must be considered government revenue, that gave a tremendous boost to the plan's opponents.

Somehow, Americans are so fundamentally antistatist that it seems to makes a terrific difference whether to pay for health insurance through taxes or through premiums. Yet, in practice, there probably is not a great deal of difference in the amount of red tape, arbitrary rulings, and compulsion between dealing with Blue Cross and dealing with Medicare. Indeed, the administration of Medicare may be more efficient than the administration of private insurance. So a searching debate may be in order about the distinction between taxes and premiums and about whether the distinction makes a difference.

I want to emphasize that these sorts of debates do not take place in a realm that is separate from "politics" as we usually think of it. Indeed, deliberation over such ideas is very much at the center of political struggles. Even if health policy debates were not cast primarily as ethical issues, we would still be very much involved in the world of ideas.

Long Periods of Discussion

When a window opens, when officials are receptive to a new idea, the opportunity must be seized before the window closes. People who wish to have their ideas considered cannot wait to develop ideas, orientations, and proposals until the opportunity arises. At that point, they are too late. A long period of discussion, research, writing, deliberation, and softening up is needed well in advance of the policy-making opportunity in order to be ready to take advantage of it when it (sometimes unpredictably) presents itself. As one respondent said, you have to be ready to paddle.

This means that advocates must be willing to invest time in their ideas. Just getting the attention of government officials is a major accomplishment, even under the best of circumstances. Using open windows takes skill, knowledge, and luck, to be sure. But of all the attributes of successful policy entrepreneurs that I could name, sheer persistence is probably the most important.

The gradual reorientation of world views, perspectives, and categories within which people think makes a tremendous difference. Within a community of health policy specialists, for instance, a major difference exists between using health insurance simply as a device for paying the bills and using health insurance as an instrument for redirecting incentives in health-care delivery. A long process of discussion within such a community can sometimes contribute to the reorientation of whole approaches, so volumes like this one, even if they do not have a short-term impact on health policy, are not just wasted motion.

REFERENCES

Baumgartner F and Jones B (1993) *Agendas and Instability in American Politics.* Chicago, IL: University of Chicago Press.

Cohen M, March J, and Olsen J (1972) A garbage can model of organizational choice. *Administrative Science Quarterly* 17:1–25.

Daniels N (1985) *Just Health Care*. Cambridge: Cambridge University Press.

Holland J (1995) *Hidden Order: How Adaptation Builds Complexity*. New York: Addison-Wesley.

Kingdon J (1989) *Congressmen's Voting Decisions*, 3d ed. Ann Arbor, MI: University of Michigan Press.

Kingdon J (1993) Politicians, self-interest, and ideas. In: Marcus G and Hanson R (eds) *Reconsidering the Democratic Public*. University Park, PA: Pennsylvania State University Press.

Kingdon J (1995) *Agendas, Alternatives, and Public Policies*, 2d ed. New York: Harper Collins.

Kingdon J (1999) *America the Unusual*. New York: St. Martin's.

Lindblom C (1959) The science of muddling through. *Public Administration Review* 14: 79–88.

White J (1995) *Competing Solutions: American Health Care Proposals and International Experience*. Washington, DC: The Brookings Institution.

7

When public opinion counts: inserting public opinion into health policy

STANLEY B. GREENBERG AND MARION DANIS

This book stresses the importance of giving a voice to those with a stake in policy. While the public as a whole has a great deal at stake in health policy, it is often difficult to envision how people's views might be taken into account. Polling provides a mechanism for doing so, as public opinion surveys are increasingly prominent in the American political landscape. In this chapter we present a brief history of polling, its nature, and its limitations. We then describe the way in which surveys have provided a voice for public opinion during periods of change in health policy. Finally, we consider the extent to which public opinion influences policy making and the ethical implications of this interaction for those who sponsor, conduct, and make use of public opinion surveys.

We are writing about polling because of our underlying assumption that public opinion matters. While some will be skeptical about the importance of public opinion, we do not share this view. As Jedediah Purdy writes,

> One of our leading phantoms is the word *public*. Like many ghosts, it has a distinguished—but in this case not a royal—heritage. It comes from the Latin *publius*, the people. It is the source of *republic*, the realm ruled by the people; its homeliest cousin is the beer serving *pub*, a shortened version of *public house*. Dur-

> ing the fierce debates of the 1780s over what form the American constitution should take, James Madison and other revolutionary leaders wrote their pamphlets under the pseudonym Publius. The idea of speaking for the public was important enough in the young republic that the most serious and high-minded figures tried to personify the *publius*; where the public rules in principle, its personification rules in fact.
>
> Purdy, 2000, p 78

Locating and listening to this public is no less important now. Somebody will speak for the *publius*—the question is, how well and through what means?

THE ROLE OF POLLING IN ASCERTAINING PUBLIC OPINION

The goal of polling, one would hope, is to bring ordinary people into decision making, involving them in decisions that greatly affect them but in which they might not otherwise participate. People find that they operate within institutions where their judgments, priorities, and values are barely heard. In the political process people certainly perceive that decision makers, politicians, and bureaucrats operate with many different pressures upon them—public pressure being only one, and perhaps not the biggest or loudest, among them.

At its best, polling brings people into the process. Though a fairly crude instrument on its own, polling forces awareness of some of the public's sentiments onto the country, institutions, and political leaders. It puts issues on the public agenda during elections and, afterwards, shapes legislative agendas. The historian Gil Troy (Troy, 1966) argues that polling, along with universal primaries and widespread media coverage, gives the public more exposure to candidates and more input into elections than would otherwise be possible.

Yet, despite the potential value of polling, many remain cautious. Walter Lippmann (1922) worried that politicians tailor their campaigns to public opinion, a process he thought threatened democracy. The iterative process in which experts survey public opinion and then respond to it by crafting slogans to appeal to public views could, in Lippmann's view, put political leaders in a position of slavish adherence to the advice of opinion experts and thus reduce the capacity of politicians to lead. Bernard Wiesberger advances a different worry when he suggests that while polling may facilitate the insertion of popular opinion into pubic debate, it may contribute to reduced voting (Weisberger, 2000).

HISTORY OF PUBLIC OPINION SURVEYS IN THE UNITED STATES

The growth of public opinion surveys in the political history of the United States reflects ambivalence about the value of inserting public opinion into the electoral process and public policy making. The framers of the Constitution did not intend to create a government that was directly responsive to popular sentiment, as reflected in the establishment of the Electoral College (Weisberger, 2000b). In his history of surveys in the United States, Weisberger argues that leaders did not seek to determine public opinion directly until almost half a century after the Declaration of Independence (Weisberger, 2000a).

Popular sentiment, however, gained new importance with the presidential election of 1828, when the popular presidential candidate, Andrew Jackson, won office. At the heart of the developing party system were political parties that depended increasingly on popular support for their success. The earliest polls which were called straw polls, after the habit of tossing straw in the wind to see how the wind blew, appeared in the press as these popularly based parties became dominant. This initial process was a very haphazard and unscientific endeavor.

Around the turn of the 20th century, public opinion gained added attention with intense political battles concerning the populist revolt and assault on the political machines. The progressive era brought a range of changes to broaden popular participation in government, including a constitutional amendment to allow direct election of United States senators, the institution of primary elections in many states, and the use of referendums to put propositions to a popular vote.

Public opinion polling gained much wider prominence after World War I, Weisberger argues. Propaganda drives during the war and the development of the new fields of advertising and public relations reflected a growing interest and capacity to influence public opinion. Freudian psychology helped change the concept of public opinion; rather than being viewed as a mere collection of reasoned judgments by individuals, public opinion began to be seen as a set of presumed unconscious prejudices and attitudes that could be potentially manipulated.

A decade later, surveying public opinion and determining political views became an applied social science. Survey firms and organizations developed, including the widely publicized Fortune survey in 1935. George Gallup began the American Institute of Public Opinion, Hadley Cantril began the Office of Public Opinion Research at Princeton, the Survey Research Center began in Ann Arbor, and the National Opinion Research Center opened in Denver, later moving to Chicago.

THE VALUE OF POLLING COMPARED TO OTHER APPROACHES TO HEARING PUBLIC VIEWS

Despite the improvement in techniques as polling emerged as a social science, limitations remain: polling usually has a fixed set of responses to a fairly limited number of policy options and lacks the complexity that policy issues themselves have. This is particularly true in the health-care arena. People would like the government to play a role in changing the system, but they are nervous about having the government involved in a sector they would prefer to be private. At times, polls can capture this ambivalence; other times, they force people into boxes or choices that do not accurately reflect their ambivalence.

This is why it is useful to supplement polls with techniques that better reflect conflicting views. Qualitative methodologies, particularly focus groups, allow people the opportunity to discuss their views in more depth, express their ambivalence, make trade-offs, and reflect their values.

INTERPRETING THE VALIDITY OF SURVEYS AS A REFLECTION OF THE PUBLIC'S VIEWS

A survey, to be used effectively or interpreted accurately must be evaluated in its entirety and in context. This is particularly important to appreciate when someone releases a partial set of responses. To understand the context in which respondents are answering questions, it is best to be aware of all the questions being asked, not just the ones that are highlighted. Policy makers trying to understand public opinion amid a myriad of results must rely on several surveys that reflect many perspectives. A battery of surveys, like those funded by foundations, provide a deeper understanding of public opinion on an issue.

Since the public is frequently unsure or conflicted on an issue, effective surveys must allow respondents to express these feelings; surveys simulating the public debate need to ask about opposing perspectives. A contentious issue is surveyed fairly when opposing sides think their positions are well represented in the survey instrument.

A good sample represents the whole population; every person in the population theoretically should have an equal probability of being selected for an interview. A measure of a representative sample, this is also a measure of quality in participation. To accomplish this, a survey should be conducted over multiple nights and in different time periods, and callbacks should be made to try to reach people who are not initially home or have busy phone lines. Achieving representation is costly, and some media polls are conducted over just a single night, thereby excluding people with lifestyles or work patterns that make them difficult to contact. Shortcuts in sampling methodology also shortcut participation in the public debate.

Even when surveys are representative of the population, they may still fail to represent parts of the population with very particular health-care needs, such as those with acute health problems, young people, and ethnic minorities. These segments may constitute only a small portion of the sample and thus cannot be reported separately, but because results cannot be reported, these segments are excluded from the public debate. To prevent this, opinions of these groups can be accurately captured and their views made public by special surveys targeted at such groups.

DRIVING FORCES IN THE POLLING PROCESS

Sometimes public sentiment can force itself on policy makers, with polling operating as an important vehicle. After the demise of the Clinton health-care reform plan, for instance, politicians opted to avoid major health-care initiatives rather than face new political battles. The legislative initiatives brought forward were extremely narrow and targeted. But while politicians were very cautious about returning to health-care issues, the public would not let them go away. Numerous polls revealed a great deal of frustration with the evolving health-care system, particularly with gaps in insurance coverage and the bureaucratic practices of HMOs. For example, a survey sponsored by the Cable News Network and USA Today and conducted by Gallup revealed the importance of health care issues, including HMOs, in the 1998 vote for Congress, with 21% of those surveyed responding that these issues were somewhat important, 43% citing that they were very important, and 28% reporting that they were extremely important (Gallup, 1998, see also Q. W. Ayres and Associates, 1998 and Princeton Survey Research Associates, 1998). Likewise, a 1998 survey conducted by Princeton Survey Research Associates, Newsweek had 81% of respondents indicating that protecting patients' rights in HMOs should be one of Congress's top priorities over the next two years (Princeton Survey Research Associates, 1998; see also Hart and Teeter Research Companies, 1998). Consequently, public sentiment, often voiced in polls, eventually forced politicians to address these issues again.

While the media and the press play a large role in making these private sentiments public, they frequently capture these sentiments simplistically. People will be asked, very basically, whether they are concerned about the cost of prescription drugs or whether the government should or should not provide prescription drug benefits to seniors. But the public policy debate is much more complex than the initial portrayal the media conveys. As the debate evolves, the alternatives that are proposed by congressional and presidential candidates differ in their underlying philosophies about the role of government and the diverse kinds of political goals they hope to achieve. In the presidential election of 2000, for example, the Republican program focused on using state governments and expanding benefits for the neediest; the Democratic candidate focused on broadening Medicare to provide prescription drugs to all seniors.

As the issue of health care becomes fully public, the field of public opinion research becomes more crowded. It is joined by a range of actors, particularly foundations like Kaiser, which attempt to look at the issue in more depth. The debate is likely to be joined by various parties to the controversy; these groups who sponsor polls and sometimes release the results to the public in order to try to publicize their interpretation of the public's interests, needs, and desires. Polling by candidates for political office probably overwhelms all other polling and uses more sophisticated questions to test the public's support for various health-care initiatives. Officials in government are likely to conduct surveys of public thinking as they move toward actually proposing specific health-care changes.

While this sequence of the roles played by the media, foundations, candidates, and politicians is fairly routine, the order can vary. Sometimes interest groups or politicians with strong views drive the issues, forcing them onto the agenda and getting the public involved in the process. For example, the ethics of late-term abortion only became a broad public concern after pro-life groups organized to put the spotlight on the issue. These groups thereby brought late-term abortion to the public's attention and made it a public issue (Johnson, 2000).

In general, politicians are cautious about boldly intervening in the arena of health care. Major health-care reforms involve many diverse and entangled interests from health-care professionals to the insurance companies. While leaders obviously want to address the public's health-care concerns, they are cautious about the large potential costs involved. Advocating benefits for prescription drugs or new rules for health care organizations, for example, could involve real costs. Employer mandates for health insurance may raise cost to employers and create a new set of issues.

So the public's health concerns have to reach a high level before political leaders rush to popularize the issue and move for change. Indeed, public concern with health-care issues rose in the years after the failure of the Clinton health-care reforms, ultimately ensuring a full-blown health-care debate in the last presidential election (Democracy Corps, 1999; Democracy Corps, 2000).

Who takes part in public debate, that is, who gets included in surveys, is frequently determined by the scope of the survey. Surveys on public policy usually use national random samples of the voting age population. However, when the subject becomes electoral, surveys may be confined to registered voters and those most likely to vote, further narrowing the segment of the public that is drawn into the public debate despite the infused interest in health-care issues. The use of samples of registered and likely voters, while understandable for those focused on winning elections, leaves important population segments outside the public debate. The nonvoter thus misses the opportunity to be heard twice—once in the survey and once in the polling booth. While polling serves to bring public opinion into policy making, there is always the danger of a skewed sample that reflects those who are already making their views known through the voting booth. Furthermore, if the promotion of polls discourages public interest in voting, the hope that opinion polls will promote the insertion of the public's views into policy will remain unrealized.

New electronic technology has the potential to address the sampling problems we have alluded to by providing a means to survey a broad range of individuals, including reluctant participants. Efforts by political scientists to take advantage of Web TV to access samples as large as tens of thousands of individuals on a weekly basis for years at a time provide the potential to sample broadly (Lewis, 2000).

Electronic survey methods may also make it possible to probe issues at a much more complex level than previous survey methods have permitted. While surveys are useful for revealing the opinions of large numbers of individuals, they do not provide functional approaches to asking about complicated policy issues. New programs on the Web may allow for both more complexity and more participation, with the caveat that participation will be limited to that portion of the population with familiarity and access to the Web.

THE ROLE OF PUBLIC OPINION IN HEALTH POLICY

When fundamental questions about delivery, access, and cost arise, health issues become a matter of concern and are pushed into the public realm. This is not where most people like to see these issues normally addressed; health care is very private, involving a network of relations with health-care providers. People are thus instinctively reluctant to see the government play an on-going and intrusive role in shaping medical practice or health-care delivery. Sometimes the providers themselves are public or are underwritten by public funds, but patients still tend to view these relationships as private in character. If one spends any time listening to senior citizens talk about

Medicare, then one understands the extent to which this state-supported patient–doctor relationship is viewed as private, financed by individual contributions and premiums. In a similar vein, support for health-care reform or new public guarantees has historically faltered as opponents have successfully raised doubts about the capacity of government to improve health care without undermining private care.

There are, however, notable moments when the public realm seems irresistible to those interested in having their opinion about health care heard. For the health-care issue to be forced into the public realm, a number of items must occur simultaneously. First, there must be a strong desire to change the way health care is delivered or financed. People may want to see new health-care arrangements, or they may want to protect old ones that are threatened by developing practices. In either case, the status quo in health is considered increasingly unacceptable and people want change, even fundamental change. Second, attitudes on health topics have to become concentrated around a few concerns that allow these attitudes to rise to the level of public opinion. People have varied views on many health-related topics, but there are some periods when attention narrows to a few concerns that begin to dictate the public agenda outside the health field. Third, people must begin to view a number of actors or institutions as acting badly—usually seen to be abusing their market position for unfair gain, perhaps endangering the quality of care, forcing up costs, or eroding the autonomy of other actors. In these periods, a growing sense arises that somehow these actors must be constrained. Fourth, more and more people and groups need to believe that these issues in health care can only be resolved in the public realm. And finally, political leaders, perhaps political entrepreneurs, need to step forward to champion these issues and mobilize organizations and the public around them. When all these forces converge, health care surfaces on the public agenda.

Because all these elements are necessary to push the topic of health care from the private to the public sphere, health-care reform was episodic in the 20th century. With the Progressive era in the 1920s and the New Deal era in the 1930s, reformers came close to enacting legislation in a few states that would have introduced public health insurance. They were responding to new efforts in Europe to create a social safety net, but progressive social reformers in the United States found little support in the political classes. Even so, the work of the reformers energized the medical profession and the insurance industry, who successfully pushed the idea of public health insurance off the public agenda. When President Franklin Roosevelt proposed the introduction of a national Social Security system for the retired, he stepped back from any offer in the health field (Skocpol, 1995, 141–5).

After World War II the public in most of the industrialized world wanted an expanded welfare state, particularly in the area of health. In Britain the new Labour government created the National Health Service. In the United States the public strongly favored changing privately financed health care in order to create a system of universal coverage. Indeed, Harry Truman made universal health coverage a signature issue before the Congress in 1946 and 1949 and in the campaign of 1948. He challenged a "do-nothing" Congress to enact the Wagner-Murray-Dingel Bills to create a program of national health insurance. While Congress balked at the proposition, it did pass some minor reforms and voted to expand hospital construction, which had broad support in the health industry (Skocpol, 1995, 178, 200–1). Health care then nearly disappeared as a public issue until the 1960s.

In 1965 Congress created entirely new areas of public health by enacting Medicare and Medicaid. In part, this period of health-care reform in the mid-1960s came in reaction to Michael Harrington's *Other America*, which helped concentrate public attention on poverty in general and elderly poverty in particular (Matthews, 2001; Muravchik, 2000; Wolfe, 2000). Two-thirds of the public was already in favor of using Social Security for health care for seniors. President John F. Kennedy tried to mobilize public support for Medicare, for example, by holding a rally at Madison Square Garden. President Lyndon B. Johnson used increasing concern to garner support for the greatest expansion of public health insurance in the country's history. Indeed, Johnson made Medicare the principal issue in his election campaign in 1964. His proposal was opposed by the American Medical Association and the medical establishment, which charged that the program would "destroy the [country's] . . . moral fiber" and undermine the "concept of individual and family responsibility"(Jacobs, 1993, 137–48).

In the following three decades, all the private actors in health care accommodated themselves to the new system and, in an important sense, moved the issue out of the public realm. The creation of a public system of health-care financing for senior citizens was not the opening to a new set of debates about unresolved issues. Instead, it addressed a glaring problem and then allowed the remaining health-care issues to fade from the public eye.

THE CLINTON MOMENT

All the elements that force health-care concerns into the public realm came together in the 1992–1994 period, after three decades of remission. The starting point was with the public itself. After years of rapidly rising health-care costs, squeezed health benefits and wages, and a growing number of people with no insurance at all, the public demanded change. More than three-quarters of the public (81%) said they wanted to either completely rebuild or fundamentally change the health-care system in the country (Princeton Survey Research Associates, April 1993). The public was focused on two problems—rising costs and declining access.

These growing concerns about health care did not, in themselves, create a public health issue. But, starting in 1991, politicians, particularly Democratic ones, spoke out with increasing frequency about the need for bold reforms. One United States senator and an early candidate in the race for president, Bob Kerry, voiced his preference for a Canadian-type health-care system and made health care his number-one issue. Before announcing his own candidacy, Bill Clinton met with groups of social scientists and health policy analysts to work through the issue. In his announcement Clinton, too, made clear his commitment to universal coverage. The upset victory by Harris Wofford in the 1991 special election to the United States Senate brought new force to the call for universal coverage and further raised political antennae on the issue. With blunt campaign advertisements asking questions like, "If a criminal has a right to see a lawyer, why doesn't a working person have a right to see a doctor?" Wofford helped catapult health-care reform to the top of the national agenda (Skocpol, 1996, 25–30).

Given these stimuli, any legitimate Democratic candidate for president in 1992 was compelled to address the health-care issue in a bold way. During the presidential primary in New Hampshire in early 1992, Clinton was under pressure from other candidates and the press to release his own full-blown plan for reforming the health-care system. Immediately before the candidates' debate, he released an employer-based plan for universal coverage entitled "Bill Clinton's American Health Care Plan: National Insurance Reform to Cut Costs and Cover Everybody" (Skocpol, 1996, 39–40). During the general election Clinton released his "Putting People First" plan to get national health-care spending under control, "take on the insurance industry," and "guarantee universal coverage." The plan provided for expanded health networks and employer-based insurance that, in many respects, resembled the mixed public/market plan that he would offer the following year (Clinton, 1992, 107–11).

Throughout the fall Clinton emphasized three dominant themes in his campaign advertising: an economic plan to create 8 million jobs, a plan to alter welfare policy, and a guarantee of universal health coverage. In post-election polls conducted for the incoming White House administration and funded by the Democratic National Committee, these were the three promises voters most remembered from the election campaign.

Elections matter in shaping the public agenda. Few in the administration doubted that President Clinton would soon make proposals for universal health coverage and cost containment. First Lady Hillary Rodham Clinton was chosen to head the initiative, and, after an elaborate preparatory process,

President Clinton spoke in September 1993 to a joint session of the Congress and the nation. He stated then and repeated in the State of the Union Address in early 1994 that "our health care system takes 35 percent more of our income than any other country, insures fewer people, requires more Americans to pay more and more for less and less, and gives them fewer choices. There is no excuse for that kind of system, and it's time to fix it" (Skocpol, 1996, 1).

The "villain" of the piece was the insurance companies, which were raising prices to employers and individuals and creating new insecurities by trying their best to insure the healthiest. People feared losing health insurance, and more and more people—38.9 million in 1992—found themselves without coverage. Hillary Clinton put the spotlight on insurance companies by portraying them as greedy actors whose private interests resoundingly clashed with the interests of families and the public.

In this environment the solution had to be political, and, indeed, in surveys 60% to 72% of Americans said they supported some kind of national health insurance (Skocpol, 1996, 25). In this period few pundits or political leaders doubted that the government would act. Even the Senate Republican leader, Bob Dole, and the Senate Republican charged with health issues, John Chafee, entertained the thought of some kind of major governmental action, most likely an "individual mandate." The health issue was fully politicized.

The Clinton health-care initiative, it seems, was carried out during a period of intense public interest in health issues: the public did, in fact, have opinions on health issues framed in a public context. However, while Americans wanted change in the public and private health policies that were forcing up costs and making insurance less secure, the public was hardly unified on how best to achieve results. Opinions were aggregating around public options, but they were not aggregating around a single or dominant approach. At the time of the launch of the Clinton health-care plan, opinion was essentially concentrated around three perspectives—about a third wanted a smaller role for government, about a third wanted a comprehensive federal Canadian-like health-care system, and about a third supported major reforms of the current system, like an employer mandate.

Very few people supported the perspective that was at the heart of the Clinton plan—a state-developed structure promoting choice and competition to bring down costs and increase coverage. Most of those who favored promoting competition also preferred that the government play a smaller role, which left the Clinton plan isolated in the arena of public opinion; his concept was an orphan in the world of public opinion.

Further fragmentation of public opinion tended to undermine the possibility of developing a broad majority for any specific way to reform the health-care system. Union households, 15% of the public, were some of the strongest supporters of universal health-care coverage and were natural allies of the president and his plan. Yet the Clinton plan, by making health-care coverage universal and recommending other changes, weakened some of the primary inducements unions could offer to potential new members. The unions opposed any changes in the tax laws that shielded the most comprehensive and most expensive packages, and they argued against provisions that would allow employers to increase the premium contribution required of employees. In the end, unions were reluctant to support the plan, especially after voicing concern that Mr. Clinton was drifting away from his natural allies on this issue by conceding far too much to big business (Pear, 1994). The public, too, eventually became disenchanted with Clinton's plan, despite their strong desire for health-care reform. A Princeton Survey Research/Newsweek poll, for example, demonstrated that more than three-quarters of Americans feared that, were it to be passed, a health-care bill like Clinton's would increase their taxes while decreasing the amount of choice they would have over treating physicians and hospitals. The same poll revealed that nearly 60% of respondents were convinced that quality of care would diminish were a health-care bill to be passed (Trafford, 1994).

Additionally, senior citizens covered by Medicare, the segment of the population most concerned with health-care issues, were narrowly focused on protecting Medicare and minimizing premiums and co-payments. For them, universal coverage of the rest of the population was not a high priority, and the American Association of Retired Persons never endorsed the plan. As for poor and low-income Americans, those on Medicaid were covered fairly well under a fee-for-service system. They were never mobilized in support of this plan. Finally, there were those with good coverage—professionals and employees working for large corporate employers or for the government—who were concerned about escalating costs but reluctant to support changes that undermined what they already had.

That more than 50% of the American people supported the Clinton health-care plan was testimony to the desire for change and worries about the future. When Clinton unveiled his plan in September 1993, 59% supported the initiative, a figure well below the 67% supporting fundamental change, but still impressive. The specifics of the plan were late in coming, though, and support fell to 52% by the end of the year. Support of the plan rose to 57% when the president again took his case to the American people but fell thereafter. Support sank finally to 43% in April, where it stood at the time of the plan's death in August (Skocpol, 1996, 75). In a sense, 43% is a notable number given the lack of consensus and the rocky political process, but the health-care system was not to be changed without much broader support for the proposed changes.

The early Clinton presidency was one of those rare periods in American history when health issues moved into the public realm and when the public's views mattered to politicians and policy makers. The political collapse of the plan and the defeat of the Democratic candidates for Congress in 1994 drove politicians and political entrepreneurs away from the issue. In the next Congress, health care, except in its narrowest form, was off the public agenda. Politicians slinked away. There was nothing worse in this period than to be accused of having supported "Clinton's government takeover of the health-care system" (Trafford, 1994). In 1994 Harris Wofford lost his seat in the United States Senate, making it clear that this issue had lost its political imprimatur (Clymer, 1994).

The public itself had not walked away from the health-care issue, however. The voting public was upset with the course of health-care reform but was not finished with its desire to change the system. Public opinion surveys for the White House in 1995 showed that voters remained upset about their health care and presumed the health-care debate would continue. Younger women without college degrees had been the biggest supporters of the Clinton plan and the most disappointed with its defeat. According to post-election polls, they were the group most likely to have dropped out of the electorate as a result (Greenberg, 1994, 7). Even after the 1994 election, they expected the debate to begin again, but by then the politicians were gone. Health care was no longer the clear public issue that would attract ambitious political entrepreneurs.

THE INFLUENCE OF PUBLIC OPINION ON POLICY

In the end, the public's reticence about publicly addressing health-care issues and cautiousness about government involvement in health-care allowed interest groups to gain the upper hand in the outcome of the Clinton reform effort. What does this tell us about the influence of public opinion on policy making?

Jacobs gives some helpful insights (Jacobs, 1994). He argues, as we have, that the American public is extremely unsure of government involvement in health care, supportive of universal health insurance, but reluctant to expand government involvement. He argues, however, that while the public is ambivalent, its opinions are generally enduring. Indeed, studying trends in public opinion over a 50-year period, Page and Shapiro suggest that Americans' preferences are stable, shifting only in response to changing information and circumstances (Page, 1992). Public views are less well-informed and less constant only when rapid changes in circumstance lead to misinformation and misunderstanding. Jacobs considers the general long-term tendency of public opinion to be stable as crucial for its capacity to influence policy because it makes public opinion a reliable element in the policy-making process (Jacobs, 1994, 384).

The fact that political candidates and officials now survey the public in order to gain electoral and institutional advantage gives public opinion more influence in policy making. As Jacobs writes, "While the strategic importance of the public's policy preferences to a candidate are mitigated by voters' reliance on political party labels and candidate image, politicians remain sensitive toward highly salient, well-supported issues. They calculate that popular issues may attract independent voters" (Jacobs, 1994, 385).

To what extent does public opinion hold sway in influencing policy? Jacobs suggests that unequivocal, sustained public preferences can contribute to agenda setting—the process by which an issue moves from the margins of policy discussion to its mainstream, where executive and legislative branches assign it a high priority. If, however, public sentiment is ambivalent, interest groups' influence will overwhelm the input of public opinion and push the issue out of the public's political realm.

In assessing the influence of public opinion on policy it is important to acknowledge that public opinion is itself created and given form. The growing use and sophistication in survey techniques have been paralleled by the development of increasingly sophisticated media techniques for advertising and shaping public opinion. In the political world, where campaign spending by candidates and independent committees has risen tremendously, public opinion becomes distorted. It is consequently unclear whether polling will fare better with new technologies or whether its role will be reduced to merely reflecting, rather than shaping, the policy process.

THE ETHICS OF POLLING

Conducting public opinion polls is a quasi-political act. This act inserts public opinion into the policy-making process. Those who sponsor, conduct, and use public opinion survey data are in a position to influence the evolution of public policy on health care, as with any publicly important issue. How to conduct the survey, whom to interview, what issues to address and how to frame them, what policy options to pose as possible solutions, and how to present them, are questions with ethical ramifications. Given the public's stake in health care, it is important to provide an accurate view of public opinion so that it can be brought to bear on public policy.

A constant tension exists between the influence of interest groups and the public at large. Opinion surveys serve as a fulcrum on which a balance must be struck between serving the specific political or policy agenda of the sponsor of a survey and seeking responses in as unbiased a manner as possible.

Selecting the focus of questions, wording questions, analyzing results, and deciding what slant to take in presenting results are a matter of discretion. Polling experts have a responsibility to present results that are not distorted by reporting partial findings. Valid interpretation of the conclusions necessitates avoiding over-generalization or over-interpretation of the results. Reporting of results should include explicit acknowledgement of the survey sponsor.

CONCLUSION

We have suggested in this chapter that public opinion surveys can serve to bring public opinion to the table when health policy changes are in the making. The capacity of public opinion to influence policy is limited when public sentiment is ambivalent and interest groups are powerful but can be more substantial when opinion is strong. In endorsing a prominent role for public opinion in policy making, we have articulated a view that has its critics. Some would argue that attention to public opinion has reduced public leadership to an inordinate degree of adherence to public opinion, rendering leaders less effective. We would suggest that this view confounds two issues—the value of culling public opinion and the proper use that leaders ought to make of this information. We believe that the ascertainment of public opinion, when done in a way that presents views accurately, is always valuable. The manner in which public leaders respond to public opinion, on the other hand, is a matter of discretion that should be judged on its own merits.

REFERENCES

Clinton B and Gore A (1992) *Putting People First.* New York: Times Books.

Clymer A (1994) The 1994 campaign: Health care. *New York Times* October 22, 1994, A1.

Democracy Corps (1999) National Surveys of the American Public. Sept., 1999.

Democracy Corps (2000) National Surveys of the American Public. March, 2000.

Donelan K, Blendon RJ, Schoen C, Davis K, and Binnis K (1999) The cost of health system change: Public discontent in five nations. *Health Affairs* 18:3.

Gallup Organization (1998) Gallup Poll, C.N.N., U.S.A. Today Poll. Reprinted on *Public Opinion Online*. Roper Center at University of Connecticut. Available at http://roperweb.ropercenter.uconn.edu.

Greenberg, SB (1994) The revolt against politics. In: Greenberg SB (ed) *The Third Force. Why Independents Turned Against Democrats—and How to Win them Back.* Washington, DC: Democratic Leadership Council.

Hart and Teeter Research Associates (1998) NBC News, Wall Street Journal Poll. Reprinted on *Public Opinion Online*. Roper Center at University of Connecticut, Accn #0303617. Available at http://roperweb.ropercenter.uconn.edu.

Jacobs, LR (1993) *The Health of Nations. Public Opinion and the Making of American and British Health Policy*. Ithaca, NY: Cornell University Press.

Jacobs LR (1994) The politics of American ambivalence toward government. In :Morone JA and Belkin GS (eds) *The Politics of Health Care Reform*. Durham, NC: Duke University Press.

Johnson D (2000) Abortion foes in Nebraska take spotlight. *New York Times* January 23, 2000, A14.

Lewis M (2000) The two-bucks-a-minute democracy. *New York Times Magazine* November 5, 2000, 64–7.

Lippmann W (1997) *Public Opinion*. New York: Free Press.

Matthews C (2001) Committed crusaders. *Washington Times* February 11, 2001, B3.

Muravchik J (2000) Socialists of America disunited; Why the revolution never happened here. *The Weekly Standard* September 4, 2000, 40.

Page B and Shapiro R (1992) *The Rational Public*. Chicago: University of Chicago Press.

Pear R (1994) Business groups and labor unions attack Clinton on health plan. *New York Times* February 4, 1994, A19.

Princeton Survey Research Associates (1998) Princeton Survey Research Associates, Newsweek poll. Reprinted on *Public Opinion Online*. Roper Center at University of Connecticut. Available at http://roperweb.ropercenter.uconn.edu.

Princeton Survey Research Associates (1998) Kaiser, Harvard Medicare Policy Options Survey. Reprinted on *Public Opinion Online*. Roper Center at University of Connecticut. Available at http://roperweb.ropercenter.uconn.edu.

Purdy J (2000) *For Common Things*. New York: Vintage Books.

Q.W. Ayres and Associates (1998) Post-Election Health Care Issues Survey. Reprinted on *Public Opinion Online*. Roper Center at University of Connecticut. Available at http://roperweb.ropercenter.uconn.edu.

Skocpol T (1995) *Social Policy in the United States: Future Possibilities in Historical Perspective*. Princeton, NJ: Princeton University Press.

Skocpol T (1996) *Boomerang: Clinton's Health Security Effort and the Turn against Government in U.S. Politics*. New York: W.W. Norton and Company.

Trafford A (1994) A collective case of compassion fatigue? *Washington Post* October 11, 1994, Z6.

Trafford A (1994) What went wrong? How wonks and pols—and you—fumbled universal health care. *Washington Post* August 21, 1994, C1.

Troy G (1996) *See How They Ran: The Changing Role of the Presidential Candidate*. Cambridge, MA: Harvard University Press

Weisberger BA (2000) Taking America's temperature. *American Heritage* November 2000, 58–61.

Weisberger BA (2000) *America Afire: Jefferson, Adams, and The Revolutionary Election*. New York: William and Morrow.

Wolfe A (2000) Sects in the city. *The New Republic* April 3, 2000, 34.

8

Medical ethics in the courts

M. GREGG BLOCHE

Judges are America's health policy makers of last resort. Ambiguous statutes and contract terms, legal challenges to administrative decisions, and gridlock in Congress and state legislatures give courts a large role by default in the governance of health-care provision. Judges with cursory understandings of the ethics and economics of medical care define the environment within which market forces operate. In so doing, courts answer questions of distributive justice, disclosure and consent, and professional duty that are staples of medical ethics discussion. The managed care revolution has deepened judges' engagement in matters at the heart of medical ethics discourse about the doctor–patient relationship and the role of the market. Health plans routinely seek to manage costs by influencing physicians' clinical judgments and recommendations. Financial rewards for limiting care, prior authorization requirements, clinical practice protocols, and practice profiling aimed at identifying (and discouraging) high-cost providers are among the methods that spark legal conflict concerning the governance of doctor–patient relations and the appropriate scope of the market paradigm.

Clinical practitioners are inclined to look to ethics as much as to law to understand their professional obligations (Capron, 1999), and, increasingly, medical ethics commentators are speaking to these controversies. Ambiguities in statutory and contract terms often leave room for courts to take interpretive guidance from medical ethics principles and scholarship. To the extent that the law reinforces prevailing ethical understandings, clinicians and consumers do not face the confusion of mixed messages. However, when legal outcomes diverge from widely held ethical beliefs, conflicting messages confound practitioners, patients, and clinical institutions.

Such divergence not only sows doubt about what constitutes proper conduct; it invites skepticism about the legitimacy of both the law's outcomes and medical ethics reasoning. To be sure, such skepticism is sometimes justified. Courts may at times disregard ethics reasoning that would yield large social benefits if incorporated into the law. Conversely, professional and other groups can employ ethical norms to stifle competition, furthering their parochial interests at society's expense. Yet much is lost when both law and ethics lose their aura of legitimacy as sources of guidance concerning right conduct. People's internalization of legal and ethical obligations (Tyler, 1990) and their affirmation of these obligations to one another through imposition of reputational costs upon violators (Kahan, 1996) play large roles in empowering a society's members to resist their baser inclinations in the interest of the common good. A culture in which nihilism concerning the virtues of legal and ethical norms prevails forgoes these psychological mechanisms for containing self-aggrandizement.

This chapter considers the courts' responsiveness to medical ethics reasoning in the cases that have shaped the American system of health-care provision. I begin with a generalization sure to dismay some readers of this book: Medical ethics reasoning has made only a modest mark on the law of health-care provision in the managed care era, and judicial decisions routinely depart from prevailing medical ethics understandings. Especially when cost containment methods have been at issue, neither traditional physician ethics nor the contemporary bioethics movement has had much impact on the law governing clinical caretakers' obligations to patients, payers, and other actors. I then explore the reasons for the courts' poor responsiveness to ethics arguments. These reasons include the perceived social urgency of cost control, judges' self-consciousness about their problematic institutional role in a democracy, their skepticism about links between ethical argument and economic self-interest, and the indeterminacy of medical ethics principles as regards many concrete questions.

Inchoate, often conflicting ethical understandings are, nevertheless, discernable in judicial opinions. The ideals of market-driven efficiency, regard for personal autonomy, and professional benevolence make recurring appearances in health care caselaw, not as overtly ethical arguments but as policies and values embedded in statutory schemes and common law. I briefly review the place of these ideals in courts' treatment of the health-care system, then turn to the question of what a more self-conscious judicial reliance upon ethical reasoning might contribute to the law of health-care provision. My answer to this question is avowedly pragmatic. From an opinion-writing judge's perspective, I contend, the distinctive power of ethical arguments lies in their moral authority—and in the consequent legitimacy they can lend to social concerns not adequately supported, in politics or the marketplace, by private actors' self-regarding behavior. By presenting arguments as *ethical*, we proffer them as public-regarding, as claims that transcend private interest and therefore merit heightened deference.

This advantage of ethics as rhetoric carries at least two downside risks. First, deference to ethics reasoning fits uneasily with judicial efforts to resolve social controversies by reference to politically expressed preferences embodied in statutes and constitutional text. Judicial authority in a democracy rests on reason giving that displays fealty to these formal expressions of the popular will. Overt reliance upon ethics arguments and commentary weakens the nexus between judges' conclusions and expressed popular will. Second, when ethical claims are exposed (or cast) as cover for private aggrandizement,[1] their distinctive moral force is lost. Courts' reluctance to rely upon medical ethics reasoning reflects judges' sensitivity to these downside risks. I argue herein that this sensitivity is overgeneralized. These risks are real but selective, and greater receptivity to ethical norms can make the law of health-care provision both more humane and more efficient.

THE LEGAL IMPACT OF ETHICAL NORMS

Contemporary medical ethics draws from two principal sources—the professional ethics tradition epitomized by the Hippocratic Oath and its reliance on physician benevolence (Veatch, 2000) and the late-20th-century bioethics movement, which places paramount value on patient autonomy (Faden and Beauchamp, 1986; Rothman, 1992). These sources give rise to a wide range of norms that bear upon the organization, financing, and provision of health care, including professional conduct within the doctor–patient relationship. These norms direct physicians to safeguard their patients' autonomy and privacy, avoid conflicts of interest, maintain clinical competence and quality, and put their patients' welfare ahead of the needs of health-care payers and other third parties. Although medical ethics norms are classically aimed at physicians, they imply that health-care institutions have corresponding obligations to patients. More controversially, medical ethics calls upon individual clinicians and medical institutions to ameliorate the health effects of socioeconomic inequity (Beauchamp and Childress, 2001).

To what extent do courts draw upon these ethical norms when confronting legal disputes engendered by the new medical marketplace? In the cases that have most influenced the law of health-care provision, evidence of such reliance is slight. To be sure, courts have at times proven responsive to ethical norms (e.g., proscription of physician-assisted suicide) that reflect the larger society's mores and limit what physicians and patients can choose to do together.[2] But there is little evidence that either traditional professional ethics or contemporary bioethics thinking have heavily influenced judicial decisions concerning health-care organization, financing, and provision. To the contrary, professional ethics thinking about the responsibilities of physicians and clinical institutions has been a focus of deepening judicial skepticism in recent decades. The bioethics movement's emphasis on patient autonomy, by contrast, has paralleled the courts' sharpened focus, since the 1960s, on protecting health-care consumers' rights to make informed choices. But whether these coinciding trends result from bioethics theory's influence on the law or some common, underlying cause is difficult to discern. Moreover, even if the courts' endorsement of informed consent in the 1960s and 1970s should properly be credited to the bioethics movement, the law's subsequent support for the paradigm of consumer choice within a competitive medical marketplace cannot plausibly be attributed to bioethics thinking.

Professional Ethics

Fifty years ago the medical profession stood at a pinnacle of influence over the law of health-care provision. The profession's ethical proscriptions against advertising and corporate authority over clinical decision making were honored by courts, legislators, and licensing bodies. Its norms concerning disclosure of diagnostic information and therapeutic alternatives defined clinicians' legal responsibilities to share knowledge and decision-making authority with patients. Challenges by health insurers to physician judgment were both ethically beyond the pale and utterly without legal basis. The law's deference to physicians' ethical understandings was of a piece with the prevailing view in society at midcentury that the profession's altruism and expertise entitled it to sovereignty in clinical and ethical matters (Starr, 1982; Parsons, 1951). But beginning in the 1960s, courts became more skeptical of the medical profession's account of its ethical obligations and prerogatives. The ban on advertising, once seen as expressive of a morality higher than that of the marketplace, was recast in opposite terms, as self-protective collusion proscribed by the antitrust laws (*AMA v. FTC*, 1980). The rule against the so-called corporate practice of medicine, which enshrined the profession's objections to bureaucratic constraints on clinical discretion, fell by the wayside (Freiman, 1998) as doubts grew about the altruism and expertise said to justify this discretion.

Courts also challenged professional authority to set ethical and legal ground rules for the sharing of information and decision-making power with patients. As judicial confidence in physicians' benevolence gave way to concern about unwarranted paternalism, a series of landmark cases on informed consent in the 1960s and 1970s rolled back professional discretion to withhold diagnoses, prognoses, and information about therapeutic alternatives.[3] And, since the late 1970s, courts have given health insurers increasing license to put contractual limits on treating physicians' power to determine clinical need.[4] Even the initiation and termination of the physician–patient relationship has become less a matter of professional norms. The physician's freedom "to choose whom to serve," enshrined for nearly nine decades in successive AMA ethical codes,[5] has been trimmed by federal and state statutes, regulations, and court decisions that condition public funding on free care to the poor (EMTALA, 2001; *Baber v. Hospital Corporation of America*, 1992) and compel continued treatment after insured patients have exhausted their coverage (*In the Matter of Baby "K,"* 1994).

Even the core Hippocratic premise of undivided physician loyalty to patients and commitment to their welfare has received surprisingly little judicial deference. Courts have refrained from recognizing a professional duty of fidelity to patients, as distinct from physicians' obligation, under tort law, to provide care of adequate quality (*Neade v. Portes*, 2000), and they have eschewed ethicists' calls for the creation of a new professional duty to advocate for patients when health plans deny coverage for care that physicians deem necessary (*Pryzbowksi v. U.S. Healthcare*, 2001). In *Pegram v. Herdrich* (2000), a unanimous U.S. Supreme Court overturned a lower court holding that the federal law governing employer-provided medical insurance limited health plans' use of monetary enticements to physicians to withhold costly treatments. In upholding such enticements as consistent with federal law and as necessary tools for health-care rationing, the justices rejected pleas from ethicists and others to give effect to the ethic of undivided loyalty to patients by construing the statute at issue to limit these enticements (Brief of Health Law, Policy, and Ethics Scholars, 1999).

In 2001 the Supreme Court drew on constitutional arguments concerning privacy but ignored the ethics of divided professional loyalty in striking down a state hospital policy requiring physicians to tell criminal prosecutors about illicit drug use by pregnant women (*Ferguson v. City of Charleston*, 2001). Concerning patient confidentiality more generally, courts have been less than vigorous about either requiring or empowering health-care providers to protect it. They have rarely subjected physicians to liability for its breach, and the doctor–patient privilege (the protection courts afford physicians against use of legal process to compel breach of confidentiality) is laden with exceptions that force physicians to break faith with patients to serve the interests of the state and other third parties (Slovenko, 1998).

Bioethics

The erosion of professional ethics' influence over the law of health-care provision coincided with the advent of bioethics as both an academic field and a program for reform. The bioethics movement's greatest apparent influence upon the law governing physician–patient relations has been in the area of informed consent. Prior to the 1960s, the notion of an obligation to obtain a patient's informed consent to clinical interventions had no place in American law. To be sure, the law of battery required doctors to obtain consent, absent emergency, to surgery and other invasive procedures (*Bang v. Charles T. Miller Hospital*, 1958; *Mohr v. Williams*, 1905), but disclosure and discussion of clinical risks and benefits was not legally required and was, in practice, a matter for physician discretion. The disclosure obligations set out by the Nuremberg Tribunal in the 1947 Nuremberg Code (Trials Of War Criminals Before The Nuremberg Military Tribunals Under Control Council Law No 10, 1949), which governed medical research on human subjects, introduced the idea of *informed* consent into international law at a time when neither U.S. law nor prevailing clinical practice norms called for doctor–patient conversation about risks and benefits.[6]

American courts were slow to adopt the informed consent paradigm. In the early 1960s only a few jurisdictions required informed consent (Faden and Beauchamp, 1986), and these deferred to professional standards of disclosure (at a time when *nondisclosure* was often the prevailing professional standard). Only in the 1970s did informed consent sweep the field, with many jurisdictions—but not a majority—rejecting deference to professional standards of disclosure in favor of the requirement that physicians reveal all risks and benefits that a "reasonable" lay person would find "material" to the consent decision (*Canterbury v. Spence*, 1972; Schultz, 1985). During the same period (the 1960s and 1970s), the contemporary bioethics movement emerged, challenging the professional ethics tradition with a proliferation of commentary, rooted in analytic philosophy, on patient autonomy and the requisites for informed consent (Rothman, 1992).

To what extent did this new bioethics movement spur the courts to adopt the informed consent paradigm? Citations to bioethics literature in the judicial opinions that imposed informed consent requirements were rare. These opinions typically made the case for informed consent in the language of *legal* rights and duties. By itself, this proves little about the legal influence of bioethics thinking. The bioethics movement's emphasis on patient autonomy could have shaped judicial understandings of legal rights and duties without appearing in judicial opinions in the form of citations to scholarly literature. Indeed, the judicial preference for presenting legal innovation in conservative terms, as the product of established principles applied to new circumstances, could have discouraged overt reliance on the new bioethics scholarship. Thorough assessment of this scholarship's influence on the path-breaking informed consent decisions of the 1960s and 1970s must await comprehensive review of briefs and other lawyerly advocacy documents submitted to the courts, as well as, perhaps, interviews with a representative sample of judges and lawyers in these cases.[7] But the absence of an overt bioethics presence in judicial opinions, coupled with the fact that informed consent jurisprudence emerged in parallel with the bioethics movement rather than afterwards, suggests that the causal connection between the bioethics emphasis on autonomy and the courts' embrace of informed consent is weak.

Indeed, to some degree, causality may have gone the other way. Bioethics scholarship in the 1970s and 1980s was often critical of judge-crafted informed consent doctrine on the ground that it failed to fulfill hopes for robust protection for patient autonomy. Bioethics commentators criticized some courts' deference to professional standards of disclosure and others' reliance on the "reasonable person" standard (Katz, 1977), both of which they said failed to take seriously the varied fears and wishes of actual patients. The emerging law of informed consent may thereby have contributed to the sharpening of the bioethics movement's autonomy-based critique of clinical (and judicial) practice. At a minimum, it is clear that the courts did not push informed consent doctrine as far as many bioethics commentators hoped, toward deference to individual patients' feelings, values, and preferences.

More probably, the emergence of autonomy-centered bioethics and the legal doctrine of informed consent are traceable to common origins. The post–World War II rights revolution, in large measure a reaction to Nazi and Stalinist contempt for the individual, swept broadly through international (Henkin, 1990) and U.S. law (Dudziak, 2000), political theory, and applied ethics, including the ethics of the professions. The paternalism inherent in traditional medical ethics and sociological thinking (Parsons, 1951) about patient ignorance and dependence and professional benevolence was cast into doubt by the rights revolution generally, by accounts of Nazi medical atrocities, and, later, by American researchers' exploitation of unwitting clinical subjects. Judges and medical ethics commentators reacted along parallel lines, by moving personal autonomy to center stage in the governance of medicine.

Both as doctrine and as Zeitgeist, the paradigm of informed consent spread from the bedside throughout the health-care sphere in the 1980s and 1990s. Consent, variously obtained, became the legal basis for forensic use of clinical findings; disclosure of personal health information to insurers, employers, and even marketers (Bloche, 1997); and use of human tissue for commercial purposes (*Moore v. Regents of University of California*, 1990). Courts invoked consumer consent as justification for managed health plans' utilization control procedures (*Sarchett v. Blue Shield of California*, 1987), limits on choice of providers (*Ward v. Alternative Health Delivery Sys.*, 2000), and financial rewards to physicians for frugal practice (*Shea v. Esensten*, 2000). But judges framed their arguments for reliance upon consent in contract law and statutory terms, eschewing overt dependence upon ethics rationale. Contract law's acceptance of market outcomes despite large inequalities in resources and bargaining power made contract doctrine a potent means for extending the consent paradigm to cover health plans' utilization management, provider selection, physician payment, and health information privacy practices, so long as plan–subscriber agreements contained at least cursory descriptions of these practices.

WHY MEDICAL ETHICS HAS HAD SO LITTLE WEIGHT

Why have courts given such short shrift to medical ethics considerations when addressing the law of health-care provision? Judicial sensitivity to the self-serving potential of traditional physician ethics has been a major factor, as has judges' concern about the paternalistic implications of reliance upon Hippocratic benevolence. Until a quarter century ago, the law treated physicians' self-imposed bans on advertising and price competition as socially desirable safeguards against professional self-aggrandizement and exploitation of patients' medical ignorance. But the antitrust revolution in medicine recast these restrictions as self-serving restraints on trade, supportive of physicians' incomes and status at consumers' expense.

The sense that professional norms ostensibly protective of patients in fact serve physician self-interest became more generalized in the 1980s and 1990s, spreading beyond bans on advertising and price competition to encompass protections for physician autonomy. The growing influence of the law-and-economics movement on judicial thinking over the past few decades fed this skepticism. Judges inclined toward the economist's preference for market ordering looked askance at constraints on the contractual redesign of health-care provision. Market-oriented health law commentators lent support to courts' skepticism about professional ethics in articles that presented legal safeguards for physician self-governance as barriers to clinical efficiency (Hall, 1988). Public choice theorists portrayed the law's adoption of rules favored by particular groups as use of state power to advance parochial interests at society's expense. Since the early 1990s, a new school of law-and-economics commentators has argued that social groups (including professions) commit to ethical norms out of collective self-interest (Bloche, forthcoming). Physicians' self-serving behavior as entrepreneurs (Bloche, 1998) and their self-interested public advocacy concerning economic matters (Sharfstein, 1994) heightened judicial, scholarly, and popular skepticism about the profession's conception of its ethics.

Judicial dismay over the paternalism inherent in traditional physician ethics contributed to the courts' skepticism. In an age of rights, the Hippocratic tradition's emphasis on doctors' benevolence and benign intentions (Veatch, 2000) seemed, at best, quaint and, at worst, antagonistic to personal autonomy. Hippocratic ethics asks doctors to be virtuous and patients to reciprocate with trust. This moral transaction is of a piece with the classic understanding of the "sick role" as calling for patient passivity and unquestioning faith in physician judgment (Parsons, 1951; Bloche, 1996), but it is at odds with the post–World War II rights revolution's insistence on regard for personal autonomy. The rights consciousness that crystalized in response to the war's atrocities, deepened with the civil rights movements' successes and spread to most areas of American life in the 1960s and 1970s, fits better with an account of doctor–patient relations that relies less on physician virtue and more on sick people's participation in clinical decision making.

Revelations in the 1960s and 1970s that American physician–researchers breached their patients' trust by putting them at unknowing risk for their lives in medical experiments (Rothman, 1992) cast further doubt on the Hippocratic paradigm of professional benevolence. Reports, since the 1970s, documenting wide variations in medical practice patterns and weak empirical support for many clinical practices fueled rising skepticism about the soundness of even well-intentioned professional judgment. Clinical outcomes research, centralized management of medical decision making through implementation of evidence-based practice protocols, and use of new information technologies to empower health-care consumers emerged as attractive alternatives to protection for independent physician judgment.

These challenges to the relevance of the Hippocratic ethical tradition point to an opening for bioethics reasoning in the courts. The fit between law's individual rights consciousness and the bioethics movement's emphasis on patient autonomy has produced some synergy, most notably in the areas of informed consent and end-of-life decision making. Leading court decisions in these areas have drawn upon bioethics scholarship,[8] and bioethics commentators have sought to influence judicial constructions of constitutional (Dworkin, 1997) and statutory (Brief of Health Law, Policy, and Ethics Scholars, 1999) provisions bearing on medical care. But the law has not embraced the robust conceptions of individual autonomy at the bedside championed by many bioethicists. The law's separate institutional concerns—about reliability and accuracy in fact finding, consistency in constitutional and statutory interpretation (Dworkin, 1986), efficiency in decision making, and relationships between branches and levels of government—have pushed judges to discount many bioethics arguments.

In matters of informed consent, for example, the bioethics ideal of deference to individuals' varying, idiosyncratic values and preferences (Katz, 1984) has been compromised by courts concerned about the difficulty of discerning a person's authentic preferences after the fact, during litigation, when she has powerful motives to say whatever it takes to win. Most jurisdictions define doctors' obligations to reveal risks and benefits in terms of what a "reasonable physician" would tell patients. Although this standard leaves ample room for courtroom disagreement, it cabins this space (and protects the integrity of the legal process) by limiting the scope of inquiry to the range of disclosure practices extant in the medical profession. Those jurisdictions that define disclosure obligations in terms of what *patients* might want to know before giving (or withholding) consent pursue a similar containment strategy by limiting the disclosure duty in objective terms, to those risks and benefits that a "reasonable patient" would find "material" to her consent decision. Judicial concerns about both accuracy and efficiency in legal decision making favor this containment strategy despite its plain disregard for individual variation in health-care preferences.

In its end-of-life decision-making cases, the U.S. Supreme Court confronted questions of constitutional interpretation involving both federalism concerns and the Court's jurisprudence of individual rights beyond the health sphere, in addition to questions about substituted decision making and personal autonomy that animate bioethics debate. In *Cruzan v. Missouri Dept. of Health* (1990), the Court needed to locate its consideration of an asserted right to withdrawal of life-sustaining treatment within the larger context of its Due Process Clause jurisprudence concerning the balance between individuals' liberty interests and relevant state interests. The Court also was compelled by governing principles of federalism to defer to a state supreme court's construction of state law. Missouri's high court had required "clear and convincing evidence" of a mentally incompetent person's wishes, while competent, concerning treatment withdrawal. To be sure, as the *Cruzan* dissent evinces, the legal framework left room for different views about whether the state's "clear and convincing evidence" standard passed muster under the *federal* constitution—i.e., whether was supported by a state interest (in preserving life) sufficient to outweigh liberty interests that might support a lesser standard of proof. But the imperative of interpretive integrity—of "fit" with prior Due Process Clause jurisprudence (mostly involving cases outside the health sphere)—pushed the justices to argue for their conclusions in terms that permitted room for bioethics values but put bioethics theory on the periphery. Had the justices not done so, had they instead stated their cases in pure bioethics terms, they would have been vulnerable to the charge that they had acted without legitimacy by failing to root their reasoning in the principles of our constitutional democracy.

The law's separate institutional concerns also shape courts' approaches to their expanding load of cases arising from disputes over the contractual and regulatory governance of managed care. Efforts to extend the paradigm of disclosure and consent beyond the bedside to the realm of health-care organization and financing have been hindered by a federal statute, the Employee Retirement Income Security Act (ERISA), that shields the administration of employer-provided health plans from most state law. Bioethics commentators have urged robust disclosure requirements, covering financial incentives to physicians to withhold care, the cost–benefit tradeoff policies that underlie plans' "medical necessity" determinations, limits on provider choice, and measures of health-care quality and consumer satisfaction. But ERISA tightly restrains judges' hands. ERISA imposes few federal obligations on health plans, giving courts little legal basis for the crafting of disclosure duties aimed at bringing the paradigm of informed consent to health-care administration and financing.[9] Were a court to invoke bioethics scholarship, without statutory grounding, as its justification for introducing new disclosure duties, it would invite charges of illegitimacy due to the disconnect between these duties and Congress's expressed will. And were a court to draw upon bioethics commentary as a basis for attaching new disclosure duties to some vague clause in ERISA with applications beyond the health sphere, the court would risk interpretive inconsistency between this clause's meanings within and outside the health sphere.

A further difficulty with judicial application of the consent paradigm to health-care organization and financing is intrinsic to the concepts of autonomy and consent. Proponents of extending the consent paradigm to health plans' administrative and financial practices have urged competing sets of disclosure obligations and taken different approaches to defining the minimum range of medical coverage options that must be available to subscribers to offer an adequate set of choices. Specification of prerequisites for informed consent to a health plan's practices—or to anything else—requires moral judgments about the circumstances necessary for autonomous choice. These circumstances include the information the chooser has at her disposal, her resources and options, and the consequences attached to these options. Arguments over whether autonomous consent has been given reflect underlying disagreements about the morality of the circumstances of choice. Informed consent, in other words, is a plastic concept, dependent for its normative content upon answers to these underlying questions (Bloche, 1996).

At the bedside bioethics provides content to the informed consent requirement through consensus resolutions of some of these underlying questions and limits on debate about others. By consensus, bioethics treats all *medical* circumstances (e.g. pathophysiology and prognosis), however ominous, as morally *acceptable* constraints or pressures on choice. Thus, for example, a patient with a mouth tumor for whom disfiguring facial surgery offers the only prospect of survival can, consistent with bioethics thinking, give autonomous consent to surgery so long as her physician's disclosure of risks, benefits (a chance of averting death), and alternatives (none) passes muster. The intense pressure on her decision (certainty of death without surgery) is of no moral import or, at least, not enough import to qualify as "coercive" from a bioethics perspective. Similarly, conventional bioethics thinking treats a patient's financial circumstances as irrelevant to her ability to give adequate consent to treatment, however much these circumstances might narrow her range of alternatives. Bioethics commentators differ, to be sure, over the nature of bedside disclosure duties: Some urge that disclosure be custom-fitted to each patient's subjective thinking about which risks and benefits might be material to her consent decision (Katz, 1984), while others tolerate more generic disclosure requirements out of regard for administrative efficacy (Faden and Beauchamp, 1986). But the materiality of risks and benefits to the patient's decision is a common touchstone, narrowing bioethics debate over disclosure duties to the question of how much space they should allow for individuals' subjectivity and idiosyncracy.

In the realm of health-care organization and financing, by contrast, ethicists (and society in general) are nowhere near to agreement on the underlying moral questions that must be answered to specify the prerequisites for autonomous consumer consent. Bioethics and health policy commentators have put forward competing ideas about what health plans should tell prospective subscribers about their restrictions on choice of treatments and providers (Daniels, 1998), financial incentives to physicians (Rodwin, 1993), cost–benefit tradeoff policies (Havighurst, 1995), and performance on indices of clinical quality and consumer satisfaction. Commentators have also differed over whether health plan bureaucrats, physicians, or others should make these disclosures and over the minimum range of coverage options (and economic resources) that must be available to prospective subscribers to create morally acceptable conditions for choice. Animating these differences are competing moral views about such core matters as the roles of efficiency and market exchange in medicine, the place of patient trust, the relative import of emotional support and biological efficacy, and the extent to which health-care financing should abate society's larger distributive inequities.

Without consensus, or at least a cabining of disagreement, on these underlying matters, the paradigm of informed consent cannot provide governing rules for the managed care industry's administrative and financial practices. The paradigm's plasticity makes it adaptable to a wide range of legal governance purposes, and its affirmation of individuals' responsibility and dignity makes it appealing within our legal culture. It appeals also because legal focus on the adequacy of disclosure averts our gaze from moral judgments—and painful compromises among deeply felt values—that undergird its application. But it cannot guide the law absent these moral judgments. Its plasticity makes it of little use to judges who confront the task of crafting a legal governance scheme for managed care, since neither the bioethics movement nor American society has resolved the poignant, often bitter moral questions that such a governance scheme must mediate.

THE INCHOATE ETHICS OF HEALTH-CARE LAW

Although American health law has not self-consciously embraced any ethical paradigm as its conceptual basis, inchoate ethical understandings inform the courts' treatment of health-care disputes. Because courts submerge these understandings beneath their discussions of legal doctrine and legislative policy, the law's patchwork of ethics models defies easy portrayal. These understandings, moreover, are at war with each other across a broad range of health policy controversies. Analytic confusion, even chaos, results from the law's ad hoc mixing of these models. The ethics models that tacitly inform health-care law can be grouped into three categories for discussion purposes—professional duty and prerogative, personal rights, and market exchange. These categories overlap: Economists of a Chicagoan bent root their commitment to markets in a robust conception of personal liberty (Freedman, 1962), and Kenneth Arrow and others have analyzed physician prerogative and Hippocratic obligation as a market-driven response to consumer need (Arrow, 1963; Bloche, 2001). But they capture three core themes that judges must often choose among. Inconsistency in these choices accounts for much of the conceptual disarray that besets health law.

Professional Duty and Prerogative

More than many proponents of the minimally regulated marketplace would prefer (Havighurst, forthcoming), the Hippocratic paradigm of professional duty and prerogative persists in the law. In medical malpractice cases, courts continue to look to professionally set standards of care as touchstones for liability. Except in rare cases of egregious, obvious wrongdoing, malpractice plaintiffs must produce expert medical testimony to get their cases to a jury. By eschewing calls from some for a shift in the doctrinal ground for medical malpractice claims from tort to contract (Epstein, 1976), courts have, in effect, barred health-care providers and plans from adopting standards of care below those widely adhered to by physicians. As mentioned earlier, most jurisdictions also defer to physician-set standards for disclosure in informed consent cases. Independent review of health plans' medical coverage decisions typically relies upon professional standards, at the courts' insistence (*Bauman v. U.S. Healthcare, Inc.*, 1999), despite managed care industry efforts to persuade judges and legislators to require that independent review defer to contractual definitions of medical necessity. Even in the antitrust law arena, where the market paradigm has made the most inroads upon professional prerogative, the courts—most notably the U.S. Supreme Court in a 1999 decision on professional self-regulation of price advertising (*California Dental Ass'n v. FTC*, 1999)—have created doctrinal space for arguments that collaborative ethical and clinical standard-setting by physicians can advance consumer welfare. Undergirding this continuing deference to physician prerogative is the persisting belief that the profession's ethical commitments to patients often better protect them than do the market and regulatory pressures to which other industries are more vigorously subjected.

Personal Rights

That the rights revolution has recast the law of health-care provision since the 1960s is evident to the most casual observer. Whether understood in utilitarian terms or as Kantian recognition of human dignity and capacity, respect for each person's right of self-determination has become the basis for an array of constraints on professional and institutional prerogative. As discussed earlier, the paradigm of informed consent has spread beyond the bedside to the financing and ordering of our health-care system. But the plasticity of the consent paradigm renders it a vessel for myriad, sub rosa normative premises. These competing premises—concerning matters of distributive fairness, efficiency, the merits of professional authority, and the place of individuals' subjectivity and idiosyncracy—shape judgments about the sufficiency of disclosures and about the adequacy of choices that consumers confront.

By submerging these competing premises beneath a doctrinal formulation (informed consent) that avows self-determination, a near-sacred value in American political culture, we finesse the painful task of choosing among these premises; instead, we argue in court over the surface question of whether valid consent was given. But this procedural finesse has a crucial limitation. It works by distracting us from our core, substantive disagreements, not by resolving them. It is thus ever at risk of being subverted by the seepage of these disagreements into our discussions of the prerequisites for valid consent (Bloche, 1997). Beyond this, it leaves the normative basis for legal governance ill-defined.

Market Exchange

The expanding role of market exchange has been one of the central storylines in health law since the 1980s. The market paradigm, and its undergirding ethic of efficiency grounded in expressed preferences, now reaches beyond the antitrust realm. Most notably, courts have treated ERISA, the federal statute governing the market for employment-based health insurance, as a far-reaching deregulatory scheme, one that shields health plans (and employers) from many state requirements while imposing few federal restrictions in their place (Jacobson, 1998). Although ambiguous language in ERISA left room for courts to craft a more robust regulatory approach, the U.S. Supreme Court (*Pilot Life Ins. v. Dedeaux,* 1987; *Metropolitan Life Ins. Co. v. Massachusetts,* 1985) and an array of lower courts (*Corcoran v. United Health Care,* 1992; *Jass v. Prudential Health Care Plan,* 1996) had, by the mid-90s, construed the statute to give plans and employers free rein in defining the scope of coverage and immunity from suit for denying benefits in particular cases. Language in some of these opinions explicitly embraced labor markets as the preferred way to set health benefits,[10] treating medical insurance as no different than other employee compensation.

Outside the ERISA context, courts moved more gingerly toward the market paradigm in disputes involving denial of benefits. Whereas in the 1960s and 1970s courts were inclined to accept treating physicians' assessments of medical need as binding on insurers (despite these physicians' obvious financial interest in the outcome) (*Van Vactor v. Blue Cross Association,* 1977), by the 1980s judges were deferring to insurance contract terms that allowed health plans to make their own medical necessity decisions[11] and set forth criteria for these decisions. To the dismay of some market proponents, however, courts in these cases required that such contract terms be free of ambiguity and insisted that they be construed in accordance with the "reasonable expectations of the insured." In effect, the courts thereby made deference to treating physicians' assertions of medical need the default assumption. Health plans could override this assumption only through contract language that highlighted—and clearly explained—the plan's power to decide medical need.

This approach to medical coverage disputes reflects tension in the law between the paradigms of market exchange and professional prerogative. Were courts entirely comfortable with the market approach to medical coverage, they would do what the market model's most vigorous proponents urge: They would construe coverage contracts without a presumption in favor of treating physicians' conclusions concerning medical necessity. This presumption is an awkward compromise, defended in judicial opinions by reference to off-the-shelf doctrines of insurance contract interpretation. This legal formalism obscures the core normative questions at stake, concerning the proper scope of market exchange vis a vis professional authority (and the values that professional authority serves).

Judicial discomfort with the market's operation in medical coverage matters has influenced the most recent developments on the ERISA front. Since the late 1990s, courts have been shrinking the scope of ERISA's preemption of state tort and contract law actions against health plans for denial of coverage and care. In a series of cases, courts have recast such denials as clinical judgments (*Bauman v. U.S. Healthcare, Inc.*, 1999) or mixed clinical and administrative decisions subject to state law (*Pegram v. Herdrich,* 2000), rather than administrative judgments beyond the states' reach. This recharacterization pushed back the boundaries of ERISA preemption (binding in matters of plan administration), exposing plans to state liability for withholding coverage and care. Insofar as state liability hinges upon judicial review of plans' medical necessity decisions, physician practice norms—and thus professional authority—play a central role. Thus the market paradigm's place in the legal governance of employment-based health benefits has been substantially reduced over the last several years. That this reduction coincided with popular backlash against managed care and revived confidence in professional authority as a safeguard against health plans' skimping was rarely noted in judicial opinions,[12] which largely limited themselves to doctrinal formalism disconnected from the normative matters at stake.

TOWARD A PLACE FOR ETHICS REASONING IN HEALTH LAW?

What, if anything, might be gained from making more of a place for medical ethics reasoning in the judge-made law of health-care provision? An important limitation needs to be acknowledged at the outset. Judicial legitimacy, as discussed earlier, rests on courts' sensitivity to the law's separate institutional concerns—about efficiency, interpretive consistency, and relationships between branches and levels of government. Above all, judges' moral authority is tied to their deference to public preferences as expressed through political institutions. Courts depart from these constraints at their own political peril. Ethics arguments that fit poorly within these constraints are unlikely to find their way into judge-made law.

What, then, does medical ethics have to offer to judges and the law? For starters, a distinctive feature of ethics reasoning and rhetoric is its credibility as a public-regarding exercise, in pursuit of a conception of the good that is well-insulated from base, private interests. The very feature of ethics reasoning that fits most awkwardly with democracy—its avowal of disconnection from factional interests—lends it particular cache amidst competing, self-interested legal arguments. There is a yin-yang quality to the courts' relationship to parties' and citizens' self-interest. As pieces in a democratic governance scheme, courts are constrained by the balances among parochial interests that the political branches strike. The adversary system magnifies the role of self-interest by giving litigants the first take at framing issues for decision. Yet as institutions insulated from parochial concerns and charged with the task of disinterested judgment, courts reach beyond the balance of competing interests toward a public-regarding basis for action.

Beyond this, ethics reasoning at its best probes beneath the law's formalism, toward the gist of what is normatively at stake when disputes reach the point of legal conflict. This potential for clarity carries a downside. With moral candor about hard decisions comes the visible sacrifice of cherished values (Calabresi, 1978)—and the risk of social discomfort, even discord. Cost–benefit balancing decisions that entail the sacrifice of life to save money, or the differential valuation of lives based on social and economic status, can wound and anger. But the social solidarity we preserve by avoiding moral candor is at best hollow and at worst oppressive. Its inauthenticity invites cynicism—and erosion of public confidence in the law. The candor about normative matters that ethics discourse brings can push courts to see painful choices and to make them visibly, empowering democratic politics to act as a check on what courts do.

The distinctive credibility of medical ethics as a public-regarding enterprise offers courts a medium for championing values not adequately sustained by private actors in either politics or the marketplace. When our public-regarding concerns clash in court with our self-centered preferences (Sunstein, 1986), the law must mediate between the two. Ethics reasoning and rhetoric can weigh in on such occasions. They can encourage judges to interpret ambiguous political outcomes (and to adjust troublesome market outcomes) in line with public-regarding conceptions of the good. Such a role for ethics, however, raises the stakes when private actors make ethics claims as cover for their pursuit of self-interest. A crucial task for courts (and scholars) is to screen out such claims (Bloche, 2001) so as to maintain the credibility of ethics discourse as voice for conceptions of the public good.

This account of possibilities and limits suggests a self-consciously pragmatic strategy for incorporation of ethics into judge-made law. It begins with an effort to identify public-regarding values expressed in ethics discourse but ill-supported in the medical marketplace and health-care politics. Ethics reasoning and rhetoric that give voice to these values merit a place in the law to the extent that they can be squared with the law's separate institutional concerns, especially the need to tie judicial interpretation to public preferences expressed via democratic institutions. Efforts to discern public-regarding values, assess the sufficiency of market and political support for these values, and square ethics thinking with law's institutional concerns will inevitably engender disagreement. Consensus on public-regarding values is beyond our reach, competition between medical ethics paradigms is robust, and the fit between these paradigms and the law's institutional concerns is deeply subjective. But this line of inquiry frames, and thus narrows, deliberation concerning medical ethics' role in judicial decision making.

A variety of public-regarding concerns are candidates for incorporation via medical ethics into the judge-made law of health-care provision. The ideal of undivided professional loyalty to patients is central to traditional medical ethics, but it is routinely compromised today by contractual arrangements that reward physicians for cost savings regardless of the quality or efficiency of the care they provide. The self-serving features of physician-prescribed ethics have invited appropriate judicial skepticism, but the ethic of fidelity to patients meets core emotional needs that market and political outcomes may not adequately incorporate. The mostly healthy people who sign up for medical coverage—and who vote—may not fully anticipate their feelings of neediness and fear of abandonment when they become seriously ill; thus, they may not adequately anticipate their needs for professional trustworthiness (Bloche, forthcoming). By incorporating the ethic of professional fidelity to patients into the law governing physicians' duties and limiting what health plans and other institutions can, by contract, press doctors to do, courts can meet human needs to which markets and politics may not give enough weight.

Similarly, contemporary bioethics thinking about the informational prerequisites for sufficiently informed choice among health-care coverage options could both clarify the normative choices that underlie competing legal claims concerning disclosure duties and bring public values (and disinterested perspective) to resolution of these claims. ERISA's opaque provision concerning employee benefit plans' fiduciary duties leaves ample room for bioethics perspectives on disclosure of physicians' financial incentives; medical information privacy policies; and approaches to cost–benefit balancing, clinical practice protocols, innovative treatments, and other coverage issues. Ambiguous state statutes and common law leave similar interpretive space for bioethics thinking about the question of disclosure.

Bioethics approaches to questions of distributive justice are also candidates for incorporation into the judge-made law of health-care provision.

The overarching distributive injustice of America's more than 40 million uninsured is beyond judges' reach. The U.S. Supreme Court long ago held that the federal constitution does not require public provision of medical or other social benefits (*Harris v. McRae,* 1980), and no federal statutes or state laws impose such a requirement. Courts must work within these institutional constraints. But where judges have interpretive options (e.g., in cases involving ambiguity in statutes requiring hospitals to provide free emergency care) they can and should draw upon the widely accepted bioethics premise, also embodied in international law (International Covenant on Economic, Social and Cultural Rights, 1966), that all people should have access to at least a basic level of care.

To be sure, distributive questions can be complicated. For example, the financing of so-called "free" hospital care for the poor is highly regressive by comparison to income taxes. This is because revenues from insured patients cover the cost of "free" care, and the fraction of insured Americans' incomes that goes toward medical coverage (and thus "free" care for the poor) is highest for those who earn the least (Bloche & Carolina, 1992). Thus, court decisions that expand uninsured people's rights to "free" care have harsh distributive consequences for poor and middle-class families who buy insurance. Ambiguity regarding the scope of statutory "free care" obligations cannot be resolved by the courts without trade-offs between these two sets of distributive concerns. This example underscores the importance of institutional and financial arrangements: Bioethics divorced from an understanding of organizational and economic complexity in health care is as likely to lead courts astray as to assist them.

Other legal questions with a distributive justice dimension involve the range of health-care and coverage options that should be available to consumers in order to treat their decisions concerning care and coverage as binding choices. Contract law offers judges a range of off-the-shelf doctrinal tools for relieving consumers after-the-fact from responsibility for disappointing outcomes. Judicial decisions to invoke these doctrinal tools entail underlying judgments about the fairness of choice situations (Kronman, 1980). An example is the current controversy over whether courts (and independent medical reviewers) in cases arising from denials of payment should apply contractual definitions of "medical necessity" or make their own judgments about medical need, based on medical expertise, without reference to contractual restrictions. Those who see restrictive contractual definitions of medical necessity as chosen by consumers from a fair set of options want courts to hold consumers to these definitions. Another example is the courts' refusal to permit health-care providers to contract out of common law approaches to the setting of standards of care in medical malpractice cases. Judicial deference to contractual options that permit clinical quality to drop below professional standards of care (the metric of liability under common law) would permit much greater distributive inequity in clinical care than medical tort law currently sanctions.

CONCLUSION

Neither traditional professional ethics nor the contemporary bioethics movements should become mere adjuncts of the law: Ethics entails distinct psychological and social means for encouraging behavior deemed socially desirable. Feelings of guilt arising from the internalization of ethics norms, shame arising from high public regard for the content of these norms, and the power of private institutions to reward and punish behavior play crucial roles in shaping professional conduct. But neither should judicial development of the law of health-care provision occur in isolation from those ethical norms that serve the social good. The principal challenge for those who wish to see a larger, more explicit role for ethics in the law of health-care provision is to separate out such norms from the chaff of ethics claims that cover for narrow self-interest. Ethics reasoning that expresses public values slighted in politics and the marketplace merits a more visible place in the law. But lawyers and scholars committed to making such a place for ethics in the courts must take account of judges' separate institutional concerns—about the courts' role relative to the political branches, relationships among levels of government, and consistency across areas of law.

NOTES

1. *See Goldfarb v. Virginia State Bar*, 1975 (holding that bar associations' prohibitions against price advertising violated the Sherman Antitrust Act, 2001).

2. *See Vacco v. Quill*, 1997 (citing longstanding professional ethics proscription against physician-assisted suicide in support of argument that past and present social and legal prohibitions against physician-assisted suicide weigh against affording it substantive due process protection under the U.S. constitution). When such norms (and the social mores they reflect) have been controversial, courts have typically been reluctant to invoke them as grounds for constitutionalizing the prohibition of professional conduct but open to drawing upon them as a basis for permitting *statutory* prohibitions of professional conduct to survive constitutional challenge.

3. *See Natanson v. Kline*, 1960 (defining physicians' disclosure obligations in terms of what a "reasonable physician," motivated by the patient's best therapeutic interests, would reveal to a patient); *Canterbury v. Spence*, 1972 (defining physicians' disclosure obligations in terms of what a "reasonable patient" would find material to his or her treatment decision).

4. Compare *Van Vactor v. Blue Cross Association*, 1977 (accepting treating physician's

judgment as touchstone for medical necessity) with *Sarchett v. Blue Shield of California*, 1987 (accepting health insurer's contract-based right to make its own medical necessity decisions).

5. The current version of the American Medical Association's *Principles of Medical Ethics* states: "A physician shall, in the provision of appropriate patient care, except in emergencies, be free to choose whom to serve, with whom to associate, and the environment in which to provide medical care" (American Medical Association, 2001). For a history of this principle in its varying forms dating back to its inclusion in the 1912 *Principles of Medical Ethics*, see Baker, 1999.

6. See Advisory Committee on Human Radiation Experiments, 1995 (arguing that the absence of an informed consent norm in professional ethics and in clinical and research practice—what the Commission termed "cultural moral ignorance"—explained the general failure of American medical researchers in the 1950s to obtain informed consent from human subjects).

7. The emerging discipline of computerized content analysis of texts might find productive application here to judicial opinions, briefs, and trial transcripts.

8. *Washington v. Glucksberg*, 1997 (citing Brief for Bioethics Professors as amici curiae).

9. Lower federal courts have differed over whether ERISA's vague "fiduciary duty" provision, which requires employee benefits administrators to act in beneficiaries' best interests, 29 U.S.C. §§ 1002(21), 1104(a)(1), constitutes sufficient statutory basis for requiring health plans to tell subscribers about their physicians' financial incentives. See *Shea v. Esensten*, 208 F.3d 712 (8th Cir, 2000).

10. See *McGann v. H&H Music Co.*, 946 F.2d 401 (5th Cir. 1991) (stating that specification of employee benefits is a task "more appropriately influenced by forces in the marketplace" than undertaken by courts).

11. *Sarchett v. Blue Shield of California*, 1987. To be sure, such deference was hardly complete. Courts scrutinized plans' medical necessity decisions for compliance with plans' contractual medical necessity criteria, and where these criteria failed to clearly answer coverage questions, courts drew heavily from professional practice norms.

12. An exception was the 7th Circuit Court of Appeals opinion in *Herdrich v. Pegram*, 1998, (reversed by *Pegram v. Herdrich*, 2000), which condemned the HMO industry for skimping on care and intruding upon professional judgment.

ACKNOWLEDGMENTS

Preparation of this chapter was supported in part by a Robert Wood Johnson Foundation Investigator Award in Health Policy Research. The author thanks Genvieve Grabman and Michael Sapoznikow for their superb research assistance.

REFERENCES

Advisory Committee on Human Radiation Experiments (1995) *Final Report*. Washington, DC: U.S. Government Printing Office 214–6.

AMA v. FTC, 638 F.2d 443 (2nd Cir. 1980), aff'd by an equally divided Court 455 U.S. 676 (1982).

American Medical Association (2001) *Principles of Medical Ethics*, Principle 6

Arrow K (1963) Uncertainty and the welfare economics of medical care. *American Economic Review* 51: 941–943.

Baber v. Hospital Corporation of America, 977 F.2d 872 (4th Cir., 1992).

Baker R, Caplan A, Emmanuel L, et al (eds) (1999) *The American Medical Ethics Revolution.* Baltimore: Johns Hopkins University Press, 346–54

Bang v. Charles T. Miller Hospital, 251 Minn. 427 (1958)

Bauman v. U.S. Healthcare, Inc., 193 F.3d 151, 162 (3rd Cir., 1999).

Beauchamp T and Childress J (2001) *Principles of Biomedical Ethics*, 5th ed. New York: Oxford University Press, 225–72

Bloche M and Carolina R (1992) Paying for undercompensated hospital care: The regressive profile of a "hidden tax." *Health Matrix* 2: 141–165.

Bloche M (1992) Corporate takeover of teaching hospitals. *Southern California Law Review* 65: 1035–1170.

Bloche M (1996) Clinical counseling and the question of autonomy—negating influence. In Faden R, Kass N (eds) *HIV, AIDS and Childbearing: Public Policy, Private Lives.* New York: Oxford University Press, 257–319.

Bloche M (1997) Managed care, medical privacy, and the paradigm of consent. *Kennedy Institute of Ethics Journal* 7 :381–386.

Bloche M (1998) Cutting waste and keeping the faith. *Annals of Internal Medicine* 128: 688.

Bloche M (2001) The market for medical ethics. *Journal of Health Politics, Policy and Law*. 26: 1099–1112.

Brief of health law, policy, and ethics scholars as Amici Curiae in support of respondent at 16–20, *Pegram v. Herdrich* 530 U.S. 211 (1999) (No. 98–1949).

Calabresi G (1978) *Tragic Choices*. New York: Norton

California Dental Ass'n v. FTC, 526 U.S. 756 (1999).

Canterbury v. Spence (1972) U.S. Court of Appeals for the District of Columbia Circuit. No. 22099. May 19, 1972.

Capron A (1999) Professionalism and professional ethics. In: Baker R, Caplan A, Emmanuel L, et al (eds) *The American Medical Ethics Revolution.* Baltimore: Johns Hopkins University Press, 180

Corcoran v. United Health Care, 965 F.2d 1321 (5th Cir. 1992).

Cruzan v. Director, Missouri Dep't of Health, 497 U.S. 261 (1990).

Daniels N and Sabin J (1998) The ethics of accountability in managed care reform. *Health Affairs* 17: 50–64.

Dudziak M (2000) *Cold War Civil Rights: Race and the Image of American Democracy.* Princeton: Princeton University Press.

Dworkin R (1986) *Law's Empire*. Cambridge, MA: Belknap Press, 225–75.

Dworkin R, Nagel T, Nozick R, et. al. (1997) Assisted suicide: The philosophers' brief. *The New York Review of Books* March 27, 1997.

Emergency Medical Treatment and Active Labor Act ("EMTALA"), 42 U.S.C.S. § 1395dd (2001).

Employee Retirement Income Security Act ("ERISA"), 29 USC §1001 et seq. Preemption: § 502(a) of ERISA, 29 U.S.C. § 1132(a)(1)(B); and § 514(a) of ERISA, 29 U.S.C. § 1144(a). Fiduciary duty: 29 U.S.C. §§ 1002(21), 1104(a)(1).

Epstein R (1976) Medical malpractice: The case for contract. *American Bar Foundation Research Journal* 1976: 87–149.

Faden R, Beauchamp T, in collaboration with King N (1986) *A History and Theory of Informed Consent.* New York: Oxford University Press.

Ferguson v. City of Charleston, 121 S. Ct. 1281 (2001).

Freedman M (1962) *Capitalism and Freedom*. Chicago: University of Chicago Press.

Freiman A (1998) Comment: The abandonment of the antiquated corporate practice of medicine doctrine: Injecting a dose of efficiency into the modern health care environment. *Emory Law Journal* 47: 697–751.

Goldfarb v. Virginia State Bar, 421 U.S. 773, 781–83 (1975).

Hall M (1988) Institutional control of physician behavior: Legal barriers to health care cost containment. *University of Pennsylvania Law Review* 137: 431–536.

Hall M (1997) A theory of economic informed consent. *Georgia Law Review* 31: 511–586.

Harris v. McRae 448 U.S. 297 (1980).

Havighurst C (1995) *Health Care Choices: Private Contracts as Instruments of Health Care Reform*. Washington, DC: American Enterprise Institute for Public Policy Research, 185–90.

Havighurst (2001) Health care as (big) business: The antitrust response. *Journal of Health Politics, Policy and Law*. 26: 939–955.

Herdrich v. Pegram, 154 F.3d 362 (7th Cir. 1998), rev'd 530 U.S. 211 (2000).

Henkin L (1990) *The Age of Rights*. New York: Columbia University Press, 16–29.

International Covenant on Economic, Social and Cultural Rights, adopted Dec. 16, 1966, 993 U.N.T.S. 3, art. 12.

In the Matter of Baby "K," 16 F.3d 590, cert. Denied, 513 U.S. 825 (4th Cir 1994).

Jacobson P and Pomfret S (1998) Form, function, and managed care torts: Achieving fairness and equity in ERISA jurisprudence. *Houston Law Review* 35: 985–1078.

Jass v. Prudential Health Care Plan, 88 F.3d 1482 (7th Cir. 1996).

Kahan D (1996) What do alternative sanctions mean? *University of Chicago Law Review* 63: 591–653.

Katz J (1977) Informed consent—a fairy tale? Law's Vision *University of Pittsburgh Law Review* 39: 137–174.

Katz J (1984) *The Silent World of Doctor and Patient*. New York: Free Press 104–29.

Kronman A (1980) Contract law and distributive justice. *Yale Law Journal* 89: 472, 485–91.

Massachusetts Mut. Life Ins. Co. v. Russell, 473 U.S. 134, 148 (1985).

McGann v. H&H Music Co., 946 F.2d 401 (5th Cir. 1991).

Metropolitan Life Ins. Co. v. Massachusetts, 471 U.S. 724 (1985).

Mohr v. Williams, 95 Minn. 261 (1905).

Moore v. Regents of University of California, 51 Cal. 3d 120 (1990).

Natanson v. Kline, 350 P.2d 1093 (1960).

Neade v. Portes, 193 Ill. 2d 433, 505–506 (2000).

Parsons T (1951) *The Social System*. New York: Free Press of Glencoe, 428–47

Pegram v. Herdrich, 530 U.S. 211 (2000).

Pilot Life Ins. Co. v. Dedeaux, 481 U.S. 41 (1987).

Pryzbowksi v. U.S. Healthcare, Inc., 245 F.3d 266, 282 (3rd Cir., 2001).

Rodwin M (1993) *Medicine, Money and Morals: Physicians' Conflicts of Interest*. New York: Oxford University Press, 179–219.

Rothman D (1991) *Strangers at the Bedside: A History of How Law and Bioethics Transformed Medical Decision Making*. New York: BasicBooks.

Sarchett v. Blue Shield of California, 729 P.2d 267 (Cal. 1987).

Schultz M (1985) From informed consent to patient choice: A new protected interest. *Yale Law Journal* 95: 219, 226–7.

Sharfstein J and Sharfstein S (1994) Campaign contributions from the American Medical Political Action Committee to members of Congress: For or against the public health? *New England Journal of Medicine* 330: 32–7

Shea v. Esensten, 208 F.3d 712 (8th cir, 2000).Sherman Antitrust Act, 15 U.S.C.S. § 1 (2001).

Slovenko R (1998) *Psychotherapy and Confidentiality*. Springfield, IL: Charles C. Thomas Publisher, 57–75

Starr P (1982) *The Social Transformation of American Medicine*. New York: Basic Books 9–29

Sunstein C (1986) Legal interference with private preferences. *University of Chicago Law Review* 53: 1129–1174.

Trials Of War Criminals Before The Nuernberg Military Tribunals Under Control Council Law No 10 (1949) 2 :181–182

Tyler T (1990) *Why People Obey the Law*. New Haven: Yale University Press 45–50

Vacco v. Quill, 521 U.S. 793, 800 n6 (1997).

Van Vactor v. Blue Cross Association, 265 N.E.2d 638 (Ill.App.Ct.1977).

Veatch R (2000) *Cross-Cultural Perspectives in Medical Ethics*. Boston: Jones and Bartlett 1–54

Ward v. Alternative Health Delivery Sys., 55 F. Supp. 2d 694, 699 (2000).

Washington v. Glucksberg, 521 U.S. 702, 733 n23 (1997).

9

Health policy making: the role of the federal government

JO IVEY BOUFFORD AND PHILIP R. LEE

In his chapter of this volume, Churchill notes that "ethics can serve the very important function of clarifying and examining the larger goals and purposes of health policies." If we accept this function for ethics, then the role of ethics in policy matters, he continues, is "fundamentally, one of identifying the ends sought in policies, examining the values embedded in these ends, [and] asking whether they are in keeping with social values." Yet, as we shall see, fulfilling these tasks when it comes to an ethical framework for health policy making at the federal level immediately leads to a series of complications, both historical and operational. The most important ones, in our view, and the ones we will explore here are incrementalism, pluralism and federalism. These are all powerful characteristics of the American political system that have made it difficult, if not impossible, to "clarify and examine the larger goals of health policies."

INCREMENTALISM

In a very real sense, the health policy we have at the federal level reflects the incremental effects of nearly 1000 different health and social programs. More than 300 of these programs provide domestic grants in aid for health programs and are administered by its lead federal agency in health, the U.S. Department of Health and Human Services (DHHS). The programs have developed incrementally to respond to political pressures, to address the needs of specific populations, the need to tackle specific diseases, and the needs of specific organizations providing services, usually personal health-care services.

The resistance to a large-scale, integrated approach to change in federal health policy was recently seen most dramatically in the 1994 failure of President Clinton's national health-care reform. This failure saw a return to incrementalism. The Kennedy-Kassenbaum Act to provide insurance coverage to workers between jobs, the State Children's Health Insurance Program (SCHIP) to provide expanded coverage to poor children, and the proposed expansion of drug benefits to Medicare beneficiaries were but a few of the "incremental" health policies that followed in the wake of the failure of the Clinton reform.

PLURALISM

The pluralism of health policy making at the federal level is reflected in the multiple executive branch actors in health, which include about 40 cabinet and cabinet-level departments and subcabinet agencies and commissions as well as the White House; multiple agencies within large cabinet departments like the DHHS, each with its own policy agenda, programs, budgets, and advocacy groups; the interdependence of the executive branch with multiple legislative entities in the House and Senate that have some authorizing and appropriating authority over health programs; and the frequent tempering of health policy by acts of the Judiciary. Each health program has its advocates among the public, and there are thousands of intermediary organizations involved in all aspects of the health sector—physicians, nurses, hospitals, health plans, insurance carriers, corporations paying for health insurance, unions, the pharmaceutical and medical device industry, state and local departments of public health and environment, and so on. This creates a very complex environment that makes developing a framework for larger health policy goals a unique challenge!

FEDERALISM

The fundamental division of powers between the states and the national government has varied over the history of this country. This has resulted in a complex interdependence in health policy that virtually precludes unilateral federal action on large-scale health policy issues.

The very idea of a common ethical framework that can help to move toward a unifying health policy goal at the federal level already seems difficult. The tasks of reconciling such elaborate competing interests and addressing the huge power differentials among these interests seems nearly out of reach. Up to now, this situation has led to problem solving on specific issues rather than the adoption of a more holistic approach, thereby perpetuating the categorical and fragmented nature of our health policy.

There may, however, be the potential for a new framework for federal health policy making. This framework would broaden the current traditional health policy paradigm driven by the biomedical model, with its focus on the science and services need to treat the diseases of individuals, for a paradigm driven by a health model that includes new evidence about the multiple determinants of health—human behavior, human biology, physical and social environment, education, socioeconomic status, as well as medical care—and their effects on the health of communities and populations. The ethical basis for such a shift assumes both the presence of a strong societal value for health and clear evidence about factors that promote health, as well as a responsibility on the part of the government to be responsive to these. As such, the federal government would have to both play an appropriate role in supporting policies that promote health as well as assure that our investments in these policies reflect the actual potential of different policy actions to effectively promote health.

THE LIMITS OF CURRENT HEALTH POLICY

Health is a "state of complete physical, mental, and spiritual well being, not just the absence of disease." This definition of health defines an ideal state for the individual and was accepted more than 50 years ago by member nations of the World Health Organization (WHO), a specialized agency of the United Nations. There is broad international agreement that the role of the state is to assure the conditions that allow all its citizens to enjoy the highest attainable level of health. This is clearly a statement of social values that, if accepted, can become a guide for decision making in federal health policy. Those who hold this view acknowledge the variability in human capacity to achieve the WHO ideal and agree that a nation's health policy must focus not just on access to health care but also on population-oriented public health, which has been described as "what we as a society do collectively to assure the conditions in which people can be healthy (Institute of Medicine, 1980).

The nation is facing a new set of health challenges, and the historic federal health policy focus on the financing of personal health-care services and biomedical research, while necessary (especially in view of the high numbers of uninsured individuals), is not a sufficient strategy for effectively meeting these new challenges. Some of these challenges are global, such as the spread of infectious diseases and epidemics like HIV/AIDS and the threat of bioterrorism. Others are more unique to the United States, such as the aging of our population with the consequent growth of chronic disease; the complex behavioral and social factors in disease that increasingly affect more and more of our people; the growing diversity of our population and the resulting need to eliminate huge disparities in health status between the poor and vulnerable populations and the rest of our people; and the growth in problems of mental health and substance abuse as well as other risky behaviors that threaten our communities, especially the young. Advances in research relating to the factors that influence a population's health (Evans et al, 1994; Marmot, 1994; Wilkinson, R. et al, 1988; Kindig, 1997; McKeown, 1976; Marmot et al, 1978) have increased our understanding of how health behaviors, as well as socioeconomic factors, experiences of work, and availability of community support all influence individual health and disease. Accordingly, the potential strategies for action to tackle these complex disease problems are now much broader than before.

Using our current categorical approach to health policy, with its emphasis on individual care and cure, the United States invests more in health care than any other country on the planet. Yet the results are not what we would expect, either in the satisfaction of our people with their health-care system or in the health status of our population. Factors such as length and quality of life are not as optimal as they could be, and we have not succeeded in eliminating the glaring inequities in the health status of the poor and communities of color. In fact, the United States has met only about 15% of the health objectives set ten years ago in the *Healthy People* report for the year 2000. While progress has been made on another 44% of these objectives, in another 20% of the objectives the health status of the population has deteriorated. (Consider, for example, the rise of obesity.) Moreover, health disparities among ethnic groups reveal that problems are growing worse (*Healthy People 2010*, 1999).

Why have our investments not resulted in higher levels of health? One reason is that medical care is not the major factor in health. McGinnis and Foege (1993) have shown that only 10% of avoidable mortality in the United States is directly related to lack of access to medical care. The vast majority (50%) is instead due to such risky behaviors as smoking, drinking, lack of exercise, poor diet, and substance abuse. Even these behaviors, however, are heavily related to other factors of socioeconomic status, education, and social cohesiveness.

The World Health Report 2000 ranked the U.S. health system 37th overall and 24th on overall health attainment, lagging behind all of the other G-7 countries (WHO, 2000). Anderson's analysis of Organization for Economic Co-Operation and Development (OECD) countries' health systems (10) shows the US health system to be the most expensive (14.2% of its gross domestic product (GDP) vs. 10.5% in Germany, the next most costly system); one of the least financially accessible (in 1995 the United States, Turkey, and Mexico were the only OECD countries that had not achieved the objective of nearly universal health insurance coverage for all of their citizens); and 23rd and 21st, respectively, of 29 countries in infant mortality and male life expectancy (1997). We would not tolerate this standing in education or national defense; we should not tolerate it in health, either.

As we enter the 21st century, the federal government has an important role to play in initiating and shaping health policy, even in a system that is as decentralized, pluralistic, and privatized as that in the United States. The current machinery for policy making and implementation in the executive and legislative branches of the federal government is not well suited to the shift from a biomedical model to a health model for federal health policy. It is nonetheless important to understand the origins of our current health policy and the institutions that implement it at the federal level in order to consider strategies for change. We turn to an examination of these elements now.

THE EVOLUTION OF THE FEDERAL ROLE IN HEALTH

The current federal role in health and health policy making is complex and changeable. It is strongly influenced by history and the evolving relationship between the federal government and state governments. Indeed, this relationship was at the center of health policy making for much of the 20th century. Unlike interstate commerce and national defense, the notion of federal involvement in health was not explicitly mentioned by our founding fathers. Nonetheless, Gostin (2000) argues persuasively that a concern for protecting the community's health and safety was clearly intended under the general welfare purposes for the national government in the Constitution.

Almost from the beginning, federal action in health has been reactive—a response to pressure from states and localities, especially large cities, reacting to a crisis large in scale or high in visibility. Federal action is usually tempered greatly by resistance from states asserting their rights, differences in approach between the executive and legislative branches, differences of opinion among the professionals in the health sector, and, often, by direct action by the judiciary.

The first federal action in health concerned "a bill for the relief of sick and disabled seamen," to be financed from deductions from their wages with federal money used to arrange for hospitalization in existing facilities and to build hospitals to serve them where none existed (Boufford, 1999). In a sense, seamen were the migrant workers of their time, not citizens or the responsibilities of any single state. During debate over the bill in the 5th Congress in 1798, supporters asserted that without federal action, the burden would fall to the states in which they were stationed. Opponents of federal action contended that this particular group was no different from other sick and disabled individuals who could not provide for themselves and, thus, should be provided for through charity, not the government.

In telling the story of the debate over this bill, Mustard (1945) recounts an interpretation by some contemporary medical historians that the ultimate passage of the bill set certain precedents for federal action in health: compulsory support for a group of nondependent persons (seamen), financing by payroll deductions and general tax revenues, and federal funding of treatment by private hospitals and private physicians. However, Mustard disagrees with this interpretation. Looking at the government's action in the context of the times, he draws a different set of lessons, which seem more likely. First, he notes, the bill was referred to the Commerce and Manufacture Committees. Consideration of the health, or medical care, element came about only because it was a problem of commerce, thus setting a precedent of approaching health issues indirectly—a pattern that, 150 years later, has resulted in health programs and functions being located in more than 40 different government departments, ranging from Agriculture to Treasury to Labor to Commerce.[1]

One year after the passage of the seamen's bill, another pattern was established—incremental expansion of coverage, as naval personnel were added to the list of beneficiaries. The progress under this act over the next 75 years was very mixed. There were corruption and influence peddling to get new facilities; broad expansions of groups using the facilities beyond those designated as eligible; and poor quality of service, with both increasing complaints and costs—a crisis, at least of embarrassment, to the federal government. In 1869 the secretary of the treasury appointed a supervising surgeon (the precursor to the modern surgeon general) to reorganize the Marine Hospital Service. This surgeon increased use and investment, improved quality, established laboratory and research services, and generally expanded the role of the service, which became the U.S. Public Health Service in 1912.

States and large cities began to develop health boards and authorities and to take on most of the responsibilities for both public health and, through charity care provisions, health care for the poor and disabled. The federal government did not take on a major population-wide public health issue until almost 100 years after its first federal action in health policy. More specifically, in 1877 a national quarantine law was passed in response to a yellow fever epidemic that killed 20,000 people in the Mississippi basin area. While an attempt 75 years earlier to create a Federal Quarantine Authority (FQA) had been defeated in Congress due to concerns over states rights, the time was ripe in 1877 for the establishment of such an authority, for there was pressure from some states for federal action in light of the failure of other states to deal with this public health threat, which put them at risk and cost them money. In addition to the FQA, a National Health Board was created and acted for a short time but became too confrontational with states' authority. It was opposed by the Surgeon General of the Marine Hospital Service and was officially dropped from the books by 1893.

Over the next 20 years, especially with impetus from the Progressive movement, a series of national actions was taken: In 1897 the Hygiene Laboratory was established in the Marine Hospital on Staten Island. In 1890 authority was given to what is now the Public Health Service to conduct health screening of immigrants, and the federal government added to its powers the authority to convene state health officers and to collect health data. The Hygiene Laboratory was moved to Washington, D.C., and its authority was expanded to conduct research and, in 1902, regulate biologics. In 1912 the U.S. Public Health Service was formed and given authority to investigate the diseases of man and conditions influencing their propagation and spread, including sanitation, sewage, and pollution.

As England and Germany established social insurance programs in the early part of the 20th century, the Progressives in the United States established a Social Insurance Commission that in 1917 proposed a model compulsory health insurance bill for workers earning less than $100 dollars per month and their families. The premiums would be divided among employer, worker, and state. Bills involving this proposal were introduced in state legislatures around the country with the American Medical Association (AMA) leaders' support, yet AMA members did not support them, and state medical societies, together with the insurance companies, scuttled them. Finally, U.S. involvement in World War I killed any remaining momentum the legislation had.

After World War I a shift in focus occurred from contentious broad health coverage issues toward federal investments in research and attention to new subpopulations, especially substance abusers and the mentally ill. Federal funding to states for projects such as rural sanitation began in 1916. This kind of swing from a highly contentious political period of national health initiatives toward a quieter one, with a focus on targeted investments in research, more categorical programs, and state funding, has repeated itself several times over, as federal action has been alternately resisted and welcomed.

In 1930 an act to establish the National Institute of Health (NIH) was passed, reorganizing the Hygienic Laboratory into the NIH, while the Veteran's Administration was created as an independent agency. The Social Security Act (SSA) of 1935 codified large, more discretionary grants to states for special populations—maternal and child health—and public health programs with matching fund requirements and allocation formulas based on population, financial need, and mortality rates from the diseases related to total mortality in the United States. There was considerable debate over the advisability of further pursuing this fragmented approach of singling out populations and issues, but it appeared, politically, the only way to move forward.

What the SSA did not do was establish a national program of health insurance. The Wagner-Murray-Dingle Bill, introduced following passage of SSA, attempted to set up a general medical care program supported by taxes, insurance, or both, but the states rights activists, the AMA, and business were strongly opposed, and the bill was not enacted. Given this resistance, President Roosevelt concluded that it was not worth the political fight.

In 1938 the passage of the Food, Drugs and Cosmetics Act expanded federal authority to act against adulterated and mislabeled food, drug, and cosmetic products, and it gave the Food and Drug Administration authority to regulate new drugs prior to marketing. In 1939 the Federal Security Agency was created by President Roosevelt to bring together the Social Security Administration, the US Public Health Service, the Food and Drug Administration (FDA, from the Department of Agriculture), and a variety of human service and welfare programs from various cabinet departments.

After World War II ended President Truman proposed a program of national health insurance. Even though 100 million Americans were uninsured, the National Health Insurance proposal could not garner sufficient backing. Organized labor, while supportive, was distracted by other activities. AMA members (100,000 physicians), most of whom were enjoying new post-war prosperity, were effective in steering public sentiment against the measure. Meanwhile, significant advances continued in federal support for hospital construction (the Hill-Burton program) and biomedical research at the NIH. In 1953 President Eisenhower transformed the Federal Security Agency into the Department of Health Education and Welfare (DHEW), which later became the current Department of Health and Human Services after creation of an independent Department of Education in 1980.

Federalism and the Federal Role

The structure and functions of the executive branch in health have also been shaped by the changing historical relationships between the national and state governments, especially beginning in the mid-20th century. The Roosevelt era marked a shift from what Walker (1981) has called "a dual federalism" (1789 to 1930), in which state and local governments retained powers and jurisdictions not expressly granted to the U.S. government and served as collaborators, if not dominant partners, with the Federal government. The new approach fostered by the New Deal, on the other hand, was called "cooperative federalism" and was characterized by a larger federal role with state and local government sharing of responsibilities.

Between 1960 and 1969, Lyndon Johnson's "creative federalism" saw the federal government bypassing states in many of its programs and linking directly to substate units of local government, especially cities as well as nonprofit organizations. In health, the Medicare and Medicaid programs were passed in the 1960's, and literally hundreds of other grant in aid programs were enacted in public health. In addition, in 1963 the authority of the FDA was strengthened to regulate the safety and effectiveness of drugs.

Nixon's "new federalism," initiated in 1970, opted for a more decentralized model of federal–state relations, with general assistance grants complimenting the more categorical approach. However, in the health arena he did take executive action to create the Environmental Protection Agency (by moving programs out of the DHEW); enacted the Family Planning legislation under Title X of the Public Health Service Amendments; enacted early legislation for health maintenance organizations; and tried but failed to implement an employer health insurance mandate. Congress, however, controlled by the Democrats, reacted to the looser relationships with states by what some have called "congressional federalism," which Walker sees as a persistent pattern. This pattern is incremental (ad hoc), confrontational (antipresidential), strongly categorical (low trust), heavily conditional (national purpose conditions vs. no strings), and politically co-optive (interest group driven). The strength of one element or another in this set of characteristics varies depending on whether Republicans or Democrats control the White House and/or Congress and according to the degree of tension between the executive and legislative branches.

President Carter took a middle ground between Nixon and Johnson. As a former governor, he valued simplification of the state and federal partnership. He also appreciated the critical role of the private sector and hence the government's need to leverage private sector involvement in its programs. However, he also sought more precise targeting of federal action to the most hard-pressed communities.

The Reagan administration saw too much "government as the problem," and his version of new federalism again saw a shift to block grants with considerable flexibility left to states. Toward the end of the Reagan administration, general revenue sharing grants were ended due to concern about accountability for them. The Bush administration implemented little change in the pattern of federal–state grant making but began to use the federal regulatory role to implement national goals (DiIullio, Jr. et al, 1995). This regulatory approach to federal action led to strong reactions from states against so-called unfunded mandates that, in turn, led to greater attention to state roles and authority in 1990s health policy making.

David Osborne notes that many of what he calls "the new Governors" resisted unconditional decentralization, like that of Reagan, and sought a more "intelligent sorting of the appropriate state and federal role" (1998). Osborne's new governor saw a middle ground between government as the solution and government as the problem, seeing it more appropriately as the partner, letting the market lead but channeling it to achieve greater equality of opportunity, if not necessarily of outcomes.

In 1992 Bill Clinton, one of these new governors, laid out his administration's policy blueprint in "Mandate for Change," identifying his conception of the foci of federal involvement: (*1*) on interstate issues where problems cannot be solved without federal action, because state and local governments lack either leverage or incentives; (*2*) when solutions require uniform standards (e.g., Social Security); (*3*) to counter destructive competition among units of government or within the private sector; and (*4*) to redistribute national resources to poor regions that lack them (DiIullio, Jr. et al, 1995).

DiIullio and Kettl, however, characterize this effort to limit the federal role as nothing new. First, federal action is always subject to politics. In fact, in an early statement Clinton said that crime was clearly not a federal issue, but public outcry at the rising crime rates led to a major federal program to put 100,000 police into communities to combat it. Second, the federal government is already using intermediaries for almost everything it does with states and local government and through grants and contracts with the private sector. A decreasing federal workforce is attempting to manage these relationships with an increasing state and local government workforce and myriad private sector providers. The movement toward performance measurement reflects the fact that the national government has almost no direct hand in administering its domestic programs, except for Social Security, but must use the tools it has to shape and guide implementation by others.

Walker argues that often a "disconnect" occurs between an expansionist national policy agenda, on the one hand, and the realities of state and local government resources that determine whether these governments are able to implement the policies, on the other. A serious question also arises as to whether government at any level is currently able to assure accountability for implementation of government programs by nongovernmental entities

(1981). The differential ability of states and localities to manage the devolution of welfare reform, use federal waivers to implement state health-care reform through Medicaid managed care, and develop effective programs to implement the State Child Health Improvement Program (SCHIP) enacted as part of the Balanced Budget Act of 1997 is, in some cases, ideological, but in many instances it reflects a lack of administrative resources and/or management expertise.

The Judiciary and the Federal Role

The judicial branch can also affect health policy by modifying the legal basis for public health initiatives. These decisions are rendered by state and federal courts and the U.S. Supreme Court. At the federal level, the greatest public health power is the power to "regulate Commerce . . . among several states." This has been the basis for national government action in environmental protection, occupational health and safety, and food and drug purity, among other areas (Gostin, 2000). At the state level, police powers have been used to promote and preserve the public's health in areas ranging from injury and disease prevention (smoking, safety helmets) to mandatory vaccinations, sanitation, and waste disposal. The Supreme Court has rendered many decisions of fundamental importance to the public's health. These include their interpretations of the Constitution concerning the commerce clause and the welfare clause (e.g., for Social Security and Medicare) and a woman's right to privacy (for abortion services). Gostin notes that while the courts have generally been permissive on matters of public health, they have scrutinized more closely issues in which they might otherwise appear to be discriminating against a historically oppressed class or invading a fundamental right, such as that of bodily integrity. He also notes the tendency of the current Supreme Court to return authority to the states as outlined in the 10th Amendment after several decades of decisions that had increased federal authority.

While some still seek a clearer delineation among federal, state, and local government roles, most students of American government believe this to be unrealistic in a general sense, though specific roles must be clarified in specific laws and programs in order to assure effective implementation. As Lee notes, this changeability and overlap are workable as long as: (*1*) administrative and regulatory responsibility and financing and accountability are consonant and (*2*) the various levels of government possess the appropriate capacities (and political will) to assume the responsibilities assigned to them (1997). This holds true for the government's relations with nongovernmental partners as well.

A truly effective health policy that achieves real gains in the nation's health status depends not only on investment in certain health programs but also on rationalizing the organization at the federal level and developing effective linkages across levels of government and with the private sector in order to effect change in other determinants of health like education, environment, and the economy. Administrative resources must be invested in government to manage these partnerships and assure that the entities responsible for implementation have the resources and capacity they need to attain program goals.

THE STRUCTURE AND FUNCTION OF FEDERAL HEALTH POLICY ORGANIZATIONS

In order to understand how health policy is made, it is important to understand the structure of the Department of Health and Human Services and the other major participants in health policy making in the executive branch of government. The congressional committees that ultimately determine the legal basis for health policy through legislation and the myriad interest groups that seek to influence the outcome of the process round out the complex group of federal stakeholders in this process.

Department of Health and Human Services

The Department of Health and Human Services (DHHS) and, within it, the U.S. Public Health Service, is the lead federal agency in health. It plays this role through activities in six major areas: policy making, financing, public health protection, collecting and disseminating information, capacity building for population health, and direct management of programs. Figure 9–1 shows an organizational chart of the current U.S. Department of Health and Human Services. The secretary and the deputy secretary are chief executive and chief operating officers, respectively, of the department.

Around the outside of the diagram are the staff divisions that support the secretary in her work on behalf of the entire department. Policy functions are led by the assistant secretary for planning and evaluation; overall budgetary and management oversight is led by the assistant secretary for management and budget. The department's legislative agenda is managed by the assistant secretary for legislation, and press relations are handled by the assistant secretary for public affairs. The general council, the Office of Civil Rights, and the inspector general also operate across the department.

The twelve boxes in the center of the diagram represent the operating divisions of the department. Each has its own organizational structure and annual budget and is responsible for administering a wide variety of pro-

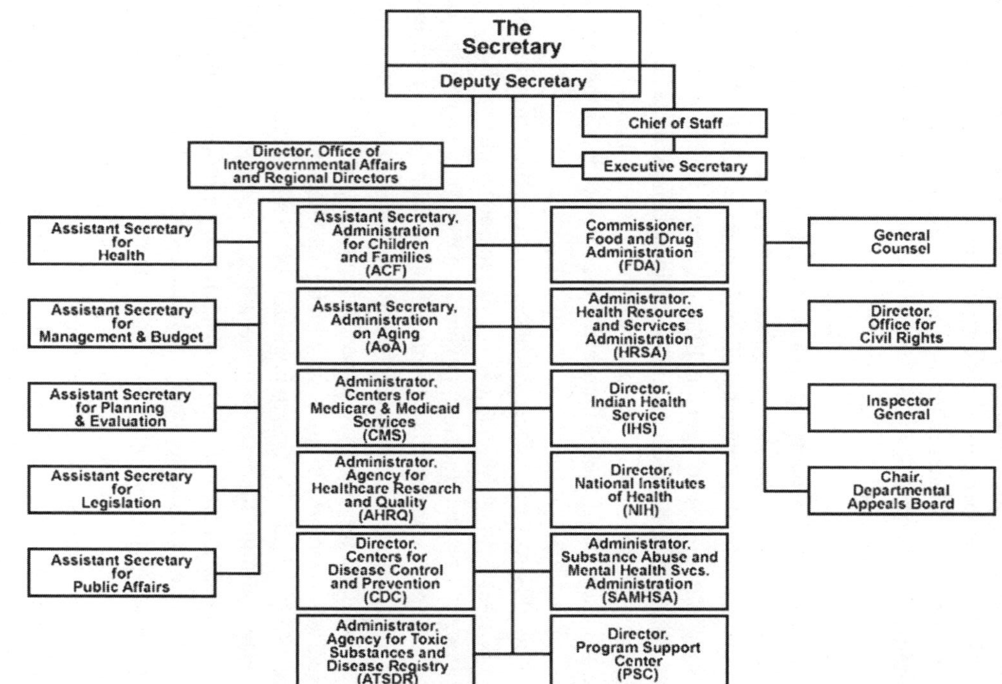

FIGURE 9–1. Health and Human Services organizational chart.

grams authorized by Congress. Each agency also has its own management, budget, planning, legislative, and public affairs staff, often structured in a way that mirrors the organizational arrangement at the department level.

The department is large and complex and, over a period of years, has become highly decentralized, with each of the working divisions operating relatively autonomously within a policy and budgetary framework set by the secretary. Each individual operating division also has constituencies composed of one or more special interest groups advocating for and seeking to shape its programs. These groups are much more closely tied to the individual operating divisions than to the department as a whole. They may serve as advocates to Congress for additional budget support for programs in the particular operating division regardless of the overall department's priorities for the role and size of that program. Each of the operating divisions must defend its individual budget before Congress, which ultimately decides the resources that division gets and the programs it will administer. The staff of various congressional committees also becomes quite loyal to the individual operating divisions, often because the services there are much more concrete for their constituents than are those of the department as a whole.

To see just how this sort of advocacy works, consider the following examples. The Food and Drug Administration is the major regulatory body to assure safe blood, drugs and medical devices, and certain categories of foods. It has a complex constituency ranging from public interest groups that want it to protect the public's health to institutions such as drug companies, device manufacturers, and blood banks regulated by the FDA who may wish to see less oversight in areas in which they feel federal intrusion is unwarranted. As well, the National Institutes of Health (NIH) has the major federal responsibility for financing the nation's biomedical research. It currently manages about half of all the discretionary funding in the Department of Health and Human Services. Its constituents include the scientific community and medical schools, who have been extremely successful in gaining major congressional budgetary support for the NIH. Finally, the Substance Abuse and Mental Health Services Administration (SAMHSA) manages block grants to states. States as constituents want more flexibility in their use of these funds, while advocacy groups for substance abusers and the mentally ill may wish to see the agency operate with more federally driven policy initiatives in the face of what they see as unresponsive state bureaucracies. All will clearly fight for increased resources for this agency. This pattern is repeated for all the operating divisions.

The connection among the senior staff of the operating divisions, the congressional staff, and the special interest groups and constituencies are often called the "iron triangle." While the administrators of the operating divisions and the senior staff in the department are political appointees who may change with presidential administrations, the senior civil servants in the operating divisions tend to continue in their roles, and they develop long-term relationships with special interest groups and the congressional staff. Many of the staff at this operational level take jobs in Congress, special interest groups, and the executive agencies over a period of years, carrying their information and expertise in certain programs with them.

Other Executive Branch Actors in Health Policy

Alongside the DHHS, the White House is the other major actor in the executive branch in health policy. The involvement of the White House begins with the Office of Management and Budget, the president's budget office, which reviews the financial requests of each agency on an annual basis and oversees their managerial competence. It must also approve all major regulatory decisions proposed by departments and agencies before these become effective. Depending on the issue and the priority of health on a president's agenda, a number of other health related entities in the White House may play a role in the health policy process. The Office of Policy Development (composed of the Domestic Policy Council and the National Economic Council) was established in 1993. It advises and assists the president in the formulation, coordination, and implementation of domestic social and economic policy, which can include public health policies such as those addressed by one of its components, the Office of HIV/AIDS Policy. The president may have one or more members of the Domestic Policy Council watching and acting on health issues. Other groups include the Council of Economic Advisors (created in 1946), the Council of Environmental Quality (created 1969), and the National Security Council (created in 1947), which deals with such international public health issues as bioterrorism. The Office of Science and Technology Policy (created in 1976) serves as a source of scientific engineering and technological analysis and expertise for the president; the Office of National Drug Policy, established in 1988, coordinates federal efforts with state and local programs to control illegal drug use and devises national strategies to assure effective coordination of drug policies and programs. The Office of the U.S. Trade Representative, which was created in 1963, was made an agency within the executive office of the president in 1974. This office represents the United States for all activities of the General Agreement on Tariffs and Trade (GATT) and in other conferences and discussions in which trade and commodities are at issue for example, for the World Trade Organization. Recent public health issues handled by this office include food safety, prescription drug regulations, and tobacco product promotion and control.

President Clinton, for example, tended to articulate his priorities and lead high-profile efforts from the White House. In the case of the 1993 health-care reform effort, the legislation was largely developed within task forces led by Mrs. Clinton and Ira Magaziner from the White House with the DHHS both analyzing data and offering policy advice. That reform failed in 1994 due to strong interest group and congressional opposition. In the case of welfare reform in 1996, while the DHHS played an analytic role, many of its senior officials opposed the proposal and left the administration after its enactment. In this case, it was direct negotiations between Congress and the White House that resulted in legislation acceptable to the president. After 1996 Clinton used the mechanism of a senior health adviser to the president as his lead on health policy. This individual, who is also a deputy director of the Domestic Policy Council, serves as liaison with cabinet agencies on health issues to coordinate efforts among the White House entities and the DHHS and other cabinet offices as needed. President Bush has continued this pattern.

Congress and Special Interest Groups

The other major force in health policy making is Congress. Each house of Congress, the Senate and the House of Representatives, has a set of committees that deals with health issues. Two types of committees act on a given piece of health legislation. The first are the authorizing committees, which approve the substance of the legislation. The second are the appropriations committees, which decide whether to fund legislation and, if so, how much money will be appropriated for the particular activity outlined in the authorized legislation.

Jurisdiction over health-related issues is dispersed across many different congressional committees because of the complexity and scope of the underlying policy area. Lawrence Evans (1995) contends that virtually all authorizing committees in the House (except for the Select Committee on Intelligence) have some type of jurisdiction over health issues, and most authorizing committees in the Senate have some health related jurisdictions. The House and Senate parliamentarians determine which bills proposing policy changes and new programs will be referred to which committees for action. In looking at Library of Congress records on the percentage of health bills referred to House authorizing committees, Evans notes that the dominant committee is Commerce, since it has authority over Part B of Medicare and hundreds of programs within the Public Health Service dealing with a variety of issues. It also has jurisdiction over Title V (the Maternal and Child Health Act), Title XIV (Medicaid) of the Social Security Act, as well as those parts of Title XVIII (Part B of Medicare) not funded by payroll deductions. Second-most-important is the House Ways and Means Committee, which has major authority over Medicare Part A and some parts of Part B, as well as the entire tax code, which gives it authority over health insurance mechanisms related to tax income.

The other major health related authorizing committee in the House is the Economic and Educational Opportunities Committee, which handles 8% of health bills. Its major jurisdiction is over ERISA, the Employment Retirement and Security Act, which would place it squarely in the midst of any discussions of changes in health insurance benefits. Five other committees get a total of 5% each of the legislative referrals on health.

In the Senate, there are two dominant committees. The Senate Finance Committee has authority over health programs under Social Security, Medicare and Medicaid, and the Maternal and Child Health Act. The Labor and Human Resources Committee has jurisdiction over public health, biomedical research and alcohol, employee health and safety, ERISA, and special populations of children and elderly persons. Other committees receive less than 3% of bills on health.

In recent years approximately 20% of all House bills have been referred to more than one committee, but for health legislation this percentage is higher, with more than 40% percent of health bills referred during the 102nd Congress going to multiple committees. In the Senate, multiple referrals constituted less than 1% of bills referred during the 102nd Congress. Following the "Republican Revolution" in 1994, House Republicans moved to ban multiple referrals in the House, although some primary and secondary referrals to committees with overlapping jurisdiction still occur.

Each committee has specific subcommittees, and the potential for dispersed jurisdiction compounds the current fragmentation of the executive branch on health issues. Evans sites the example of the Clinton Comprehensive and Health Reform plan transmitted to Congress in the fall of 1993, for which Mrs. Clinton testified before five different House and Senate committees in a single week. After jurisdictional debates, the three key committees, Energy and Commerce, Ways and Means, and Labor were designated to have lead jurisdictions, but seven other panels wished to have testimony and hearings on a variety of issues within the bill nonetheless. On the Senate side, a similar power struggle broke out between the Finance Committee and Labor and Human Resources Committee. The committees eventually reviewed bills with the segments having to do with overlapping jurisdiction deleted. This diverse and controversial legislation would have required considerable consensus to move along, and such consensus could never be developed. It is evident that the differing jurisdictions could make passage difficult even for simpler legislation.

In the late 1990s, the major vehicles for legislative action were annual budget bills, which must be considered and passed by Congress to continue government funding. As a result, these jurisdictional conflicts among authorizing committees were less salient, as details were hammered out in appropriations committees.

Figure 9–2 shows the steps of the legislative process for a bill to become law. Initial action in both the House and Senate begins when legislation that is facing expiration must be renewed or when new legislative proposals are filed. Bills can originate in the executive branch, legislative branch, or in a constituency group. They must be filed in either the House or Senate, although eventually a bill must be filed for consideration in both houses in order to have a chance of becoming law. Once filed, a bill is referred to an authorizing committee or subcommittee by the House or Senate leadership. Hearings are held

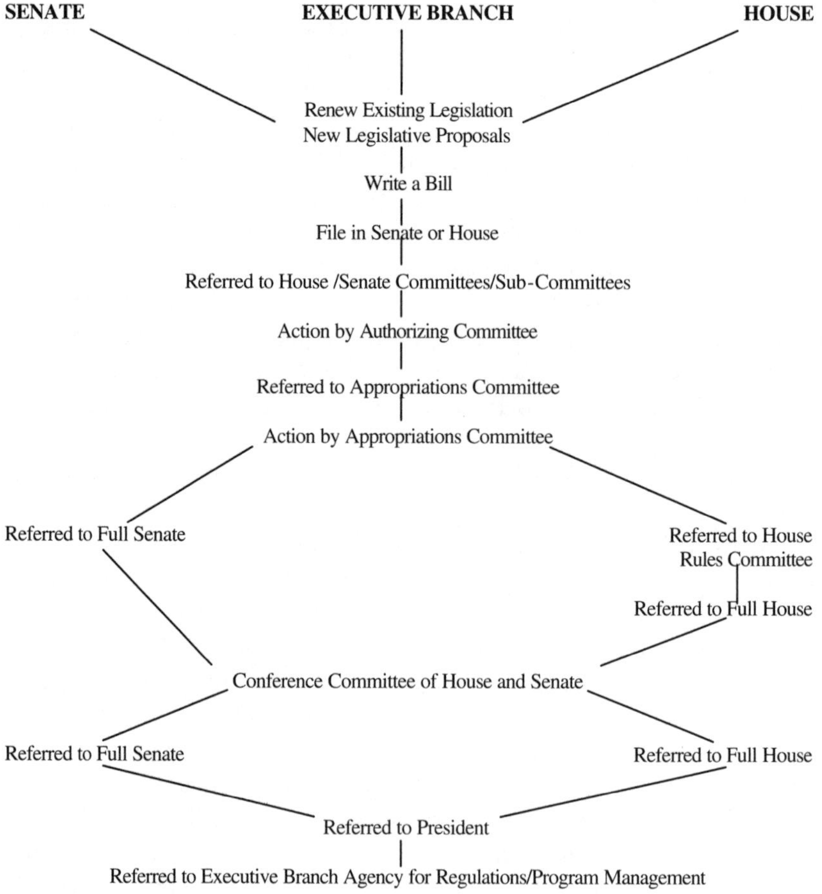

FIGURE 9–2. Legislative process.

and, if the authorization is approved, it is forwarded to the appropriations committee, which determines the level of budgetary support.

If both the authorizing and appropriations committees approve the bill, it is referred to the full Senate (via the House Rules Committee for a decision on how it will be handled) and the full House. Assuming the bill is passed by both houses, it is then referred to a conference committee. Members of the House and Senate are selected for this committee by the leadership of each of these bodies to reconcile any differences between the two bills. Once the committee agrees on a version, the bill is referred back to the full House and Senate and, if passed, sent to the president for his signature. After the president's approval, the new law is returned to the executive branch agency for development of regulations and/or program management guidance for its implementation. At any point during this process, special interest groups may be very active in requesting a change in one or another provision of a bill or in the amount of funding appropriated.

What Should Be Done

Given myriad organizations and interests that must be included in achieving a health policy goal, the reasons the categorical, issue-by-issue approach predominates and perpetuates fragmentation should be obvious. Each activity can be examined in its own right for the ethical values embedded in its goals and the methods chosen for its implementation. Yet it is possible to envision a way in which a comprehensive ethical framework that seeks to promote population health could help evaluate the appropriateness of actions in each area: policy making, financing, public health protection, collecting and disseminating information, capacity building for population health, and direct management to achieve this goal and reshape our health policy and programs accordingly. In the following sections, current problems and some opportunities to achieve such a change will be explored.

Policy making

Policy making is a critical function of a national health authority. It involves creating and using an evidence base that is informed by social values, so that public decision makers can shape legislation, regulations, and programs to achieve the agenda of the national leaders. In the United States, there is obviously a combined process of executive and legislative branch interaction influenced by a variety of stakeholders in the nongovernmental sector that is also tempered by judicial action. The major policy function of the DHHS is to initiate, shape, and, ultimately, implement and monitor the effects of legislation passed by Congress and signed by the president. It does this, as we have seen, in coordination with the White House and in consultation with Congress and interest groups.

The signature example of a policy effort to promote health is the program for setting national health goals, the Healthy People process, begun 20 years ago and led by the Office of Disease Prevention and Health Promotion in the Office of Public Health and Science (OPHS) of the Office of the Secretary of DHHS. The effort now involves all DHHS operating divisions and a number of federal departments and includes partnerships with state and local public health officials as well as more than 350 national membership organizations, nongovernmental organizations, and corporate sponsors. The program goal is to set and monitor progress on health goals for the American people. While the effort is voluntary, the activity and regular widespread public consultation involved has proven to be one of the department's most effective nonlegislative policy vehicles for promoting action on population health at national, state, and local levels.

Its vision, "Healthy People in Healthy Communities," centers around two goals: increasing quality and years of healthy life and eliminating health disparities. A menu of 467 scientifically based objectives in 25 focus areas was developed for the Healthy People 2010 cycle, which was launched in January 2000. Data from the National Center for Health Statistics is used to monitor progress on the chosen objectives and provide periodic reports to the American people on health status, health threats, and promising interventions. Ten leading indicators have been selected after wide public consultation and reviews by the Institute of Medicine on measurement feasibility: physical activity, overweight and obesity, tobacco use, substance abuse, responsible sexual behavior, mental health, injury and violence, environmental quality, immunization, and access to health care. All of these complex indicators are linked to underlying issues of education, income, and community support.

Forty-seven of the fifty states have published their own Healthy People objectives, and hundreds of community coalitions are involved in the process. Within the federal government, work groups led by various agencies are organized around key objectives and serve as ongoing vehicles for interdepartmental and cross-governmental collaboration. Regular public hearings and public meetings on specific objectives also include state and local health officials as well as academic experts and representatives of the private sector. This example of an inclusive policy process is fundamental to the kind of policy making that promotes broader health goals.

Financing

The major attention of the DHHS is on the financing of personal health care through the entitlement programs the of federal Medicare program and the federal/state Medicaid program. Other DHHS discretionary programs provide direct financial support for health services to particular segments of the population judged to be at risk. For instance, the Indian Health Service is the major provider of personal health care and public health services on Indian reservations and in Alaskan native villages, although 40% of these programs are now administered by tribes under contract and self-governance agreements. The uninsured receive care through Health Resources and Services Administration (HRSA) grants to community health centers. Care for individuals with HIV/AIDS is funded through Ryan White grants and preventive and care services for drug abusers and the mentally ill through Substance Abuse and Mental Health Services Administration (SAMHSA) block grants to states. Other departments provide federal funding for health-care services for specific beneficiaries. These departments include the Veterans Administration, the Department of Defense, and the Office of Personnel Management for federal employees and their dependents.

The other financing for health programs in the DHHS comes from discretionary budget funding for research, health work force development, and all other categorical programs largely targeted to population groups, diseases, and organizations. By far, the major portion of this discretionary budget (about half) goes to the National Institutes of Health for biomedical research. To date, federal financing priorities have not included a similar provision for systematic funding of the so-called public health infrastructure. This includes the people, information systems, research capacity, and organizational structures at national, state, and local levels that assure well-functioning programs exist for measuring a community's health status; disease surveillance and crisis intervention; assurance of safe water, food, pharmaceutical, and blood supply; waste disposal; population oriented disease prevention and health promotion education; and quality assurance of personal health services—all elements in a strategy for promoting population health. The Public Health Threats and Emergencies Act passed by Congress in the 2000 session begins the process of making such an investment.

Public health protection

This is perhaps the classic public health function, and it covers the areas in which the federal government uses its surveillance capacity to assess health risks as well as its standard setting and regulatory powers to protect the public from these risks. Because this health protection function is for the whole population, it can be a unifying activity in promoting health. Nonetheless, creative mechanisms that can develop and sustain effective working relationships and harmonize regulations within the DHHS, with the DHHS and other federal departments, and with state and local government are critical for effective action and require special management attention.

Standard setting and regulation at the federal level involves four broad areas of activity: (*1*) provider certification, for example, for clinical laboratories through the Clinical Laboratories Improvement Act (CLIA) and to permit health care providers to meet the standards of the Joint Commission on Accreditation of Health Care Organizations so they can receive Medicare funding in lieu of a separate federal survey process; (*2*) purchaser and insurer certification, for example, through collaboration with states to establish criteria for financial viability of health plans and insurance entities that permit them to operate in the marketplace; (*3*) standard setting, for example, for age appropriate preventive health schedules, immunization schedules, clean water and air, and work place safety as well as for the use of broad social marketing campaigns on issues like exercise, diet, and antitobacco campaigns, all supported by scientific research and expert advisory groups convened by the NIH, CDC, and FDA. Quality standards are also set by HCFA for providers of health care to receive Medicare payments; and (*4*) regulations, for example, for the quality of foods, the safety and efficacy of drugs, biologics like blood products and tissues, medical devices, and cosmetics. Several other departments have regulatory authority in various areas of health like food, environment, occupational safety, transportation, and consumer products.

Some of the major challenges to the effective use of DHHS regulatory and standard-setting powers to promote and protect population health more effectively involve the need to address inconsistencies both within DHHS agencies that have overlapping jurisdictions, as well as those between DHHS agencies and other science-based regulatory agencies. Another challenge involves the integration of standard setting and regulations in health at the federal level with equally varied jurisdictions of state and local health departments or other health related agencies. The President's Food Safety Initiative, for example, is attempting to tackle this challenge, and the Environmental Protection Agency has developed models for directly working with state and local governments on environmental standards. The federal government's interaction with foreign governments on health issues is also increasing.

COLLECTING AND DISSEMINATING INFORMATION

The federal government is also responsible for the collection and dissemination of information relating to the health status of the population and the health-care delivery systems. The U.S. Census, part of the Department of Commerce, has the most basic data collection responsibilities. The National Center for Health Statistics (NCHS) within the Centers for Disease Control (CDC) is the primary agency collecting and reporting health information for the federal government. Data gathering for public health purposes is a shared responsibility with state and local governments. The collection and dissemination of information includes at least six functions: (*1*) national vital and health statistics, (*2*) population health surveys, (*3*) health-care delivery cost and utilization information, (*4*) disaster surveillance, (*5*) research findings, and (*6*) reporting requirements for federal grant and aid funded programs.

The National Committee for Vital and Health Statistics (NCVHS) is the key external advisory body to the secretary on data activities across the entire DHHS. Its membership has recently been broadened to include multiple stakeholders in the department's data systems. Working with the DHHS Data Council and the NCHS and through a broad national consultative process, it developed a draft report issued in June 2000 entitled "Shaping A Vision for 21st Century Health Statistics." This is a plan to "provide the information needed to enable the American public to achieve and maintain the best possible health." Principles were provided to guide the development of the vision. Among them are initiatives intended to arrive at:

- A conceptual framework using broad determinants of health;
- Data that is useful at different levels of aggregation to reflect local, state, and national concerns;
- Maximum access and ease of use;
- Broad multisectoral collaboration and sufficient resources.

This plan is linked to another NCVHS project to develop the National Health Information Infrastructure (NHII). The NHII is the health component of the National Information Infrastructure (NII), sometimes called the Information Super Highway that evolved from the Telecommunications Act of 1993. The Internet is central to the NHII, and the Next Generation Internet (NGI) is a series of projects supported by a public–private sector partnership. The NIH is the lead health agency, yet the DHHS must support identification and financing of the resources needed over a sustained period of five to ten years to develop a comprehensive health information infrastructure that effectively links federal, state, and local government health entities with one another and with the critical entities in the private sector to assure that we have the health data and the ability to process and consider the data to develop effective health policy for individuals, providers, and the public.

CAPACITY BUILDING FOR POPULATION HEALTH

Infrastructure

The capacity building function of the federal government must ensure that the government's own agencies can effectively discharge their responsibilities to assure and promote the health of the communities they serve. It must also ensure that other levels of government that share responsibilities in health have the resources—human, financial, and organizational—to carry out their responsibilities, whether delegated to them by the federal government or for which they are responsible by law.

The major federal investments in capacity building have been aimed toward research, human resources development, and capital development of facilities within the personal health-care and biomedical research systems. These foci mirror the emphasis in federal health policy and health-care financing. A series of annual DHHS reports to Congress have called for enhanced funding of the public health workforce, citing inadequacies emphasized in the 1988 Institute of Medicine study on the "Future of Public Health" (1998). Specifically, epidemiologists are needed to conduct surveillance and to track disease incidence, as are physicians trained in occupational and environmental health. Gebbie and Tilson are completing the first national survey of the public health workforce in 20 years. Absent a significant investment in human resources, the United States will not meet the Healthy People 2010 objective for the public health workforce (personal communication). An investment is also needed in other components of the public health infrastructure, for example, federal, state, and local information systems for surveillance and detection of health threats, clinical laboratories, and environmental monitoring systems needed for water quality, waste disposal, and air quality monitoring at the state and community levels.

Management Reforms

Management attention is another important aspect of capacity building that is critical to achieving population health. This aspect is necessary to achieve successful collaboration within and across government agencies, between government and the corporate sector, as well as between nongovernmental organizations and communities. Such collaboration is critical because an effective health policy that addresses the multiple determinants of health must integrate action across government departments and with entities outside government that promote education and economic development as well as environmental, health, and social policy. The collaborative effort must have clarity of purpose if it is to achieve a public health policy that includes specific negotiation of methods to be used, as well as the resources—human, financial, and organizational—to manage these relationships in both formal and informal structures. We must move from a vertical focus on managing myriad specific programs to a horizontal focus on the linkages needed to make these programs work for people in the communities in which they live—in order to promote and protect their health. The same challenge exists for multi-agency collaboration on international health policy.

Of course, cross-cutting issues have always been the real problem. What is different now is the large number of them. This creates a greater and greater pressure for network management, or managing at the interface. If we do not undertake this sort of management, we will fall short of achieving all that we can. We thus need to ensure that management reform is supported and rewarded as a primary function of government.

DIRECT MANAGEMENT OF SERVICES

Except for health services for the military through the Department of Defense and the work of the Veterans Health Administration, only an extremely small part of health care is directly managed by the federal government, due to both the significant levels of decentralization in the U.S. system and our high use of intermediaries to deliver federal funds and services. One example of such a directly managed service that combines personal health care and population oriented services is the Indian Health Service (IHS). Funded as a federal delivery system for Indian peoples in federally recognized tribes, it provides personal care and public health services primarily to those living or seeking care on reservations. The program is changing dramatically as the policy of support for tribal self-governance sees tribes taking their shares of funding for health services and managing them directly through contract arrangements. One can imagine a future in which the IHS becomes a payer/ purchaser instead of a provider. The IHS has also played an important role in providing elements of the public health infrastructure to reservations. It has trained community health workers who promote programs of community education on major health threats like alcoholism, drug abuse, diabetes, and accidents. It has provided information systems to track community health status and the use of health services, and it has furnished the capital investments needed to create systems for safe water and effective waste disposal. These roles will be key elements in promoting and protecting health among Indian peoples and Alaska natives. Nonetheless, enhanced investments in these systems are badly needed.

CONCLUSION

The federal role in health has evolved over many years, and it is complex and increasingly important to the country's well being. The science and health expertise in the United States that serves as the basis for health action within the federal government and through its partnerships with state and local health departments, universities, and nonprofit organizations is unique in the world and increasingly called upon as a global resource. It should be apparent that enormous opportunities exist for the federal government to play an increasingly effective role in promoting and protecting health in both the domestic and international arena. To do this, however, we must overcome obstacles inherent in both the current emphasis of our health policy and the current balance of resource investments in its implementation. The elements for the necessary changes are already present within the system but need greater focus and support to play a more effective role. By using an ethical framework that advocates a health policy that promotes population health, we can analyze the relative effectiveness of our current health policies and investments. Based on this analysis, we can sustain the best of the current priorities and build on them to broaden the potential for even greater improvements in both our nation's health and the ability of the United States to contribute to health improvement globally.

NOTES

1. One proponent of the bill, Alexander Hamilton, did advocate care for a needy group, but there was greater emphasis on the fact that the availability of care "would attract men into service to the country" and therefore would be in the national commercial interest. The financing structure supported self-reliance and kept care in the private sector.

REFERENCES

Anderson G (1997) In search of value: An international comparison of cost, access and outcomes. *Health Affairs* 16:163–71.

Boufford JI (1999) Crisis, leadership, consensus: The past and future federal role in health. *Journal of Urban Health: Bulletin of The New York Academy of Medicine* 76: 192–206.

DiIullio, JT Jr. and Kettl DF (1995) *The Contract with America: Devolution and The Administrative Realities of American Federalism.* Washington, DC: Center for Public Management, Brookings Institution.

Evans L (1995) Committees and health jurisdiction in Congress. In: Mann T and Ornstein N (eds) (1995) *Intensive Care: How Congress Shapes Health Policy.* Washington, DC: Brookings Institution, American Enterprise Institute.

Evans R, Barer M, Marmor T (1994) *Why Are Some People Healthy and Others Not? The Determinants of Health of Populations.* New York: Aldine de Gruyter.

Gostin LO (2000) Public health law in a new century, parts I, II, III. *Journal of the American Medical Association* 283: 2837–2p41, 2979–2984, 3118–3122.

Institute of Medicine (1998) *The Future of Public Health.* Washington, DC: National Academy Press.

Kindig D (1997) *Purchasing Population Health: Paying for Results.* Ann Arbor, MI: University of Michigan Press.

Lee PR and Benjamin AE (1998) Health policy and the politics of health care. In: Williams SJ and Torrens PR (eds) *Introduction to Health Services*, 4th ed. New York: Delmar Publishers.

Marmot M (1994) Social differentials in health within and between populations. *Daedalus: Journal of the American Academy of Arts and Sciences, Special Issue, Health and Wealth* 123: 197–217.

Marmot M, Rose G, Shipley MJ, and Hamilton PHS (1978) Employment grade and coronary heart disease in British civil servants. *Journal of Epidemiology and Community Health*. 32:244–9.

Healthy People 2010. July 13, 1999. http://www.health.gov/healthypeople/2010fctsht.htm

McGinnis J and Foege W (1993) Actual causes of death in the United States. *Journal of the American Medical Association*. 270:2208.

McKeown T (1976) *The Role of Medicine: Dream, Mirage, or Nemesis?* London: Nuffield Provincial Hospital Trust.

Mustard HS (1945) *Government in Public Health*. New York: Commonwealth Fund.

Osborne D (1998) *Laboratories of Democracy*. Cambridge, MA: Harvard Business School Press.

United States Department of Health and Human Services (2000) *Better Information for Better Health: Towards a National Health Information Infrastructure*. Washington, DC: USDHHS.

Walker DB (1981) *Towards A Functioning Federalism*. Cambridge, MA: Winthrop Publishers.

Wilkinson R and Marmot M (1988) *Social Determinants of Health—The Solid Facts*. World Health Organization.

World Health Organization (2000) Health systems: Improving performance. *The World Health Report 2000*. Geneva: World Health Organization.

10

Health policy and state initiatives

JONATHAN OBERLANDER AND LAWRENCE D. BROWN

As the polity grows impatient with the status quo in health care but fears "too much government," the states are repeatedly invited to lead and innovate. Several distinctive features of American political life lend recourse to the states a hardy, if not perennial, appeal. The United States is a federal system whose constitution honors states' rights in several social spheres. Political culture—traditional American distaste for big, central government and the corresponding affection for checks and balances—powerfully reinforces these formalities. American lore contends that states are "closer to the people" and hence more responsive than national government to the demands of the people. States are also said to be "laboratories of democracy," valuable testing grounds for policy innovations that may wax or wane incrementally in the clarifying light of subnational experience (Leichter, 1996). And devolution—turning back power to the states—is a staple of the conservative agenda that understandably enjoys much political "prime time" when, as in the last 30 years, conservatives have been powerful.

Health-care policies are very much formed of this political mold and mind-set. American physicians have long insisted that the professional judgments of private practitioners should run the show, a claim that critics have long derided as "provider dominance." Voluntarism—leadership of local health care arrangements by nonprofit hospitals and insurers working cooperatively with employers and physicians—enjoys enormous legitimacy among the many Americans who cling to the tenet that "health is a community affair." Yet, with rare exceptions, most notably the National Institutes of Health and Medicare, unapologetically national programs are not politically credible solutions to the unmistakable falterings of the private and professional organizations and actors who run the "community affair." When the call to arms grows loud, states are regularly drafted into battles to expand hospital capacity (Hill Burton legislation), constrain hospital capacity (certificate of need), deter overuse of services by physicians (peer review organizations), plan resources in light of needs (health planning agencies), regulate health insurance plans, and supply medical coverage for the poor (Medicaid).

Critics often charge that the celebrated civic virtues of state discretion obscure glaring ethical liabilities. If health care is in some sense a human or civil right, then subnational disparities in the terms on which it is made available should be viewed as objectionable inequities. The states' fabled "closeness to the people" likewise begs a crucial ethical question, namely, which people? If state policies are disproportionately shaped by people with the money, time, skill, and organization to advance their interests in the political process, less resourceful citizens may get short shrift, or, at any rate, shorter shrift than equity demands. Finally, federalism itself arguably has anti-redistributive features. States compete with one another for the good things of economic life—business, jobs, tax base—in a ceaseless pursuit that generosity to the disadvantaged does nothing to promote. On each of these three counts, so the critical argument goes, equity counsels that the discretion of the states in health policy be checked and balanced by firm national rules that honor the rights and claims of American citizens (Sparer and Brown, 1986).

Though this debate is often waged globally as a matter of abstract principle, it is best illuminated locally by close inspection of concrete issues contemplated in policy time and political space. Here we try to make practice speak to principle by examining two very prominent health policy issues on state agendas: the replacement of Medicaid's traditional fee-for- service system with managed care and the adoption of new public regulations governing managed care organizations (MCOs) that serve not only Medicaid beneficiaries but also much of the privately insured population.

State health policy making in the decade of the 1990s wavered between promoting market-based health care and reigning it in. States have aggressively enrolled their Medicaid populations in managed care. Meanwhile, an increasing number of states are enacting restrictions on the practices of health maintenance organizations (HMOs) and other managed care plans. Managed care regulation, ranging from mandated external appeals processes for patients protesting denials of care to asset requirements for health plans, is now widespread, though far from uniform, at the state level.

These policy innovations—promotion of Medicaid managed care and adoption of managed care regulations—arguably represent the two most important movements in state health policy during the 1990s. They thus raise many of the critical issues facing American health policy makers: how to control the costs of public insurance programs, what role should the market play in health-care delivery in public programs, and what responsibility should the government take in shaping the medical market?

From the perspective of policy making, these two policy innovations also offer a striking contrast. Philosophically, state health policy making appears to be bipolar, at once promoting and limiting managed care. Furthermore, these two policies have diverged in terms of process, as well. The movement en masse of Medicaid recipients into managed care has attracted scant attention and produced rather modest public debate and legislative struggle. In contrast, the debate over managed care regulation has enjoyed prime time in the public spotlight, garnering substantial media, public, and legislative attention.

We highlight these two policy innovations and their contrasting development with the aim of shedding light on the ethical implications of state health policy and how it is made. The contrasting trajectories of Medicaid managed care and managed care regulation reveal much about the different ways that ethical considerations influence state policy makers and the limits as well as opportunities of principled thinking in the making of public policy.

GOVERNMENT AND HEALTH POLICY IN THE UNITED STATES

Before examining these policy areas, it is worth considering the broader context of health policy and ethics that influences state action. The central issue in American public policy is what constitutes a legitimate basis for governmental intervention in private activities. This is not to say that government does not intervene a lot, nor to deny that it has done so all along more than official ideology suggests (principle has often yielded to pragmatism), nor even to discount substantial intervention even in antigovernment regimes (witness the adoption of Medicare prospective payment for hospitals by the Reagan administration). It is to say that this question of the legitimate bases of intervention is often a central issue and that it is fundamentally ethical, a question of what constitutes "good" or the "right" public policy. Health care in this nation is not viewed as a right, but as a good that should be supplied privately insofar as possible and publicly insofar as private provision is not possible.

The government (mainly the federal government in the United States) threw itself into modern health policy after World War II because there was general agreement that the production of medical technology, research, hospitals, and physicians would fall below what the public wanted absent public subsidies. More spending was, quite simply, assumed to result in better medical care; thus the expansion of the National Institutes of Health, Hill-Burton legislation to fund hospital construction, and various measures to adjust the medical workforce (Starr, 1982). Next came the hard part, the part that other societies view as the core of health policy, namely, deciding on the terms in which government should intervene in the employer-based health insurance system to help parts of the population pay their medical bills. Other countries have answered that question with relative ease. Coverage secured by the state is either a universal right of citizenship or a right extended to those below a certain income ceiling, who presumably cannot afford to make their own arrangements. In the United States, by contrast, this has been a troubling question, answered only with difficulty and still not conclusively.

The nation's most successful encounter with this question yielded the enactment of Medicare and Medicaid in 1965 (Marmor, 1973). These two programs rested on quite distinct principles of legimitacy, or ethical frameworks. Medicare targeted a group, the elderly, portrayed as both needy and deserving. The aged were vulnerable, unable to work, had paid their dues, and faced high costs if they became seriously ill—a burden to themselves and, of course, to their children, as well. Medicare was also suffused with the ethical imagery that developed Social Security and social insurance: One gets back what one pays in through payroll taxes—benefits are *earned*—in contrast to welfare, whose benefits are widely viewed as a handout. Social insurance thereby conjures up a normative image of the relations between citizen and state in contractual terms. The strategic image is officially anti-redistributive, which is key to its popularity (albeit highly misleading) (Derthick, 1979).

The key ethical issue is precisely the legitimacy of redistribution and the cross-subsidies it entails. By what right does government stick its hand into the pockets of some and create entitlements for others? This question is far less vexing in most industrialized democracies that understand such transfers as the essence of what is fair and right: There should be transfers from the better-off to the less affluent, from the healthier to the sicker, from younger to older, from the working to the unemployed, from small families to large ones, and so forth. And there must be such transfers if the welfare state, including universal health coverage, is to work. One can do it by means of general revenues (taxes, as in the British National Health Service) or by means of social insurance (such as in Germany), but subsidies there must be, and on a wide scale.

In the United States, the politics of these moral questions works differently: Social insurance was crucial to answering "handout" objections (i.e., opposition to the government providing benefits to individuals or groups who have not earned them or are otherwise deemed undeserving), and so Medicare was successfully grafted onto Social Security (Jacobs, 1993), but the poor were another story. Only those poor who could not work were judged worthy of governmental support. Social insurance therefore was out of the picture a priori. The medical assistance supplied by Medicaid was grafted onto welfare and entailed transparent redistribution of taxpayers' money. Medicaid was not enhanced by any legitimacy derived from contractual imagery. Quite the contrary, Medicaid was saddled with the stigma of welfare and, rather than the highly successful Social Security program, its programmatic anchor became the politically troubled Aid to Families with Dependent Children (AFDC). The vocabulary of American social assistance reflects and reinforces this distinction. Medicare enrollees are commonly referred to as "beneficiaries," connoting a sense of deserved entitlement, while Medicaid enrollees are "recipients," suggesting they are the objects of government largesse.

Meanwhile, the debate continued (and still does) over what to say and do about Americans who qualify neither for these public programs nor for private coverage. Evidently, the uninsured fit no culturally recognized principle of legitimate intervention, and the continuing debate can be viewed as, among other things, an endless effort to postulate such a principle in politically acceptable terms. Thus far, every effort has failed.

MANAGED CARE AND PUBLIC PROGRAMS

Federal promotion of HMOs began as the Nixon administration's answer to cost increases in Medicare (Brown, 1983). There would be a Medicare Part C that would give beneficiaries the chance to join efficient prepaid plans. (Kaiser Permanente and Group Health were the models for these plans). In the early 1970s the Senate Finance Committee opposed this proposal bitterly, contending that free choice of provider was a crucial value to Medicare that had been clearly ensconced in the statute. Subsequent administrations kept pushing, however, and in 1982 a formal risk-based (i.e., capitated payment) managed care program was added to Medicare. However, the initiative avoided heavy pressures and sharp-edged incentives to move the elderly into HMOs, for a hard sell for HMOs was not viewed as compatible with the social contract character of the program—nor, of course, with the electoral and organizational power of the aged. The 1997 legislation that introduced market reforms into the program was called Medicare + Choice—hype, to be sure, but also revealing. In a social insurance program, beneficiaries have rights and are entitled to choice. They are not to be pushed around by the state and forced into HMOs. Accordingly, mandatory Medicare managed care has never been a serious possibility.

Medicaid is a very different matter. As with Medicare, costs rose at a worrisome rate in the 1970s, 1980s, and early 1990s (Coughlin et al, 1994). But, as a welfare-based program, Medicaid fell into the laps of the states, which had to cope with the fiscal burden. The moral claims of the money issue were politically disquieting: The program was taking ever-larger sums of taxpayers' money and redistributing it to poor welfare recipients. It did so at the expense of other political priorities that were ostensibly of more "general interest," such as schools, jails, and roads, and it used up political capital on groups that were unorganized and seldom voted.

The issue therefore became what to cut—eligibility, benefits, or payments to providers—and in what combination. Debate on these options reflected ethical judgments quite directly: Should fewer people be made eligible for equal or greater benefits, or should those eligible be more numerous and the benefits fewer, as proposed by the state of Oregon, whose rationing plan pledged allegiance to the principle of the greatest good for the greatest number (Jacobs et al, 1999)? Should providers bear the brunt of cutbacks? If so, eligibility and benefits for the poor would be preserved, but reduced provider reimbursement and diminished willingness of providers to participate in the program with concomitant decreases in access might turn these benefits into formalities.

As ethical judgment, political ideology, and group influence played out, in general, in the following fashion: (*1*) eligibility went up and down—down to Medicaid covering only 40% of the poor under the Reagan administration and back up to 50% by the end of the 1990s; (*2*) benefits stayed constant—mainly because federal policy makers held the line; and (*3*) payments to providers were constrained and access to medical services for recipients became more difficult. Fee-for-service Medicaid consequently came to be widely derided for providing poor access to care and bad value for money.

MEDICAID MANAGED CARE

Into this context came Medicaid managed care. Policymakers favor MCOs because they embody the right incentives (Brown, 1983). In theory, they provide better access and quality, and at lower cost. But could one legitimately take free choice of provider from the poor when the middle class had it? Only Arizona had done this forthrightly since 1982 by requiring its Medicaid enrollees to join prepaid, capitated managed care plans. Under these circumstances, then, the right thing to do is to make it voluntary for the poor and try to induce them to join MCOs. When managed care became mainstream and middle class, the imposition of managed care on Medicaid enrollees had a different moral implication: Now it would be fair for the public sector to require the poor to join the same kinds of plans private employees had to join.

The ethical underpinnings of the issue, however, go well beyond the intuition that "if the middle class has to suffer managed care, the poor should, too." The positive theory of Medicaid managed care reassured political leaders that everything would be for the best in this best of all possible worlds. If managed care plans could be induced to enter the Medicaid market, they would bring along doctors to serve it. Medicaid recipients could then choose among plans and among the doctors in those plans—a victory for access and quality, indeed a victory for choice itself, given the sad state into which fee-for-service Medicaid had fallen. Moreover, according to managed care theory, plans would hold physicians and hospitals accountable, and the states, in turn, would hold the plans to account.

This is an attractive and not absurd theory, but to make markets work as postulated, states have to do substantially more managing. This management entails new agency tasks (Sparer, 1996, 1998). Not all are up to the challenge; indeed, one wonders how many see the challenge clearly. Once the doubts regarding the equity issue of imposing managed care on the poor faded, states found it all too easy to fall back on the literal theory of Medicaid managed care and, accordingly, to undervalue management and organizational considerations. After all, the theory of managed care paints a clear and straightforward image of how incentives and market forces balance quality, access, and cost for the best. On the other hand, the "theory" of organizations, management, and public administration mainly offers arcane and murky images of how things go awry in "bureaucracies." The interests of the poor may get caught in an unequal contest between these two analytic images, between the theory of managed care and the reality of implementation. As such, policy makers who want to do the right thing may be lulled by soothing theoretical assurances that obscure the practical complexities in making certain that managed care keeps its promises (Brown, 1983).

States had good reason to take the theory and run with it. Medicaid spending consumed a growing share of state budgets in the 1980s and early 1990s, earning the program the unflattering moniker of "Pac-man," or alternatively "the monster that ate the states." Nationwide, Medicaid spending rose from $74 billion in 1990 to $168 billion in 1997; between 1988 and 1992, expenses rose at an annual average rate of 22%. As spending led, managed care followed: In 1991 10% of Medicaid recipients were in MCOs; at the end of the decade, more than half—54%—were (Kaiser Commission on Medicaid, 1999; HIAA, 1998).

Medicaid managed care, then, held out the promise to solve a dual dilemma in Medicaid: controlling costs while improving access to quality care. The argument for how managed care can square this circle has been elaborated elsewhere and does not bear repeating here. Yet there is little doubt that fiscal considerations were the primary motivation for state health policy makers in moving toward managed care. In fiscal terms, managed care did not simply offer to slow down Medicaid expenditures; it held out the promise of budgetary control. To the extent that states moved toward Medicaid systems based on capitated payment, policy makers found comfort in the notion that program spending would be predictable, providing a measure of budgetary certainty. To be sure, in addition to improved access, other reasons beyond fiscal savings and budgetary control were cited for the move to managed care: "mainstreaming" Medicaid recipients by bringing them into the same health plans as middle-class populations, assuring continuity of care, increasing the efficiency of Medicaid service delivery by relying on the business expertise of commercial health plans rather than on traditional arrangements with safety-net providers, improving the quality of care through case management of chronic illness and integration of services, and reducing the regulatory burden on state administrators by changing their role from micromanaging the program to contracting with health plans who would set fees and clinical protocols and organize delivery systems (Grogan, 1997).

Medicaid managed care also seemed to make good financial sense for MCOs. By the mid-1990s, the managed care industry dominated insurance coverage for the employed population, and only two large bastions of unmanaged care remained: Medicare and Medicaid. Capturing the Medicaid market promised an expanded market share and a new source of revenue. To be sure, doing business with state Medicaid plans had potential down sides: dealing with public bureaucracies rather than private employers, exposing contracts to public scrutiny, and managing care for patients who presented more complexities and challenges than did relatively healthier privately employed enrollees. Yet the real burden of these risks was only to be realized later. In the halcyon days of the early to mid-1990s, Medicaid managed care resembled a gold rush, as health plans often willingly absorbed short-term financial losses in exchange for new "covered lives." Medicaid was a critical component of many health plans' growth strategies. Between 1998 and 1999, increases in Medicaid HMO enrollment accounted for 38% of total HMO growth in the United States (Interstudy, 1999).

Although a comprehensive review of the performance of Medicaid managed care is beyond the scope of this discussion, it is fair to say that managed care has not served as the magic bullet that health plans had promised and for which states had hoped (Holahan et al, 1998; Sparer, 1998). This much is clear: Savings, though tangible in some states, have been lower than originally expected; managed care has increased rather than diminished the regulatory role of state governments by enlisting them in a whole new set of responsibilities, such as management of risk selection and supervision of marketing practices; and improvements in access and quality of care have been sporadic, as evidence accumulates that many plans have done little to manage the medical care of program enrollees. The future of Medicaid managed care has also grown uncertain as commercial plans, mirroring trends in Medicare, have started to leave the program. Ironically, they cite as reasons for exiting the Medicaid market insufficient payments and excessive state regulation, precisely the two problems that the introduction of managed care was supposed to fix in traditional Medicaid. Finally, an unintended consequence of Medicaid managed care and the redirection of state dollars to commercial health plans has been to further jeopardize the precarious position of the nation's network of safety net clinics, as they lose revenues to care for the most vulnerable and costliest enrollees in the Medicaid population as well as the uninsured (Gray and Rowe, 2000). None of this, however, should obscure the reality that the older fee-for-service Medicaid was riddled with serious problems.

For our purposes, there are four intriguing points relating to the emergence of Medicaid managed care. First, there has been only limited controversy associated with moving Medicaid recipients into managed care. Legislative debates generally focused not on whether to adopt Medicaid managed care, but rather over which model to select. The desirability of Medicaid managed care, in other words, was largely taken for granted by state policy makers. Evidence that poor, chronically ill patients may not fare well in HMOs, as well as questions about the scope of expected financial savings and the capacity of commercial plans to take care of populations with different needs than their employed market, could have given legislators pause, but they rarely did, and Medicaid managed care became a policy consensus in short order.

Second, there has never been a national public debate over the wisdom of enrolling Medicaid recipients into managed care plans. In part, this quiescence reflects a structural feature of Medicaid politics. Since there are 50 separate Medicaid programs, there is rarely national debate over Medicaid policy. Neither has there been a great deal of public debate within states regarding Medicaid managed care. For example, many surveys have measured public attitudes regarding dissatisfaction with managed care and support for various consumer protection proposals (Kaiser Family Foundation,

2000). In contrast, how many surveys have been commissioned to measure the public's reaction to Medicaid managed care? In an era in which political discourse is dominated by polling, to be left off public opinion questionnaires in the United States is to be truly invisible in the body politic. In terms of public opinion, the Medicaid population is often not counted and consequently does not count politically.

A third point is that the constituency targeted for Medicaid managed care has never enjoyed any significant voice in the decision-making process. Medicaid policy has been made on behalf of the poor, but never by the poor.

The relatively quiescent, noncontroversial, and client-absent politics of Medicaid managed care contrast sharply with Medicare's experience. As with Medicaid, health plans have sought access to the Medicare market, and policymakers have viewed managed care as a solution to Medicare's problems of rising costs and inadequate benefits. However, the pace of managed care growth in Medicare has been far slower than in Medicaid. In 1999 17% of Medicare enrollees were enrolled in managed care, compared with 54% in Medicaid (Interstudy, 1999). Moreover, while 40 states have implemented mandatory Medicaid managed care for specific regions or populations, the decision to join a Medicare HMO remains voluntary for the elderly and disabled program beneficiaries. Nor has the politics of Medicare managed care been quiescent. When the Republican Congressional leadership proposed Medicare reform legislation in 1995, including provisions designed to encourage more Medicare beneficiaries to enroll in HMOs, the plan triggered an outcry about the propriety of forcing seniors into managed care. Finally, unlike low-income Medicaid recipients, political organizations representing the elderly played an active role in the debate over Medicare reform. In fact, Medicaid managed care has thus far been limited predominantly to low-income adults and their children (recipients of the cash-assistance program formerly known as AFDC). In contrast, elderly and disabled beneficiaries, who together consume roughly 70% of all Medicaid spending (Coughlin et al, 1994), have, for the most part, not been targeted. Presumably, policy makers have shied away from the controversy that would come with mandating managed care for these more politically organized and sympathetic populations. Altering health care arrangements for welfare recipients comes with far less political baggage.

A fourth point, and one that is crucial to the ethics of health policy making, is that the move to Medicaid managed care represents much more than a change in the type of medical care provided by the program. Put simply, in key respects it embodies the privatization of public policy. By adopting managed care for their Medicaid populations, public policy makers have effectively ceded operation of critical components of the program to private policymakers: HMOs and other insurers. There may be a corresponding reduction in accountability to the public and to legislators. Privatizing Medicaid policy serves several aspirations of politicians, including blame avoidance. Decisions on how to control costs and ration care are left to health plans as Medicaid policy is moved out of the public arena.

Proponents of Medicaid managed care prefer to view the growing role of private health plans as a public–private partnership that improves accountability. Instead of setting recipients adrift in search of fee-for-service physicians who decide for themselves whether and how to treat them, members of Medicaid MCOs choose among physicians who come with, and face review by, plans. Moreover, states can and sometimes do design regulations that govern both conditions according to which plans may play in the Medicaid market as well as the access and quality criteria they must meet to stay in it. It would be unfair to dismiss these putative gains as mere theory, but it would be misleading to fail to note that these enhancements in accountability are highly contingent on the commitment to rigor and know-how of complex organizations (MCOs and public agencies) whose performance is neither well understood nor uniform across states and markets (Brown, 1983).

Yet, to the extent that managed care plans become the foundation for delivering health services, establishing that accountability is one step further away. The responsibility for problems with medical care delivery in Medicaid can be placed on the plans. Medicaid patients who want to appeal denials of coverage or other problems may have to fight through the private bureaucracy of HMOs before accessing public forums. And, ultimately, key decisions about Medicaid, such as which services to prioritize and which medical care delivery institutions should be funded, are increasingly left to private policymakers.

Ethical perspectives on state health policy making should take into account the goals of policy makers, the substantive outcomes of policy initiatives, and the processes by which policy is made. The goals of Medicaid managed care—controlling costs, improving access to medical providers, and enhancing quality of care—are all praiseworthy. However, as states have discovered over time, simultaneously achieving all of these goals is a difficult enterprise. The extent to which one of these goals is preeminent varies across the states and according to differences in political culture, wealth, and partisan composition of legislatures. However, to the extent that financial savings is the central goal in many states, it threatens to crowd out concerns over quality and access as well as other ethical considerations.

Although the substantive outcomes of Medicaid managed care have not been carefully examined, the emerging picture is decidedly mixed. If protecting vulnerable populations is the core value of health insurance, the traditional Medicaid program had fared poorly, proving once again the political dictum that programs for the poor are poor programs. Medicaid managed care, though a significant step forward in some states, has not consistently improved the situation of program beneficiaries. While some program enrollees now have better access to primary care and other services through HMOs, the most vulnerable segments of the Medicaid population may not be well served by payment arrangements that make chronically ill and expensive patients financial "losers" for health plans and medical providers (Ware et al, 1996).

Finally, an ethics premised on process asks who should be making policy and what system of decision making is the most fair. Again, under traditional Medicaid arrangements, recipients enjoyed little representation in policy making, and that has not changed under managed care, though there are now efforts underway in some states to gauge beneficiary satisfaction regarding the performance and quality of health plans. The more critical development may be that of the change in who makes Medicaid policy and in what venues decisions are made. If democratic accountability is an important ethical value, then managed care further erodes its realization by privatizing policy making. The health care market is driven by the search for more patients and more profits, and, left on its own, it will not spend much time worrying about normative issues of representation, resource allocation, and procedural fairness for Medicaid recipients. How and whether ethical considerations might be made more explicit and given greater consideration in state policy making is a topic we return to at the end of this chapter.

REGULATION OF MANAGED CARE

Another cornerstone of a widely recognized moral foundation for state intervention in health care is the demand to protect consumers from excessive concentrations of economic power. This has been a long-standing theme that justifies state intervention in the United States; monopolies and unfair competitors (and other kindred malefactors) must not be allowed to trample on the little guy (producer and/or consumer), yet this has not been a prominent theme in health care, which took on industrial hues only recently. Now, with the arrival of managed care and for-profit companies, health seems to fit quite easily into this traditional regulatory rationale (Moran, 1997).

While Congress has had an interest in a patient's bill of rights, by 2000, 48 states had actually enacted some form of managed care regulation, and more than 20 states had passed comprehensive bills of rights (Stauffer and Levy, 2000). Accordingly, the backlash against managed care may be a national phenomenon, but the states are its legislative epicenter.

Managed care regulations vary widely. The most common form of regulation is a prohibition against so-called gag clauses whereby health plans do not permit physicians to discuss all treatment options with patients. Other regulations include requiring the establishment of independent review boards to which patients may appeal health plan decisions; guaranteeing access to emergency services and specialists; mandating direct access to obstetrician-gynecologists or provisions that they may serve as primary care providers; "any willing provider" laws that prohibit health plans from excluding qualified physicians from their provider panels; restrictions on financial incentives that plans use to influence the medical care decisions of physicians; and requiring HMOs to offer a point of service option that provides some coverage for patients to see physicians outside the health plan network. As of 2000 only three states had passed legislation that enables patients to sue HMOs for denial of coverage or inadequate care, a provision that figures prominently in the national debate about patient protection legislation (Stauffer and Levy, 2000).

The rhetoric of managed care regulation promises to restore patients' rights, protect health-care quality, and hold HMOs accountable for their actions. The actual consequences of such regulation are less certain, however. Critics have portrayed managed care laws as mainly symbolic, arguing, for instance, that the regulations adopted to restrict financial incentives have substantial loopholes that allow plans to circumvent rules (Stone, 1999). And the most potent tool for regulating managed care practices—legal liability for HMOs—has been implemented by only a few states. On the other hand, laws that require broader access to providers may have encouraged managed care plans to develop less restrictive physician networks. And the threat of legislation may persuade plans to soften their behavior in order to forestall further public intervention.

Three points about the politics of managed care regulation warrant special attention in addressing the ethics of policy making. First, these protections aim at those who already have insurance. Whether managed care regulations actually curtail the excesses of HMOs or instead simply offer symbolic reassurance to patients, the target constituency is largely middle class, voting, and well-insured. Second, debates over regulating managed care do not provoke the questions of redistribution and cross-subsidization that grappling with the issue of coverage for the uninsured inevitably engenders (avoidance of redistributive issues is evident, as well, in the reluctance of states to enact risk adjustment schemes that would shift resources among health plans). In fact, to the extent that such laws establish patients' rights at the expense of an unpopular industry, they are politically much more expedient than would be policies that would increase access to health insurance through explicit financial arrangements that would fall directly on the insured population.

Indeed, while the late 1980s and early 1990s witnessed a surge in state efforts to guarantee universal coverage, by the turn of the century there was little evidence of enthusiasm for such efforts, despite sustained economic prosperity. The failure of well-intended states such as Oregon, Vermont, Massachusetts, and Washington to realize their aspirations of universal coverage underscored how difficult the task is. (Even Hawaii, the one American state that is commonly said to have achieved universal coverage, boasts an uninsured rate of around 8%). In short, managed care regulation allows political leaders to take credit for doing something about health care without their having to confront the political problems of universal coverage and without any need to conjure up a politically acceptable rationale for diverting resources to the uninsured.

On the other hand, and this is our third point, state stalemate on the uninsured by no means implies a stymied or shrinking state presence in health policy. Far from it: Managed care laws establish a new principle for state intervention in medical care and expand the scope of government regulation of the private sector. Since the enactment of Medicare and Medicaid, state (and the federal) governments have assumed a growing role in financing care (roughly half the dollars in the health care system are public) but have meanwhile faced political pressure to refrain from meddling with private medical arrangements. The sharp recent turn to avowedly market-based care shifts the burden of legitimacy. Reformers in government and academia who view the incentive systems of MCOs as a pleasing harmony of goods are counterbalanced by a nervous public that sees those incentives as, at best, a double-edged sword and, at worst, an overt threat to patients' interests and rights. The ensuing backlash extends to government regulation a fairly open invitation to intervene in private arrangements to straighten things out. Whether this new regulatory legitimacy presages greater public acceptance of public intervention into spheres that extend beyond just the protection of an anxious middle ground against MCOs remains to be seen.

An assessment of managed care regulation in light of the three ethical criteria noted above—goals, outcomes, and process—yields both similarities to and differences from the "findings" on Medicaid managed care. In both sets of findings, outcomes are too new and too little analyzed to sustain firm judgments. Process, on the other hand, differs markedly and predictably in the two cases: Whereas policy making for Medicaid managed care saw little participation by a core "constituency" that is vulnerable, unorganized, and disinclined to vote, managed care regulation unfurls the glorious participatory panorama of middle-class "opinion" and consumer (and provider) organization combining to compel obedience from policy makers determined to stay on the right side of a big and inflammatory political issue.

In both cases, policy goals are superficially straightforward but devilishly difficult to explicate in practice. No one quarrels with the quest for better quality and access at lower cost in Medicaid managed care, but striking an ethically defensible balance is a complex organizational enterprise. No one questions that health care consumers should be protected from insupportable "efficiencies" driven by the material incentives facing health plans and providers, but deciding when enough is enough on more ethical grounds is not simple.

Managed care might be judged ethically troublesome if one assumes that nothing, including gatekeepers, should stand between a patient and medical care in time of need. The obvious riposte is that gatekeeping and kindred managed care practices are not obstacles to medical care but rather sources of care that exist precisely to gauge and channel needs that citizens are not trained to examine and treat themselves. Ethical objections to the current state of managed care might center on the principle that the profit motive ought not to color decisions about medical coverage or care and, therefore, that there is something inherently unsavory about corporate boards of directors, shareholders, and CEOs joined together in a common quest to wax rich by running organizations geared to reducing the medical care delivered under the health insurance policies they sell. But suppose one concedes that (*1*) much wasteful care is the norm; (*2*) this wasteful care inflates health insurance premiums while also reducing workers' discretionary incomes; (*3*) organizational arrangements with appropriate financial incentives are one reasonable and efficient way to address the problem of waste and costs; and (*4*) financial rewards for managerial innovation, acumen, and hard work are necessary, proper, common, and all-American inducements to the high quality of organizational performance one needs and wants to fix the problem. The ethical verdict on the goals of managed care turns largely on whether and how far one accepts any, some, or all of these utilitarian propositions. This is not, however, the end of the story. One can accept all of these propositions and still not embrace the current *form* of managed care, as well as wonder whether managed care truly delivers on what it promises. In the end, it is vital not simply to issue a verdict on managed care in toto, but to distinguish between better and worse forms.

CONCLUSION

In both the policy arenas discussed in this chapter, ethical considerations are much in evidence, sometimes at or near the surface of state policy debates, sometimes waiting to be unearthed from beneath obscuring theoretical overlays. The problem, it would seem, turns on the quality, not the quantity, of ethical debates in the policy process. The challenge is not to get policy makers to think more often about ethical issues but rather to get them to ponder moral conundrums more clearly and sharply.

This is easier said than done, however. Politics is how society manages deep and insolvable conflicts of value and interest. Almost by definition in the political sphere, one person's intuitively obvious ethical argument is another's specious reasoning. Moreover, clearer and sharper deliberation and debate about ethical issues risks accentuating their most problematic and controversial features, thus impairing the building of political coalitions by stimulating conflict among groups whose leaders must assuage followers now freshly awakened to the power of moral claims they may not have contemplated fully before. The largely hidden and implicit system of funding services for the uninsured, for example, made for an easier arrangement than more recent efforts to explicitly fund such care. To be sure, trying to do the right thing by technocratic stealth is a patronizing and often ineffective strategy, as the saga of the Clinton health reforms demonstrates. But does anyone believe that universal coverage would have fared better if Clinton had sold it by arguing that solidarity is a crucial moral value, that universal coverage is a citizen's right, and that the extensive redistribution universal coverage requires is an ethical imperative?

No one, presumably, contends that public policy would be improved if its formulators ignored ethics, thought less about it, or grew more wooly-headed in pondering it. The very notion of "better" public policy incorporates ethical criteria in some form or fashion almost tautologously. This granted, however, the gains to be reaped from a fuller and more sophisticated moral reckoning by policy makers are surprisingly hard to specify. In the health arena, the underlying assumption seems to be that deeper ethical deliberations would lead political leaders to turn away from such affronts as nonuniversal health coverage, that anyone who "really" thought through the ethics of the issue would affirm that health coverage is a moral obligation binding on society as represented by the state. (Thus the Left; the objective moral validity of the war against abortion may be a suitable counterpart on the Right). This is not obvious, however. The Left has no monopoly on correct philosophical reasoning; for every Rawls there is a Nozick. Moreover, policy makers may insist on the pluralism of sources of ethical insight.

Philosophy in all its academic rigor is one source, but religion, "American values," strict constitutional exegesis, and social and partisan ideologies are other rich founts of policy principle. They are more accessible to the public and their elected representatives than is philosophy and, although less disciplined, are not therefore indisputably less reliably "ethical." Their diverse readings of what is right and fair may fit under the broad umbrella of ethical debate but at some point suffuses or swamps careful moral inquiry, and the "is" risks preempting or displacing the "ought." "Ethics in policy" seems to be an independent variable floating in search of a dependent variable, a solution seeking a clearly formulated problem. The key question is "ethics for what?"

REFERENCES

Brown LD (1983) *Politics and Health Care Organization: HMOs as Federal Policy.* Washington, DC: Brookings Institution.

Coughlin TA, Ku L, and Holahan J (1994) *Medicaid Since 1980.* Washington, DC: Urban Institute Press.

Derthick M (1979) *Policymaking for Social Security.* Washington, DC: Brookings Institution.

Gray BH and Rowe C (2000) Safety-net health plans: A status report. *Health Affairs* 19: 185–193.

Grogan C (1997) The Medicaid consensus for welfare recipients: A reflection of traditional moral concerns. *Journal of Health Politics, Policy, and Law* 22: 815–38.

Health Insurance Association of America (1998) *Source Book of Health Insurance Data: 1997–1998.* Washington, DC: Health Insurance Association of America.

Holahan J, Zuckerman S, Evans E, and Rangarajan S (1998) Medicaid managed care in 13 states. *Health Affairs* 17: 43–63.

Interstudy Competitive Edge: Part II HMO Industry Report (1999). St. Paul, MN: Interstudy Publications.

Jacobs LR (1993) *The Health of Nations: Public Opinion and the Making of American and British Health Policy.* Ithaca, NY: Cornell University Press.

Kaiser Commission on Medicaid (1999) *Medicaid and Managed Care.* Menlo Park, Ca: Kaiser Family Foundation.

Kaiser Public Opinion Update (2000) *The Public, Managed Care, and Consumer Protection.* Menlo Park, Ca: Kaiser Family Foundation.

Leichter HM (1996) State governments and their capacity for health reform. In: Rich RF and White WD (eds) *Health Policy, Federalism, and the American States.* Washington, DC: Urban Institute Press.

Marmor TR (1973) *The Politics of Medicare.* New York: Aldine.

Moran M (1997) Regulating managed care: An impulse in search of a theory? *Health Affairs* 16: 7–21.

Sparer MS (1996) *Medicaid and The Limits of State Health Reform.* Philadelphia: Temple University Press.

Sparer MS (1998) Devolution of power: An interim report card. *Health Affairs*:7–15.

Sparer MS and Brown LD (1996) States and the health care crisis: Limits and lessons of laboratory federalism. In: Rich RF and White WD (eds) *Health Policy, Federalism, and the American States.* Washington, DC: Urban Institute Press.

Starr P (1982) *The Social Transformation of American Medicine.* New York: Basic.

Stone D (1999) Managed care and the second great transformation. *Journal of Health Policy, Politics, and Law* 24: 1213–8.

Stauffer M and Levy DR (2000) *State by State Guide to Managed Care Law*. New York: Aspen Publishers.

Ware JE, Bayliss MS, Rogers WH, Kosinski M, and Tarlov AV (1996) Differences in four-year health outcomes for elderly and poor, chronically ill patients treated in HMOs and fee-for-service settings. *Journal of the American Medical Association* 276: 1039–47.

11

Private sector incentives and ethical health care

STUART BUTLER

When we, as a society, ponder how to assure an affordable level of basic health care to everyone, we have to determine the most effective role of different institutions and players, from government agencies to doctors and nurses, in achieving this goal. All too often, policy makers assume that because the goal is social or collective in nature and requires the transfer of resources within society, the self-interest of private individuals in the health-care industry will tend to be in conflict with the goal. This assumption leads many policy makers to advocate approaches based heavily on public sector agencies and employees, in which the private sector in health care—the hospitals, doctors, insurers, drug companies, and others not directly employed by the government—is seen as lacking the institutions and incentives for anything more than a supporting role to government programs.

Behind this assumption is a mistaken vision of the private sector that overlooks how private markets tend naturally to channel the individual interests of producers toward actions that lead to innovation and improve the condition of consumers. To be sure, government can and must create a framework of laws and incentives if markets are also to be harnessed to achieve certain social objectives and if inherently unethical behavior is to be curbed. But today many government-created incentives in health care actually discourage institutional innovations in the private sector that would help achieve the very goals of health-care policy. Worse still, by forcing many practitioners to choose between economic self-interest and the objectives of public policy, these incentives encourage essentially ethical people either to act in dishonest ways or to sacrifice their own interests. Moreover, private insurance markets in health care cannot naturally reconcile certain public goals while managing commercial risk, and we require carefully crafted legislation if they are to do so. If we recognize these realities, it is possible to envision a set of policies that would channel private sector players and institutions to take the lead in achieving the goal of adequate health care for all in society.

The seeming conflict between private and public interest is not unique to health care. We constantly confront the interaction and conflict between self-interest, the notion of the public interest, and what we would consider ethical behavior in relationships and transactions. Recognizing this, societies have sought to create an environment of customs and rules in which individual self-interest is reasonably consistent with what people collectively consider to be the public interest.

The goal of creating an environment in which individual and collective goals are consistent shapes public policy affecting most economic transactions, just as it does other spheres. Some economists and policy makers believe the tension between individual and collective economic interests is so great that there must be stringent controls on the producers of goods and services to avoid economic exploitation. They also believe there must be a large measure of collective decision making over the production and distribution of goods and services if there is to be efficiency and fairness, particularly for goods and services that may be deemed essential, such as health, education, and housing.

But this view misunderstands the nature of private markets and their potential for achieving public goals more effectively than can the institutions of the public sector by channeling individual self-interest rather than by suppressing it. A characteristic of private markets, as the economist Adam Smith long ago emphasized, is that efficiency and consumer satisfaction do not depend on producers of goods and services placing the public interest above their individual interests. On the contrary, one reason why competitive markets generally work so well is that individual gain actually requires suppliers to provide their customers with the best value for money, and doing so helps promote the public interest.

In addition, competitive private markets transmit and use information differently and more rapidly than do centralized economic systems managed by governmental institutions, enabling markets to be inherently more innovative and efficient. As the economist and philosopher Friedrich Hayek pointed out in a seminal essay, for there to be improvements and corrections, centralized economic systems require enormous amounts of information about transactions to be gathered in the field and transmitted to a central place. A decision must then be made by planning officials, and then instructions must be distributed back to the field (Hayek, 1945). This process takes time, during which conditions may change markedly. Moreover, this process works only if the decisions and instructions are correct and clear. If they are not, the entire system may end up operating less effectively. By contrast, explained Hayek, markets continuously adjust as individuals in the field act quickly on the information they receive, most importantly through the signal of changing prices. Taken together, he argues, millions of these individual decisions, constantly being made by people responding to the economic information immediately affecting them rather than to some regulation or grand plan, enables the system as a whole to innovate rapidly and improve. And because of competition and the decentralized nature of decision making in a market, a poor decision is quickly penalized or corrected and does not hamper the entire system.

To be sure, Smith and later economists such as Hayek recognized that for markets to function in this positive way, marrying individual gain with the public interest, there must be a framework of rules governing behavior in transactions. While self-interest can be a force for public good, dishonest individuals who are prepared to cheat and steal can exploit markets just as they can other systems. Thus, private markets still depend on "outside" factors if they are to be successful. For example, there must be a reasonable commitment to basic ethical conduct and social or legal rules requiring honest transactions.

The legal and political framework in which markets function is not a benign "given," however. It is the product of political decisions and may be influenced by a number of factors. For instance, individual players with large economic stakes are constantly trying to stack the deck in their own favor. In America this leads to thousands of lobbyists descending on Congress every day seeking special advantages in the rules governing markets. Moreover, well-meaning policies can have perverse effects on individual behavior in a market, driving a wedge between individual and collective interest where perhaps no such conflict previously had existed. Economists understand, too, that there can be many instances in which unfettered markets may work against both individual and social interests, requiring institutions and rules to achieve efficiency. The policy of issuing patents for pharmaceuticals and other innovative products, for instance, recognizes that without legal protection from competition markets will not necessarily reward those who undertake the large costs of developing new products for the benefit of both customers and stockholders.

Such factors influence the environment in which daily decisions are made by physicians, hospital administrators, and other health-care providers. And, as we shall see, some policies in health-care actually add to the difficulties of private individuals trying to reconcile their own views of ethical behavior with the economic and regulatory incentives they face. The result very often is that health-care professionals face frustrating dilemmas and feel forced to press for policy changes to protect their interests, the consequence of which may be to make public and private objectives even harder to reconcile.

This does not mean that there are no bad apples in health care, only bad government incentives, and that our social goals in health care would be achieved if government simply would get out of the way. Steps are needed to combat inherently unethical behavior in health care just as they are needed in other areas. Moreover, certain technical features of health-care insurance lead to perverse results by discouraging what we would consider ethical behavior and require government policies to enable the health-care market to function efficiently. There are also widely held public objectives, such as the availability of a certain level of medical care for everyone that cannot realistically be achieved today without government intervention to reallocate resources. So collective, government-sponsored actions are needed to achieve our health-care goals. But it must also be recognized that these goals are more likely to be reached within a new policy framework based on a better understanding of the potential of private competitive markets, in which practitioners are not forced routinely to choose between their own interests and the interests of their patients.

ETHICAL ISSUES FACING THE PRIVATE SECTOR

While health care does share many basic similarities with other goods and services in the economy, some features of health care raise more vexing ethical issues for practitioners than is true of other services in the private sector. These often pit self-interest against ethical instincts and social objectives.

Allocating Scarce Health-Care Resources

For most goods and services, such as washing machines and meals at restaurants, we generally accept that the combination of our own financial resources and prices resulting from the interplay of supply and demand should determine who will receive the products that are available. In health care, however, it is broadly agreed that the goal should be to make sure that everyone receives at least a certain level of care, using taxpayer resources when needed to reach that goal. This idea of a community's obligation to the social welfare of its individual members is deeply rooted in our society. Admittedly, there are some people, such as libertarians, who reject the idea that government should be the instrument to pursue social welfare, but even they usually accept the notion of individuals living in voluntary associations with ethical or contractual obligations to provide mutual assistance.

The idea of obligation forces the private medical practitioner to confront a number of ethical dilemmas. One is how to balance the health interests of the patient with the financial limitations of that patient and society at large. This task is only apparently made easier if the patient has generous resources thanks to insurance or access to public programs. The physician in that case may feel able to care for the patient without regard to cost. But with a limited total supply of program or insurance funds, taking the view that cost can be ignored simply means forcing another practitioner and patient to confront the financial reality he or she is avoiding. While physicians may constantly seek to escape the practical need to determine how to distribute resources, in a world without infinite resources, they have to engage in rationing, either based on their own judgment or on the instructions of others (Churchill, 1987).

Another dilemma for the practitioner is how to balance his or her own values in supplying care against the values of the patient and—even more common today—the values of the third party making the immediate payment decisions. Physicians often have to deal with a range of insurance companies and government programs that provide very different guidelines on what procedures will be reimbursed.

Like it or not, then, practitioners must ration in some way, in the sense of withholding some services that could be offered with benefit to the patient. The issue is whether there are mechanisms in the private sector that can resolve these pressures in ways that are reasonably compatible with the ethical instincts of the practitioner and the values and desires of the patient. Given the complexities and value judgments involved in such decisions, most people would want the physician to be at the center of such decisions. But, as discussed below, the rising cost of health care in recent decades, combined with unwise features of public policy, makes granting the physician this central role much more difficult today. However, there are policy changes that could enable the private sector to resolve the pressures in much more sensible ways.

Dealing with Wide Differences in Medical Risk

Even prudent individuals who try to save for every eventuality can be devastated financially by an unexpected turn of events, such as a house fire or a serious accident. Within the private sector, insurance has grown up as the principal way for individuals to deal with such risks. But there are characteristics of health care that limit the effectiveness of insurance as a tool for spreading risk. In particular, as a society we are reluctant to accept that health insurance should be priced in the way markets normally set premiums in insurance, even though many insurers warn that to do otherwise can undermine the economic basis of the protection they supply. This reluctance raises special challenges for health insurance. In most other forms of insurance, such as automobile insurance and life insurance, the insurer assesses the probability that a claim will be made and charges a premium accordingly. That is why a driver with a string of speeding tickets will be charged more for car insurance than will a driver with a spotless record. Some people will pose such a high risk to an insurer that they cannot obtain insurance at all or can get coverage only at a very high premium. This may be irritating to the reckless driver, who may have to give up driving because of the financial risk. But someone with a chronic heart disease cannot decide not to be ill because of the cost. Yet if we decide, either as a society or as individual health-care professionals, that we should not deny costly medical services to patients because they were unable to insure themselves against the medical problems that befall them, who is to shoulder the cost? In particular, is it possible for the private sector to solve this problem, or must we always resort to governmental solutions such as social insurance or public health programs?

To some extent, the private sector absorbs these costs in the form of charity. Most physicians and hospitals voluntarily provide some pro bono services, and see it as a professional obligation, as physicians always have. But this is sufficient only for a minority of severe cases. Society could insist, either as a moral responsibility or as a legal requirement, that health-care practitioners treat the high-risk individual, charging only what the patient can afford and absorbing the rest of the cost. But this often presents the practitioner or hospital with an unattractive ethical choice because their economic self-interest is in direct conflict with their instincts as humanitarians and health-care professionals. For example, hospitals that accept Medicare patients are under a legal obligation to provide services to stabilize anyone who shows up (not just Medicare beneficiaries) without regard to their ability to pay. Yet, as many inner-city hospitals and their doctors have found, this can lead to financial difficulties. Worse still, announcing that you are prepared to act according to professional obligations, rather than doing only what the law requires, is an invitation to enormous financial losses.

Private health insurers have reduced the problem of high-risk and uninsurable individuals by the use of group health insurance. The premium for each individual in the group is then based not on the actual insurance risk of the person but on that of the group as a whole. This allows the potentially high costs of one individual to be shared by the whole group, but group rating is by no means a complete private sector solution. For one thing, much depends on the size and continuity of the group. The average premium for a small group can change dramatically if a very high-risk individual joins it to obtain a less expensive premium than he or she would face in the individual insurance market. The result can be an unstable pool in which very healthy individuals start to leave the group because they find it less expensive to buy individual coverage. It is for this reason that group insurance tends to be based on large preformed groups, such as the employees of a business, where a few high-risk individuals will not significantly raise the average risk and where even low-risk individuals can effectively be required to be part of the insurance pool as a condition of employment (Custer et al, 1999).

NEW ETHICAL TENSIONS IN TODAY'S HEALTH CARE SYSTEM

Despite the limitations of private insurance, for decades it provided significant protection to both patients and doctors from many of the financial pressures that otherwise would have interfered with the desire of doctors and other health-care professionals to practice medicine in line with their ethical values. For the most part, doctors charged prices for their services according to a schedule developed by their specialty that was broadly accepted as fair (the term *"usual and customary" charges* entered the lexicon of medicine). Insurance plans would almost automatically accept those charges, paying hospitals on a "cost plus" basis and using the pattern of these charges as the basis for calculating the next year's premium for the group (Whetsell, 1999).

With this approach to insurance, doctors and hospitals knew their insured patients were largely insulated from the potentially heavy cost of an illness. Even if patients were not protected in this way, as long as health insurance was not a large element in a family or company budget, it was generally acceptable for doctors and hospitals to "pad" the bills of wealthy or well-insured patients to provide reduced-cost or free services for needy patients. To be sure, it was no ideal world. Many segments of the population and poorer communities were chronically ill served, prompting the creation of various publicly funded programs, and the debate over these shortcomings of the health-care system continues today. Still, to a large extent, employer-sponsored group insurance meant the financing and insurance infrastructure of the private sector was broadly in line with the values of patients and medical practitioners.

In the last two or three decades, however, certain trends have severely strained this arrangement, forcing changes in the way doctors and hospitals practice medicine and balance costs. These trends have sharpened the ethical issues facing the private sector. They have also constrained the ability of players in the private sector to deal with these issues, often introducing conflict between the ethical instincts and self-interest of physicians and prompting private sector pressure for policy changes intended to reconcile those conflicts.

Trend 1: The Rise in Cost of Medical Care

The most important trend, which has triggered other trends, is the sharp rise in medical costs over the last forty years. U.S. health-care spending as a percentage of gross domestic product jumped from 5.1% in 1960 to 10.3% in 1985 and is projected to top 16% by 2005 (Health Care Financing Administration, 2000). While opinions differ over the exact causes of this rise in prices and total spending, there is general agreement about several of the factors. One has been the remarkable breakthroughs in medical technology, which means that more illnesses can be treated successfully today—but often only with expensive equipment, intensive and expert procedures, and costly new drugs—that were beyond the range of medical practice just a generation ago. A second reason is that the very success of private insurance as a means of insulating physician and patient from most considerations of cost has made physicians more inclined to offer costly new treatments and patients more inclined to demand them. That, in turn, has raised the cost of insurance. Another reason is the introduction of large-scale public programs, most importantly Medicare and Medicaid in the mid-1960s. These programs succeeded in reducing the cost barrier to poor and elderly patients but thereby increased the provision of costly services.

The surge in medical costs has caused those faced with paying these surging costs, including employers and individuals paying for insurance as well as governments financing programs, to take steps to curb the rise. These steps have served to restrict the discretion of doctors and hospitals to prescribe treatments while setting prices according to their estimate of the value of their own services. To be sure, the restrictions have appropriately limited the opportunity for less scrupulous practitioners to exploit the financing system in health care by ordering expensive tests and treatments when the benefit to the patient is marginal. But the techniques used to limit the rise in costs also limit the flexibility of doctors and hospitals to practice medicine in ways they feel to be in the best interests of their patients.

Price controls

Consider, for example, the government's wide use of price controls in an effort to hold down physician and hospital charges in such programs as Medicare. These controls directly limit the ability of honest doctors to vary their charges according to the financial means of the patient and the additional services they feel they must devote to a particular patient, such as taking the time to fully explain a procedure to a nervous elderly patient. So doctors and hospitals routinely face an unpleasant choice. They must act against their own financial self-interest, or they must limit the care they give to the patient.

The choice of some practitioners is to place the ethics of professional practice above the ethics of abiding by the letter of the law and to resort to a variety of "creative accounting" techniques to evade price controls (Butler, 1993). These include "upcoding" (that is, choosing a diagnosis for an ailment that will allow an increased charge) and "unbundling" (that is, maximizing the charges by breaking down a patient's condition into its multiple elements and charging for each as a separate condition). Needless to say, most doctors are uncomfortable with these tricks of the billing trade but feel compelled to use them if they are to preserve their own financial interest while caring for patients to the standard their professional ethics demand.

The policy incentive of the professional organizations in medicine is to counter controls by lobbying legislators and regulators for increases in the permissible charges. In the case of Medicare, every congressional bill to finance or modify the program unleashes an avalanche of lobbyists seeking to gain higher prices for medical services.

Managed care

The other major response to the rise in health-care costs has been the introduction into the private sector of a range of techniques that fall under the rubric of *managed care*. The term includes devices ranging from highly structured health maintenance organizations (HMOs), which may employ salaried doctors and other medical staff, to indemnity insurance plans that merely negotiate charges with doctors and require preapproval of certain procedures and referrals. These techniques are used by health-care organizations serving public programs as well as private insurance. The critical feature of managed care is that it introduces a new individual into medical decisions. The job of this person is to question or limit physician discretion with the aim of constraining the total costs associated with patient care and hence slow the rise in premiums and other medical costs. But managed care means that medical decisions ultimately are made by a person who has no direct knowledge of the patient or the case. Thus, many physicians feel that the private sector's response to rising costs—introducing in health care the kind of hard-nosed cost management that typifies private industry—directly interferes with the physician–patient relationship needed for the professional care of patients.

Even when managed care plans are most careful to pursue the best interests of the patient, there is still a subtle change in the relationship between the patient and physician—decisions increasingly are made by someone other than the attending physician. And those making the decisions or developing practice guidelines for hospitals and doctors have to rely on supposedly objective tools to measure the quality and effectiveness of care, often making their decisions on the basis of data rather than a physician's judgment and subjective considerations. The New York Academy of Medicine's Bradford Gray says this means that "[a] system based on trust in the competence and fiduciary ethics of individual physicians is being replaced by a system based on alternatives to trust. Hopes about trustworthiness of physicians' patient care decisions are increasingly being supplemented by evidence" (Gray, 1997).

Many doctors disdainfully refer to this change as leading to a world of "cookbook" medicine, in which treatment guidelines take the place of physician judgment. Not surprisingly, the spread of managed care has not been welcomed by most doctors and hospitals, even though economic pressures have forced them to accept its restrictions in order to retain their insured patients. For instance, a 1997 survey of more than 1500 physicians in mid-career by Daniel Sulmasy and others found that only 17% believed financial incentives to limit services are ethically acceptable. Half the physicians worried that changes in the health system in the preceding five years had reduced the degree of trust in them felt by their patients, and more than 80% believed that these changes had diminished the commitment and loyalty of physicians to their patients (Sulmasy et al, 2000). According to the authors, "Physicians with financial incentives to reduce services may be experiencing especially acute moral tension and confusion."

While many doctors use their discretion to determine a diagnosis and treatment to act on behalf of their managed care patients when a coverage decision is involved, there are professional dangers in this. Physicians' treatment and referral patterns are routinely tracked by managed care organizations, and unusually costly patterns can result in physicians being excluded from the network. On the other hand, the managed care industry does seem to be groping toward a greater balance between financial limits and physician control, in large part because of patient pressure but in some cases also because micromanagement of doctors may not be particularly efficient. In 1999, for instance, America's third largest insurer, United HealthCare, decided that it would no longer require physicians to seek permission before hospitalizing patients, saying that the cost of reviewing requests was greater than the amount saved. Meanwhile, it may well be that over time an increasing number of doctors will find financial limits more acceptable as the rise in medical costs leads them to conclude that economies must be made, especially if managed care plans take steps to combine limits with a reasonable level of physician discretion.

Whether or not individual physicians can reach an accommodation, ethically and financially, with steps to control costs, organizations representing doctors generally have been aggressive in their reactions to managed care. For instance, the American Medical Association and many specialty associations have sought legislative changes to limit the operations of managed care plans. These efforts have been aimed at two chief targets. One is the restriction on referrals to specialists. The other is the practice of excluding doctors from plan networks who are considered by the plan to conduct too many tests or to prescribe excessively expensive treatments. Excluded physicians claim they are being singled out because they treat patients to a high standard and that managed care is antithetical to quality care and good medical ethics.

Among the legal protections sought by lobbyists for physician groups are "any willing provider" laws. These require managed care plans to include in their network any doctor or hospital that is allowed to practice in the state. The lobbyists also push for laws to give patients greater legal rights to be reimbursed for certain treatments and receive care by a specialist even if the plan otherwise would not give approval. The aim is to avoid patients effectively being denied access to services because insurance companies will not reimburse patients for the cost. These "mandated benefits" laws are most pervasive at the state level, where most health insurance is regulated. In addition, physicians' organizations have been urging passage of federal legislation that would establish a "patients bill of right" allowing patients to appeal decisions by managed care plans to limit their access to care.

Trend 2: The Changing Nature of Insurance

The nature of health insurance itself also has been changing the practice of medicine in ways that pose ethical challenges to practitioners. In part, this is a direct result of the general rise in medical costs, or at least the demands of purchasers of insurance that premium increases be moderated. Thus, instead of the more relaxed form of insurance management of the past, in which insurers typically accepted the treatment decisions and charges of doctors and hospitals, insurers have become much less accommodating because they must be more competitive in setting premiums. This has led to more aggressive review by private insurers of charges and treatment decisions and means that doctors and hospitals have far less freedom to practice medicine in the way they feel is best for the patient—unless they are willing to forgo reimbursement or risk being dropped as a recognized provider by the insurer.

Also because of cost pressures, insurers are now much more inclined to employ techniques to avoid accepting people as enrollees who pose especially high risk, meaning the private sector is less able to accommodate certain sicker individuals. This is especially the case in the market for individual policies, where insurers have greater opportunities to select the individual enrollees. Insurers do not even have to overtly exclude people to avoid higher-cost enrollees. They can, instead, use more subtle techniques, such as varying the package of benefits to attract younger and healthier enrollees and discourage older and sicker individuals from enrolling.

Improvements in the ability of medical experts to predict illness from such information as case histories, family medical histories, genetic testing, and even simple observation (such as weight and ethnicity) could have profound effects on the insurance market. Access to this information allows insurers, not just doctors, to assess the probability of patients being afflicted by certain dangerous and expensive diseases, such as breast cancer. Whether that information should be made available to insurers raises a number of troubling ethical and practical issues (O'Connor, 1998). For example, if insurers receive the results of genetic tests or family histories as part of the medical background information they use to assess risk, a currently healthy individual with a predisposition could find himself or herself virtually uninsurable and vulnerable to catastrophic medical costs. Fear of this causes many people to avoid such things as genetic screening. The result, of course, is that their doctors do not possess information that may be critical to effective care.

Insurers respond that if they are denied such data, yet prospective enrollees possess it, individuals could seek out the insurers with the best benefits for the disease they are at risk of contracting. The worry is that the resultant adverse selection would mean "good" insurers would unknowingly attract a portfolio of bad risks, and the insurance market would break down. In fact, the more we can predict likely future medical developments for an individual, the less viable health insurance becomes. This is because pricing insurance requires uncertainty. If you know with a high degree of certainty that an event will happen, you cannot in practice insure against it because the insurer will demand a premium that is virtually the full cost of the event. Imagine the cost of a homeowner's policy if you and the insurer both knew with near certainty that your house would burn down next July.

Despite the concern of insurers, many states and the federal government have considered or enacted legislation to regulate the use of specific information, particularly genetic information, by insurers in assessing insurability and premiums. But as Jon Beckwith and Joseph Alper point out, it is difficult or impossible to draw a meaningful distinction between genetic and nongenetic information in predicting diseases (Beckwith and Alper, 1998). It is arguably also unfair to rule out certain predictive information but not other, except perhaps behavioral patterns over which the enrollee might have control (although even many of these, such as alcoholism and obesity, may in some cases be attributable to genetic factors). Beckwith and Alper argue persuasively that the only logical legislation is thus a ban on the use of *any* predictive information. With such restrictions in place, they recognize that this might make it difficult for the existing insurance system to remain stable. As such, they believe the optimal solution to that problem would be a single-payer universal system. But, as we shall see later, an alternative would be to combine restrictions on predictive information with a modification to the insurance system to adjust for risk selection.

Trend 3: The Reaction of Employers to Rising Insurance Costs

The rise in medical costs over the last few decades thus has prompted responses by insurers and the government that have made it increasingly difficult for doctors and others in the private sector to deal with the issues raised at the beginning of the chapter. This pattern has been exacerbated by the institution of employer-sponsored insurance for employees and their families. This system grew rapidly after World War II and functioned well for many years. For employees who worked most of their lives for the same firm, an employment-based plan was a convenient way to pool risk for group insurance. A long-term relationship between employer and employee also meant that it was in the self-interest of the employer to consider the long-term health of the worker. Moreover, in the complex field of health care, the mutual interest of employer and employee meant the employee could have confidence in the employer acting as an intermediary and advocate between the worker and the health-care system. And as long as health costs remained relatively low, health insurance was a cost-effective fringe benefit for employers to include as part of a worker's compensation package.

In recent years, however, deficiencies of employer-sponsored coverage have become more apparent, especially for workers employed in the small business sector. The core of the problem is the tax treatment of employer-sponsored plans (Arnett, 1999). When employers use a portion of an employee's compensation package to buy health insurance for the worker and his or her family (or, in the case of larger companies, acts as the insurer itself), that part of the compensation is completely tax free to the employee. When health insurance was relatively inexpensive and tax rates low, this tax advantage was small. But as the cost of health care has risen and tax rates have increased, the value of employer-sponsored insurance has risen dramatically, especially for upper-income workers in relatively high tax brackets. In 1998 the value of the tax break was an annual average of $1031 for all families, but for families with incomes in excess of $100,000 the average value was $2357 (Sheils and Hogan, 1999).

Yet, in order to receive this large tax benefit, the employees must allow their employers to choose, own and control their health insurance. This in turn means that it is in the financial interest of the health system to respond to the values and goals of the employer rather than those of the employee or family member actually receiving care. Thus, unlike the situation in almost all other economic relationships, the economic interest of the supplier of health services is not primarily to satisfy the consumer, but ultimately to satisfy a third party. As health costs have risen and the relationship between employers and employees has grown weaker in a turbulent economy, the goal of many employers has been to find ways of controlling total costs rather than to seek the best health-care value for their workers. This has encouraged employers to press insurers to intervene even more aggressively in the practice of medicine to limit the discretion of doctors and hospitals in order to save money.

Employees could, in theory, choose another method of organizing their health care. They could ask for the compensation now devoted to their health care to be given to them in cash and purchase care or insurance directly. But that normally means giving up the risk pooling associated with group insurance, and so higher-risk employees would face prohibitive costs. Moreover, even if employees and their families were to seek group coverage through a large organization whose interests and goals seemed to coincide with their own, say a union or a church, the tax system does not give individuals with insurance arranged by these alternatives the same tax relief as it does for employer-sponsored plans. If a worker's employer does not sponsor insurance and the worker is not eligible for a publicly funded health program such as Medicaid, the worker and family normally receive no tax breaks or other financial assistance to offset the cost of insurance or care. This explains why more than two-thirds of the uninsured are full-time workers or their dependents.

Tax policy supporting employer-sponsored insurance thus creates two artificial and perverse incentives affecting the relationship between patients and the health care system. First, it places ultimate control over insurance and hence medical decisions into the hands of employers rather than doctors and patients. Since the financial and other goals of employers frequently differ from those of the insured families, both doctors and patients tend to be frustrated by the constraints placed upon them. Doctors often feel unable to practice medicine according to their ethical values, and patients feel they are often denied care that they and their doctor believe is needed. Second, tax policy creates significant financial obstacles to the emergence of large nonemployer organizations that could address rising costs in ways that better reflect the values of patients and could sponsor affordable insurance to many of the uninsured. It does so because most of their potential customers are denied the subsidies available to employer-sponsored plans. Moreover, state insurance laws make it far more difficult for nonemployment based associations, such as churches, to organize large pools for insurance purposes. And while multistate employers enjoy considerable opportunities to assemble insurance pools—and exemptions from state insurance regulation—under federal employment laws, associations do not enjoy a similar degree of freedom.

One might assume that workers and health-care professionals would campaign for policy changes to end the tax discrimination against nonemployer organizations. Some groups, such as the American Medical Association, have indeed urged this kind of policy change, but so far there has been little general political pressure to make this change. Perhaps the main reason for this is the widespread belief among the public that the cost of health insurance is somehow paid for by employers, almost as an act of charity, rather than being merely an earmarked part of a worker's total compensation. This leads most families and doctors to the flawed conclusion that, despite its drawbacks, employer-sponsored insurance must be superior to alternatives because it is "free." Moreover, patients and doctors do not tend to appreciate that the restrictions imposed by insurers are the response of perverse incentives in an artificial market maintained by a huge tax subsidy and assume instead that they are due to the perfidy of insurers and the executives of managed care companies. Thus, the legislative changes generally demanded by doctors and the general public consist of ever more detailed requirements on insurers and managed care companies to provide specific services and levels of service to patients under the threat of litigation by patients. Insurers and managed care companies, not surprisingly, mobilize to oppose such changes.

HELPING THE PRIVATE SECTOR TO ACHIEVE A MORE ETHICAL HEALTH-CARE SYSTEM

From the discussion above it might seem that the ability of the private sector to address the complex ethical and financial issues in health care is limited and declining. Certainly the way in which private insurance has responded to rising costs has made it more difficult for doctors and hospitals to be sensitive to the medical needs and financial situation of their working-age patients, but it is also important to remember that public policy creates a framework of incentives in which private actions are carried out. If this framework consists of perverse incentives, such as the way tax policy causes employer-sponsored insurance to function, then the private sector's response may be perverse. But creating a different framework can facilitate private sector conduct in health care that would be more in line with accepted values and ethical conduct. In other words, it can help the private sector to function in a more rational and ethical way, just as a sound legal structure of contract law stimulates transactions in a private market by making it far more likely agreements will be honored even by those whose ethics leave something to be desired.

Two sets of policy changes could significantly improve the ability of the private sector to function more in line with the values of patients while resolving many of the ethical tensions facing providers. One of the changes would shift the locus of control in the health care of individuals, bringing it more in line with the pattern in other parts of the economy. The second would begin to resolve the technical difficulties facing private insurance as a means of distributing risk in health care.

Policy Change 1: Ending Tax Discrimination Against Alternatives to Employer-Sponsored Insurance

Providing the same tax relief to individuals regardless of whether they obtain health care and insurance through organizations other than their employer or through their employer would have a profound effect on the health-care system for workers and their families. In particular, it would sharply increase the number of plan choices open to them, which is artificially limited by existing the tax code, and give individuals direct ownership and control of their health insurance. Only 65% of working Americans with employer-sponsored health insurance have any choice of plan at all, and even that is only among plans selected by their employer (Kaiser Family Foundation, 1999). In small firms a choice of plans is rare. In addition to wider choice, if the new tax relief were structured in the form of a tax credit or some other design that provided a larger subsidy to lower-income families than to upper-income families, the ability of lower-income families to afford care would be increased.

If families were able to pick and own health plans without tax discrimination, they could join a group that reflected their interests and values, rather than those of their employer. In doing so, they would, of course, be faced with trade-offs between cost and methods of delivering care, as well as self-imposed limits in the total amount and cost of care. Doctors and hospitals would not be free to practice medicine exactly as they wished without regard to cost, but they and the insurer would have to deliver care in a way that was, on balance, most satisfactory to the patient, or they would lose that enrollee to another plan.

In this arrangement the organization sponsoring the plan would act as a broker and not as the owner of the plan. The covered individual would own the plan, but the organization would fulfill the important function of acting as an intermediary by pooling a group of individuals seeking insurance and care who held similar values and bargaining on their behalf with health care providers. Having such an intermediary chosen by the individual is a rational arrangement in health care, where the technical nature of the service makes it difficult for ordinary individuals to be knowledgeable enough to act as informed buyers and negotiators themselves.

The most logical organizations to play this role would be the normal community-based mediating structures of society, such as churches, unions, school associations, elder organizations, tribal groups, and similar bodies. Church-based health plans would be a likely development if church members could obtain tax or other assistance to purchase coverage through these groups. Black churches, for example, have a long history of involvement in social services for their congregations. In addition, fraternal and mutual aid societies in America played a large role in providing hospital and physician services, including within the African-American community, until the combination of tax-free employment fringe benefits and government health programs undermined their economic base (Beito, 2000).

The "friendly society" role of unions also has a long history in this and other countries and could be expected to be prominent in a health system allowing choices beyond employer-sponsored plans. In the United States, the Federal Employees Health Benefits Program (FEHBP), with 9 million covered federal employees and their families, allows organizations to offer plans directly to employees. It is notable that unions such as the Mail Handlers organize several of the leading FEHBP plans. Moreover, the relationship between insurers and patients is quite different in the FEHBP, where there are often more than a dozen competing plans to choose from. To be financially successful, the plans must provide value for money to the consumer, not simply cut costs for the employer. For example, plans and consumer organizations routinely provide detailed satisfaction information to enrollees to help them make the best choice (Butler and Moffit, 1995).

With this change a more direct and traditional relationship would reemerge between patient and health-care provider. It is not the case that there would be no economic constraints on the ability of doctors and hospitals to treat patients according to their view of best medical practice and the interests of the patient. But enrollees would be able to choose an intermediary organization they felt would set guidelines for practitioners that would best represent their values given the economic limitations faced by the family. With employees rather than employers making this choice, the financial well-being of the physician, hospital, and insurer would depend primarily on their ability to satisfy the patient rather than the employer. To be sure, insurers would continue to question decisions by practitioners that led to unusually costly tests or treatments in order to restrain future premium increases. This would discourage doctors and hospitals from ignoring cost or placing their economic interests above those of patients, but unlike an employer-sponsored insurance system, the ultimate pressure on insurers would be to achieve the best value for money for the enrollee.

Policy Change 2: Establishing a Reinsurance Market with Risk Adjustment.

As noted earlier, the traditional role of private insurance as a mechanism to spread risk is breaking down under the pressures of cost control, improved information regarding risks, and other factors. If the private sector is to be able to handle a wide array of health risks in ways that do not make the costs prohibitive to patients, or require doctors and hospitals to act against their self-interest if they provide appropriate care, a new policy framework is needed to enable the insurance market to function effectively.

Creating such a framework means making it feasible for insurers to profit from enrollees they know will cost them a great deal to care for and yet can only charge approximately the same premium as everyone else. This seeming impossibility can be achieved through a structured reinsurance market. Insurance companies buy reinsurance as their own insurance against an unusual string of costly claims. The reinsurer covers a large number of "front line" insurers and so can spread the risk widely and at a relatively low cost to the original insurer. This works well for health insurance if there is randomness to the string of costly claims. But if an insurer covers a group of individuals it knows will be costly, the cost of reinsurance will be very high and so it must still charge a high premium.

It would be possible to solve this technical problem through what has become known as risk adjustment. This mechanism is by no means perfected, but it holds promise as a reinsurance tool (Blumberg and Nichols, 1998; Newhouse, 1998). A risk adjustment system permits the price of insurance to be similar for enrollees irrespective of their health risks and yet enables the insurer to allow doctors and hospitals to treat enrollees' illnesses appropriately without incurring a large financial loss, to the insurer. Such a system would work as follows. All health insurers in a large region would be required by law to contribute to a reinsurance pool an amount of money based only on the size of their insurance portfolio. Under a "retrospective" risk adjustment, the managers of the reinsurance pool would make a payment out of the pool to each insurer based on the actual claims paid to their enrollees. In this way, the total revenues received by an insurer for each covered individual would be the combination of two elements: a premium (which could be approximately the same for each enrollee without regard to medical history) plus a payment from the reinsurance pool based on the costs of treating its group of enrollees. In this way, normal random risks would be covered directly by the insurer in the traditional way, but large, predictable risks would be shouldered by the pool.

This change in the organization of insurance, like the tax reform described earlier, would also have a beneficial effect on the relationship between the practitioner and the patient. Because insurers would not face a financial penalty by attracting a disproportionate share of higher-risk enrollees, the private sector insurance system would be far more able and inclined to handle the burden of chronically sicker individuals. As a result, insurance plans would have much less economic incentive to interfere with the medical decisions of doctors and hospitals. Just as in the proposed tax change, the ultimate pressure would be to deliver good value for money to enrollees.

OBSTACLES TO AND OPPORTUNITIES FOR REFORM

For such tax and insurance changes to be implemented, it is important to recognize the political obstacles and theoretical concerns that have so far thwarted reform and to craft proposals accordingly. Two major concerns have impeded the tax reform outlined despite widespread support among economists. One is that if the revenue cost of providing new tax relief for nonemployment based coverage is to be offset in order to achieve parity by reducing the current generous relief for employer-sponsored plans, those benefiting from the latter form of tax relief have a strong interest in opposing the change. In fact, the combined forces of unions and businesses have frustrated such proposals in the past. However, the pressure for tax reduction in America makes it more politically feasible to propose an expansion of tax relief for the uninsured without limiting the tax relief associated with employer sponsorship of insurance. In other words, the total amount of tax relief can be expanded rather than reallocated. Recent budget surpluses also helped health tax reforms of this kind to gain considerable political momentum.

The other concern about a tax change is that its very success in boosting nonemployment-based coverage might "crowd out" those employment-based plans considered successful by encouraging families to leave their current plans, causing employment-based plans to unravel. This concern has induced large employers in the past to oppose the reform, but this, too, seems to be changing. Many large companies have become so concerned about the rise in health costs and "patients rights" proposals that would limit their flexibility to manage costs that they are more open to alternatives to an employer-led system. At the same time, refinements in recent tax proposals have included options that would protect employers who wished to continue providing coverage by limiting the ability of workers to opt out of company-based plans (Butler and Kendall, 1999). For both these reasons, employer resistance to changes in the tax treatment of health care has been declining.

Instituting insurance reforms raises other issues. While insurance companies have tended to be either skeptical of restrictions on their underwriting practices or openly hostile to such restrictions, they have usually found it difficult to prevent them. In fact, there has been no shortage of legislation at the state level to experiment with changes in insurance regulation. The bigger challenge has been to enact insurance reforms that pass technical muster. States have learned the hard way, for instance, that placing rating restrictions on insurers can have many undesirable side-effects, such as the insurers eliminating coverage in certain markets or instituting price adjustments that cause healthier individuals to drop their coverage. But, as noted earlier, continuous experimentation with reinsurance and risk adjustment mechanisms has the potential to solve this problem and thus has raised the interest of insurers and policy makers in the approach, making larger-scale approaches based on the mechanisms politically feasible.

The private sector today faces limitations in its ability to reconcile the interests of practitioners within the health system and the interests of both the patient and the larger society. To some extent, as indicated in this chapter, this is because the market cannot of itself naturally incorporate the special goals we have for health care. In particular, private insurance cannot readily achieve the objective of providing affordable coverage to high-risk individuals of modest means, but there are also artificial limitations on the ability of the private sector to achieve competing goals due to the existing public policy framework. The rapid rise in underlying health care costs has exacerbated this problem, with resultant pressures on doctors and hospitals that make it more difficult for them to act ethically in the interests of patients. Many health-care professionals have responded to this frustrating situation by supporting legislation to protect their professional interests.

The private sector can be more effective in reconciling conflicting interests, but only with changes in public policy. A policy change is needed to give the insurance system a framework in which it can shoulder the cost of high-risk individuals without requiring insurers or health-care practitioners to act against their own self-interest. And a change also is needed to restore a normal economic relationship among patient, insurer, and doctor. If both these steps are taken, the private sector could achieve a health-care system for working families that would be more efficient as well as more ethical in its daily practice.

REFERENCES

Arnett GM (ed) (1999) *Empowering Health Care Consumers Through Tax Reform.* Ann Arbor, MI: University of Michigan.

Beckwith J and Alper JS (1998) Reconsidering genetic anti-discrimination legislation. *Journal of Law, Medicine & Ethics* 26:205–10.

Beito D (2000) *From Mutual Aid to the Welfare State.* Chapel Hill, NC: University of North Carolina Press.

Blumberg LJ and Nichols LM (1998) *Health Insurance Market Reforms: What They Can and Cannot Do.* Washington, DC: Urban Institute.

Butler SM (1993) The fatal attraction of price controls. In: Helms RE (ed) *Health Care Reform.* Washington, DC: American Enterprise Institute.

Butler SM and Moffit RE (1995) The FEHBP as a model for a new medicare program. *Health Affairs* 14:47–61.

Butler SM and Kendall D (1999) Expanding access and choice for health care consumers through tax reform. *Health Affairs* 18:45–57.

Churchill LR (1987) *Rationing Health Care in America.* Notre Dame, IN: University of Notre Dame Press.

Custer WS, Kahn CN, Wildsmith TF (1999) Why we should keep the employment-based health insurance system. *Health Affairs* 18: 115–23.

Gray B (1997) Trust and trustworthy care in the managed care era. *Health Affairs* 16: 34–49.

Hayek F (1945) The use of knowledge in society. *American Economic Review* 32:519–30.

Health Care Financing Administration (2000) Office of the Actuary, National Health Statistics Group.

Kaiser Family Foundation (1999) *Employer Health Benefits.* Menlo Park, CA: Kaiser Family Foundation.

Newhouse J (1998) Risk adjustment: Where are we now. *Inquiry* 35:223–39.

O'Connor DL (1998) Ethical issues in the age of genetics. *Patient Care* 32:137–44.

Sheils J and Hogan P (1999) The cost of tax-exempt health benefits in 1998. *Health Affairs* 18:177–88.

Sulmasy DP, Bloche G, Mitchell JM, Hadley J (2000) Physicians' ethical beliefs about cost-control arrangements. *Archives of Internal Medicine* 160:649–57.

Whetsell GW (1999) The history and evolution of hospital payment systems: How did we get here? *Nursing Administration Quarterly* 23:132–48.

IV

Ethical controversies in health policy

Resource allocation

12

Patient v. population: resolving the ethical dilemmas posed by treating patients as members of populations

EZEKIEL J. EMANUEL

Over the last century there have been recurring attempts to change the dominant model of American health care from an individual patient-focused model to a social, or community-focused, one. As Greenlick has reminded us, as early as 1910 Abraham Flexner had argued that "the physician's function is fast becoming social and preventive, rather than individual and curative"(Flexner, 1910; Greenlick, 1992). In the 1930s and 1940s, the early prepaid group practices, health care cooperatives such as Group Health Cooperative of Puget Sound and Kaiser Permanente, embodied another effort at creating population-focused health care (Crowley, 1996). In the 1960s, coeval with the larger liberal, social reform movement, there was yet another effort to improve health outcomes by shifting the focus of medical care from high technology, research oriented tertiary care facilities affiliated with medical schools focusing on the latest intervention for the very sickest patients to primary and preventive care in the community (Sardell, 1988; Geiger, 1984; Davis and Schoen, 1978). The goal of this shift was to improve health outcomes by preventing diseases and intervening early. The philosophy was to emphasize "the health of communities, beyond the traditional patient-by-patient focus of clinical medicine."

These earlier attempts had some successes, including the establishment of health maintenance organizations, the formation of neighborhood health centers, and the creation of departments of community health at selected medical schools. Nevertheless, there has been no fundamental transformation of American medicine. Population-focused medicine remained peripheral and marginal, championed by a few progressive (some would call them radical) health-care reformers and largely ignored or even disdained by both the prestigious academic centers and the organized professional societies of medical practitioners. The mainstream of American medicine has instead retained a focus on providing available services to the individual patients who present themselves to physicians and hospitals. Physicians continue to view their primary obligation as putting their patients first and caring for them in their offices (Levinsky, 1984). The system has emphasized reimbursement for services delivered to individual patients, thereby encouraging diagnosis and treatment of diseases and the use of high technology, tertiary care.

At the turn of the 21st century, a focus on community-based care is resurfacing. The name is different—it is now called population-based medicine. The social context is different—it is no longer liberal and social reform–oriented but conservative and business-oriented. And the advocates are different—they are no longer a few progressive physicians but academic leaders, consultants, and chief executives with leading managed care organizations. While history urges caution about claiming that such a shift will be successful, powerful supporters and financial forces make the odds of success greater than ever before.

Yet a shift from a patient-based to a population-based health care raises profound ethical challenges that could undermine the support for and legitimacy of adopting a population-based health-care system. It is important to understand the nature of these ethical challenges and to develop a conception of population-based health care that might address them.

FORCES PROPELLING POPULATION-BASED HEALTH CARE

There are at least four major developments in the health-care system that are driving the embrace of population-based health care. First is a shift in the flow of money. Fee-for-service payments are being replaced by capitation; open-ended reimbursement is being circumscribed by fixed budgets. Fee-for-service schemes permit paying as each patient presents and for each diagnostic and therapeutic intervention ordered. Conversely, capitation and budgets necessitate pooling of resources over a group of patients to cover medical services used by the entire group. As such, capitation requires thinking about the care to be delivered to the whole group and sometimes making decisions that deny patients care as extensive as that a fee-for-service scheme could provide. Second is the shift from personalized care decisions made by individual physicians who may haphazardly consult whatever research data are available to standardized care plans, guidelines, and disease management strategies. Guidelines are applied to a population of patients with a specific disease or condition. Monitoring the implementation and impact of guidelines also requires a population approach, collecting data on all the patients treated, and assessing the overall impact in terms of resource use and outcome measures of the group. Third is the shift from the delivery of care by independent practitioners working alone or in small groups and independent hospitals to organized delivery systems that integrate all types of health care providers with appropriate financial, management, and information infrastructures (Shortell, et al., 1996). Such organized systems provide services for large numbers of patients and members—a population, essentially. Finally is the shift from professional accountability, whereby physicians monitored the quality of health care provided mainly through hospital credentialing and morbidity and mortality rounds, to multiple accountabilities, especially more organized, systematic, quantitative, and routinized quality assessments (Emanuel and Emanuel, 1996; Epstein, 1996; Rodwin, 1996). These quality assessments determine how well services are delivered to a defined population—namely, the percentage of patients with a specific condition getting a specific intervention and having a specific outcome.

Clearly, these four factors are not independent. Budgets require strategies to manage care with fewer resources, leading to guidelines. Budgets also require sufficiently large pools of patients to spread financial risk. In turn, having the resources to spread risk and develop and implement guidelines requires the infrastructure of organized delivery systems.

Underlying and driving these four specific changes are two larger social trends: (*1*) the impetus to control costs for all products, health care included but not exclusively, and (*2*) the social imperative to improve quality while reducing prices and the success in manufacturing of various Total Quality Management/Continuous Quality Improvement (TQM/CQI) initiatives in achieving these goals.

OUTLINE OF POPULATION-BASED HEALTH CARE

Many commentators have argued for a population-based approach to health care (Menzel, 1990; Hall and Berenson, 1998). Among the most sustained efforts to articulate and justify population-based health care is that offered by David Eddy, a contemporary incarnation of Jeremy Bentham. Eddy, a brilliant theorist, simultaneously focuses his insights and prodigious energies on real-life issues, offering a slew of practical recommendations for improvements and reforms (Eddy, 1990, 1991a, 1991b, 1991c). One of Eddy's principles "for making difficult decisions in difficult times" states that the "objective of health care is to maximize the health of the population served, subject to the available resources" (1994). "In many ways, [this] is the fundamental principle that underlies the entire health care enterprise" (1991b). According to Eddy, population-based health care involves three critical elements:

1. Defining a population, such as all the members of a health plan or health maintenance organization, or Medicaid recipients, or people in a country.
2. Summing the health status of each individual in the population using whatever (cardinal) measure of health status is deemed appropriate, such as mortality, quality-adjusted life years, or disability-adjusted life expectancy (aggregation).
3. Choosing to fund those health services that maximize the sum of the health status of all the individuals in the population (maximization).

This means that whatever health-care services maximize the health status of the population are the services available to treat sick individuals. Further, Eddy claims that the optimal implementation of this population-based approach is one that ranks services by their cost-effectiveness.

> Ideally, we would have good information about the benefits, harms, and costs of services, about the level of health care for which people are willing to pay, and correspondingly about the level of resources that should be made available for health care. Ideally there would be some agreed-on measure of benefit per resource that would serve as a threshold for deciding when coverage of a particular service is fair. When the yield of a service is below the threshold, physicians and patients would voluntarily restrain themselves from seeking coverage for that service from the pool
>
> Eddy, 1991b, 2406

Clearly, this is an unabashed utilitarian, maximization strategy; as Eddy puts it, "[This principle] is consistent with the maxim, the greatest good for the greatest number" (1991b).

THE ADVANTAGES OF POPULATION-BASED HEALTH CARE

Population-based health care is attractive because it can have significant advantages. The overarching advantage, put crudely, is "a bigger bang for the buck." By adopting population-based health care rather than individual patient-based care, there are likely to be greater positive effects on the important health measures for each dollar spent:

> [B]y any aggregate measure of health care quality, such as morbidity rates, mortality rates, life expectancy, measures of health status, or quality-adjusted life-years, and for any specified level of resources, choices made from the [population-based perspective] can always provide as high a quality of care as choices made from the [individual patient perspective] and can often provide a higher quality of care. This means that if policies are systematically defined from the [population-based perspective] more people will live longer, with higher quality [health care] at lower cost than if policies are defined from the [individual patient perspective]
>
> Eddy, 1991b, 2405

In particular, population-based medicine is likely to lead to a complex of responses focused on improving quality. It is likely to generate more explicit quality assessments and use of quantitative measures of quality. To ensure good performance on these measures, providers are likely to adopt more care management programs and standardized treatment guidelines. Much bad medicine is the result of treatment done by old habits, intuition, and "gut reactions." While these treatments may appear to be tailored to the individual patient, they often lack any supporting research, while proven interventions are often ignored or haphazardly implemented. Population-based care that monitors whether certain proven interventions are implemented can at least reduce, if not eliminate, the low outliers. While these interventions may not raise the quality performance of all providers or that at the very finest institutions, they do present the real possibility of raising overall quality by eliminating the worst.

Not only is population-based health care likely to improve the quality of services delivered, it is also likely to change the types of services provided in important ways. In particular, population-based health care is likely to emphasize community-based interventions, such as educational efforts and the provision of certain services in community settings. It will heavily emphasize the use of preventive services, ranging from immunizations to screening tests to smoking cessation and other lifestyle changes. And population-based health care is likely to emphasize outpatient delivery of care and deemphasize hospitalization, especially in tertiary care facilities. This emphasis on preventive care and the outpatient delivery of care is likely to be viewed favorably by patients. More importantly, some key health care services simply cannot be provided when focusing on care for the individual patient but suddenly become possible when delivering services for an aggregation of such individuals. For instance, intensive home services for severely disabled patients or home monitoring for diabetic patients becomes possible because a population can justify investment both in specially trained nurses and other providers and in the delivery of infrastructure that could never be justified for isolated patients alone.

Further, a population-based focus will also attend to the health-care needs of those who do not necessarily present themselves to physicians, the so-called un- and under-treated. Population-based medicine reaches out to everyone in the population to be sure their health problems are addressed; it is proactive, not reactive, to those who seek care.

Changes involving getting more health improvement for each dollar, improvements in overall quality of care, more preventive services, more care delivered in the outpatient setting, and more care to those outside the system should be viewed as advantageous to each person. For policy makers, population-based health care has the additional advantage of affording a more rational and fair allocation of resources. Rather than paying for services that are decided upon by each individual physician working independently and treating patients as they present, population-based health care can prospectively determine where resources should be allocated and what services should receive high priority.

CHALLENGES TO POPULATION-BASED HEALTH CARE

Historically, the main problem in trying to shift to a population-based system has been that this sort of system conflicts with the dominant Hippocratic tradition of medicine. For centuries physicians have been trained to focus on the one-to-one physician–patient relationship and inculcated with the notion that their primary duty is to the patient for whom they are caring: "To the Hippocratic physician, nothing and no one was more important than his patient; this has always been a guiding principle of clinical medicine" (Nuland, 1989). Physicians view their primary obligation as one of focusing attention on the individual patient; to refrain from providing care for an individual patient because some resources need to be conserved or because services should be provided to unspecified other patients conflicts with physicians' understanding of their obligation. As Greenlick has argued, a shift to population-based health care requires that physicians integrate into the manner of their practice, their decision making, and their sense of obligations considerations of costs and resource allocation, epidemiology, and patients who are un- and under-served (1992). Physician resistance, indeed hostility, to such changes, symbolized in the past in attempts to prohibit prepaid group practices and health maintenance organizations, has been a major obstruction to population-based medicine (Starr, 1982). Because it is physicians who must ultimately deliver medical care, physician support is absolutely necessary for population-based care to succeed. Consequently, there have been significant efforts to respond to physicians. Eddy, for instance, offers a lengthy analysis of and response to the "great discomfort [of] practitioners" with population-based health care (1991b). Others have devoted significant thought and attention to "educating physicians for population-based clinical practice" (Greenlick, 1992).

A less acknowledged but no less serious challenge to population-based health care issues from the public. While there may be significant advantages to the public in terms of overall health status improvements, and while "more people will live longer, with higher quality [health care], at lower cost," many individuals are likely to be suspicious about having their care determined by rules made for a population (Eddy, 1991a). Indeed, some of the current backlash against "cookbook" medicine associated with managed care may be viewed as a rejection of population-based medical care (Anders, 1996). Why should any individual want to be treated as a member of a population rather than continue to receive the individualized care of the old model?

ETHICAL OBJECTIONS TO POPULATION-BASED HEALTH CARE

The usual conception of population-based health care articulated by Eddy clearly generates several critical problems and objections. Eddy recognizes that many people will oppose such an approach and that it will thus inevitably generate conflict, what he calls the conflict between individual and society. Individuals as patients who have illnesses requiring health-care services will desire health-care services that have a chance of curing or ameliorating their conditions. People may want MRI scans, surgical procedures, drug treatments, and so on in the hope of gaining improvements in their health, but this will consume resources that could be spent for other health-care services that have the chance of yielding greater incremental improvements of health benefit. Maximizing the care delivered to one person is likely to undermine the objective of maximizing the sum of individual health because attending to the individual could consume resources that could be used to gain larger health improvements when provided as other services. Eddy believes that "society"—decision-makers acting prudently on behalf of society—would obviously adopt his utilitarian, maximization-of-the-sum-of-individuals'-health version of population-based health care.

In addition to this problem, population-based health care as articulated by Eddy confronts at least three of the standard objections to utilitarianism, objections stemming from utilitarianism's use of aggregation and maximization (Gold et al, 1996; Ubel, 2000). One objection to aggregation focuses on whether all health benefits can be put on a cardinal scale and summed or whether some benefits, such as improved mental health, are incommensurable with other health benefits, such as prolongation of life. Another issue with aggregation is that not everyone in a population may feel she has a relationship with the other members of the population; they may not have undertaken moral obligations toward her that would warrant her sacrificing herself for them. In addition, there are objections to maximization. In particular, population-based health care often invites concerns about equity, for improvements may be maximized—thereby satisfying the goal—even while there is no guarantee that these improvements will be distributed evenly or fairly over the members of the population. Finally, while this approach may incorporate the important value of trying to maximally improve benefits for fixed costs, other critical values are ignored or minimized.

These objections have given rise to many creative approaches that attempt to address and resolve these issues. For instance, some researchers are actively examining ways of integrating a broader set of values into cost-effectiveness analysis than just that captured by quality-adjusted life years (Menzel et al, 1999).

AN ALTERNATIVE CONCEPTION OF POPULATION-BASED HEALTH CARE

The choice between traditional, Hippocratic, individual patient–focused health care and utilitarian, population-focused health care is certainly stark. And, as presented, it is hard to see how reasonable individuals will accept and affirm such a population-based system. Just as many people reject utilitarianism and maximization as the justifying philosophy in other matters of public policy, they are likely to oppose attempts to institutionalize population-based health care. In this way, a population-based model of health care based on maximization is likely to be contentious, viewed as unjust and illegitimate by many individuals. With many individuals opposed to being treated as part of a population-based health care system—indeed even viewing it as unethical—such a system is likely to be unstable, generating efforts to circumvent policies, law suits, and public campaigns, for legislative restrictions. The traditional Hippocratic health-care approach appeals to many, but it seems increasingly untenable, fraught with its own ethical problems, especially because of its inability to address the issues of resource allocation, providing services within a budget, and ensuring that all people, not just those who show up, receive appropriate health care. If the future requires population-based health care, the question becomes whether there is another, nonutilitarian conception of this sort of scheme that reasonable individuals would view as just and ethical.

The ethical challenge posed by population-based health care can be seen as parallel to the challenges posed in political theory. At its most basic, the challenge of political theory is why people should adhere to government. That is, why should a person become a member of a collectivity and permit the collectivity to make laws, regulations, and policies that govern her social circumstances and actions even in cases in which she disagrees with those very laws, regulations, and policies (Hobbes, 1962; Rawls, 1971; Kymlicka, 1990). The answer we have reached involves a set of procedural principles that safeguard certain rights and ensure decisions are made in a fair way and a set of substantive principles that guide those decisions that reasonable people should affirm upon reflection (Hobbes, 1962; Rawls, 1971). So one way to understand the challenge to population-based health care is to ask: What are the substantive and procedural principles that reasonable people would affirm to guide decision-making in a population-based health-care system of which they are members of?

It is probably beyond the scope of this chapter to delineate all the principles, as well as their justifications, for population-based health care. At best, I can outline a core set of principles and hint at their justification and some of the practical implications they have for constituting an ethically justifiable population-based health-care system. This list will not be comprehensive but should accomplish two things: (*1*) It will sketch an alternative to the utilitarian approach to population-based health care, and (*2*) it will provide basic guidance for the kind of institutional structures necessary for constructing an ethically justifiable population-based system. I will begin by delineating some broad over-arching principles, then some procedural and substantive principles that further specify these for health care, and finally anticipate some of the practical implications of these principles.

Over-Arching Ideals for Population-Based Health Care

At the simplest and most intuitive level, reasonable people would want a population-based health-care system they would enroll in to adhere to four over-arching guiding ideals. The first two are substantive ideals, while the second pair are procedural ideals used to ensure that the substantive ideals are both adhered to and properly interpreted. The four over-arching ideals are:

1. Ideal of improving health: In a population-based health-care system, decisions and policies should aim to improve the health of the population.
2. Ideal of fair sacrifice: Cost savings that result from these decisions and policies should be used to benefit the population by either enhancing

health services, offering additional health services, or expanding the number of people who provide health services.

3. Ideal of trust: Procedures should exist to assure the population members that the decisions and policies of a population-based health system actually are made based on these two substantive ideals.
4. Ideal of self-determination: Procedures should exist to offer population members the opportunity to influence and contribute to the formulation of the decisions and policies that determine the health-care services they receive.

These ideals are fairly intuitive. As such, they should be unobjectionable and elicit widespread support from people. Indeed, some of them have been endorsed by others (Dougherty, 1992; Brock and Daniels, 1994; Council on Ethical and Judicial Affairs, 1994). Like any set of ideals, they are broadly stated and can be interpreted and implemented in many ways. As stated, they do not conflict with a utilitarian version of population-based health care, such as the one proposed by Eddy. The next step requires specifying them in a way that reasonable people would affirm and that can be ethically justified. The goal here is to specify these ideals in procedural and substantive principles and, in turn, to delineate some practical policies that flow from them. At each step of specification, the aim is to ensure widespread support, while becoming sufficiently specific to influence actual policies and practices.

Procedural Principles for a Population-Based Health Care

Underlying the two broad procedural ideals is the notion that in a complex health-care system it is hard for reasonable people to know how and why fundamental decisions and policies that can deeply affect their lives are made. Decisions and policies may be made far from them; all the information and factors relevant to the decisions and policies may not be accessible to them; they may not understand how one decision or policy relates to others; and they recognize that the decision and policy makers must address multiple issues that frequently conflict, requiring complex balancing and trade-offs. Consequently, when hearing of any single decision that is not accompanied by an explanation, reasonable people can be suspicious; essentially, they want procedures that will allay their suspicions and reassure them about the integrity of the decision-making process. Further, people expect to be able to influence those decisions that are likely significantly to affect their lives. As much research on medical care indicates, most people want as much information as possible, and they want the freedom to make key decisions even if they ultimately choose not to exercise this decision-making authority. Thus, the two procedural ideals suggest the need to make decision-making accessible, to ensure that the decision makers take into account only the relevant information and factors, and to give people the opportunity to influence and partake of the decision. The following five procedural principles offer a coherent and justifiable specification of these ideals:

1. Principle of fair consideration: In making decisions and formulating policies, consideration should be given to the interests of each individual in the population. Therefore, some open mechanism should exist for individuals to express their interests, concerns, and preferences to those making the decision. This mechanism should be relatively easy to access and use.
2. Principle of openness: Decisions and policies should be made available to each individual in the population, and the information and factors used in making these decisions and policies and the reasons justifying them should also be made available to each individual in the population.
3. Principle of empowerment: Individuals who are members of the population should have the opportunity to participate in the processes of formulating decisions and policies. This requires some mechanism to provide individuals with the opportunity to participate in selecting decision makers and expressing their views to the decision makers.
4. Principle of appeal: There should be a mechanism for raising objections to the decisions and policies and their justifications. This is really a corollary to the principle of empowerment; it is one, but only one, manifestation of this principle. Therefore, there should be some open and unbiased mechanism for individuals to object to or appeal decisions and policies and to raise new information and considerations. This open mechanism should be used to appeal not only the decisions as they apply to the individual's case, but also to object to the broader policies.
5. Principle of impartiality: Those formulating and implementing the decisions and policies should not have a conflict of interest. In making the decisions and policies, efforts should be made to minimize the possibility that factors extraneous to the decisions could influence the decision maker.

Again, it is the intention that each of these principles seem fairly intuitive and elicit widespread support. The full justification of these principles is beyond the scope of this chapter. However, principles should be justified if they can be seen as the best way to assure reasonable people that decisions and policies are being made in accord with the broad ideals. For instance, by being informed about policies, the information used in the policy formulation, and the reasons for adopting the specific policy, reasonable people can determine whether the policy does fulfill the ideal of improving health. By ensuring policies that minimize conflicts of interest, policy makers can assure people who do not choose to closely evaluate each decision that factors other than the health of the population are less likely to influence decisions. Similarly, principles of empowerment and appeal are necessary to offer opportunities for people to voice their views and have them considered when major decisions and policies—those that are likely to significantly affect their welfare or even whether they live or die—are made. A more complete justification of these principles can be found in the paper by Gutmann and Thompson (1996).

While these five procedural principles are consistent with the spirit of the work of Daniels and Sabin, I believe that they go beyond Daniels and Sabin's call for accountability for reasonableness (Daniels and Sabin, 1997, 1998a, 1998b). Accountability for reasonableness is limited to requiring a mechanism for the giving of reasons behind policies. This is essentially the principle of openness. And, indeed, many managed care organizations have already implemented practices consistent with this principle. For instance, Anthem Blue Cross and Blue Shield, Tennessee Blue Cross and Blue Shield, and Aetna have all put their medical coverage policies on the Web and provided citations to the data that have informed their decisions.

While viewing the giving of reasons as necessary, reasonable people would find accountability for reasonableness insufficient. It provides limited accountability, or at least the accountability suggested is limited to providing a justification—reasons—but no mechanism for accepting responsibility. There are two differences between the sort of accountability that Daniels and Sabin advance and the five principles presented above. First, with only accountability of reasonableness operating, the individual in a population-based health system is treated as a passive recipient of the information and reasons. She is told of a decision and the reasons behind the decision, but she is not invited to participate in the decision-making process. Her perspective is not actively incorporated into the decision. In other words, while Daniels and Sabin endorse the principle of openness, they do not endorse the principle of empowerment. As they write, "The dispute resolution mechanism does not empower enrollees or clinical staff to participate directly in the decision-making bodies." Second, there is no real effector loop in which the decision makers are held responsible. Once the decision and reasons are given, there is no solicitation of reactions. The only responsibility Daniels and Sabin imagine are appeals or exit. Again, mechanisms that implement empowerment after decisions have been made, but are not just appeals, have no role in accountability for reasonableness.

Practical Implications of the Procedural Principles

What are the practical implications of these five principles? Some are obvious. They clearly support an appeals process for members who are denied services. The principle of impartiality also could be used to justify, but by no means require, the presence of an external adjudication panel. Importantly, the principle of empowerment would suggest that members of the population be included in the appeals panels. The principle of openness would require making accessible both major policies and decisions, such as those relating to coverage or exclusion of particular services, as well as the reasons behind them. This could be accomplished through letters to or open meetings of members, postings on Websites, and other forms of communications. These two practical implications have been widely discussed, endorsed, and even implemented by many managed care organizations; their widespread endorsement evinces support for the principles.

Several implications have been less widely discussed and considered. One possible way of specifying the principle of empowerment is to have a real market in which members of the population can leave, and their ability to select decision makers thus results from their selecting different population-based systems. However, an alternative way of specifying this principle is to ensure that population members are included on advisory boards, boards of trustees, or other policy-making bodies. For instance, members might be included in committees that devise practice guidelines. Similarly, population members might be incorporated into committees that make medical policy determinations, such as what services will be covered under the rubric of medical necessity. Pharmacy and therapeutics committees that determine whether certain drugs are included in the formulary could easily incorporate population members, as could committees that evaluate the adoption of new technologies or ethics committees of managed care companies that determine policies regarding whether specific patients should be withdrawn from ventilators. Inclusion of members in these committees would ensure empowerment and openness simultaneously.

Much has been written about conflict of interest as it applies to physicians and their medical decisions. But key decisions and policies are established by many other individuals, and the principle of impartiality would require scrutiny of these other decision makers, as well. For instance, members of the pharmacy and therapeutics (P & T) committees usually have significant authority over formularies and decisions about what drugs will be covered.

Their decisions must also adhere to the principle of impartiality. This principle does permit cost and cost savings to be a factor or even the primary reason, influencing these decisions. What it prohibits is the influence of extraneous factors—that certain drug representatives are friends of the members of the P & T committee or that P & T committee members get benefits, including financial bonuses, for choosing or excluding certain drugs.

Substantive Principles for Population-Based Health Care

Procedural principles are insufficient. Decision making for a population-based health-care system needs to achieve certain ends; these are given by the two over-arching substantive ideals. These ideals are vague. Clearly, one sort of ideal is a principle of maximization; this is Eddy's approach. The issue is whether there are other, nonmaximizing conceptions of improving health that might be more appealing. The problem is that beyond the banal, such as not covering cosmetic surgery, no one has been able to elaborate a set of sufficiently determinate substantive principles for health-care coverage decisions. It is for this reason that maximization seems so appealing: it at least gives a determinate, even numerical, answer. I can only delineate a very limited list of principles that fulfill the substantive ideals and elicit widespread support. Here is a first try at eight principles. They are not meant to be comprehensive or to cover the whole range of cases, but to begin, at least, the substantive discussion:

1. Collect outcomes data and support research necessary to inform allocation decisions and policies.
2. Costs and comparative cost savings can be considered in selecting health-care services for a population.
3. Cover the cheapest pharmaceutical agents, but make available other agents if the cheapest ones either prove ineffective or induce significant side effects.
4. Cover health-care services to cure and ameliorate the effects of common illnesses and to prevent common illnesses. Example: treatment of otitis media (middle-ear infection) and pneumococcal pneumonia.
5. Cover preventive health care services that can nearly eliminate illnesses. Example: DPT vaccine.
6. Cover health-care services for all illnesses that have a 15% or higher chance of being completely cured or extending life for 5 years. Example: renal transplantation.
7. Cover health-care services for illnesses and disabilities that cannot be cured but in which the impairments can be completely reversed. Examples: insulin for diabetes and eyeglasses.

8. Cover health care for catastrophic illnesses in which there is a greater than 15% chance that there can be an improvement in quality of life and function to the extent that an individual can live independently. Example: childhood acute leukemia.
9. Cover community and environmental interventions that eliminate illnesses and significantly lower health risks. Example: lead paint removal.
10. Cover health-care services for research on experimental therapies that will lead to developing new tests, preventive measures, and treatments. Example: lung volume reduction surgery.

Any substantive set of principles will be controversial because the principles are indeterminate and hence likely to engender disagreement. Thus, it is easy to object to and dismiss this set of principles. Obviously, they are neither comprehensive nor determinative and cover only a small portion of all health-care services. Hence, these principles will not be sufficient to determine important coverage choices. Further, many contain the typical qualifications "common," "significantly lower," and "nearly cured." Such words will need to be specified, and any specification will be controversial. Other principles provide a false sense of certainty by providing definitive numbers—for instance, a 15% chance of cure. Such limits inevitably will be contested as arbitrary. Further, these principles are almost entirely directed at curative and preventive treatments; interventions aimed at relieving non–life threatening conditions and symptoms are not mentioned. And even without the qualifications, people may well disagree with the content of some of these principles even in their limited realms of intended application.

Nevertheless, delineating these principles can serve several essential functions. First, without trying to justify each one, the principles as a whole do address the major objectives that people want to realize in health care. They provide for effective preventive services, treatment of common illnesses, treatment of entirely curable and reversible ailments, and treatment of catastrophic illnesses. In addition, the principles recognize the need for requiring a certain threshold of efficacy in order for treatments to be covered; just because someone believes in a treatment or it has always been done or it has marginal benefits does not provide a sufficient reason for covering it. These principles link coverage to evidence of reasonable outcomes. They also recognize that what can be treated effectively today is arbitrary and that people want progress to treat what cannot be currently cured. Finally, they recognize that costs should be one, but just one, consideration among others. All these factors reveal that the principles strive to embody deeply held views.

Second, these principles fill a void. Until now, substantive principles have been limited to allocation by cost-effectiveness calculations, exhaustive

Oregon-style lists, or vague principles of medical necessity. None of these has been or is likely to be acceptable. In part because of their shortcomings and in part because the task seems so daunting, few are willing to articulate substantive principles. Almost all discussions of allocation stop with procedural criteria. Nevertheless, some attempt at substantive principles for allocation decisions and policies is needed. After all, decision makers must make decisions about what to cover and why; they need guidance. Similarly, people need to assess the justifiability of coverage decisions and the reasons behind them; they need standards of evaluation. This is the beginning of such an attempt.

Third, these principles, or a similar set, can provide the nucleus for developing agreement on an ever more expanding set of substantive principles that can aspire to cover all health-care services. A fully articulated comprehensive set of substantive principles has not and is not likely to be proposed de novo. It is likely to be constructed through an iterative process. We should strive for a development process that begins by invoking some core set of substantive principles, then, that through the process of actual decision making and challenge, are subsequently elaborated, qualified, and refined to be consistent, coherent, and comprehensive. I believe this is what Daniels and Sabin have in mind when they call for a "case law" type of approach to allocation decisions (1997). Some set of substantive principles are indispensable to such an iterative process. This set tries to posit some core principles that we can all agree to.

Fourth, the disagreement engendered by such a list is both expected and not morally problematic. Different people and different populations will interpret the various qualifying terms differently, draw the thresholds at different places, and emphasize different priorities. This disagreement reflects different values. The different sets of substantive principles can be ethical as long as each is delineated in accordance with the procedural principles. This means that different population-based health-care systems can have different allocations of resources, cover different health services, and still be ethical. There is no single set of just substantive principles or a justifiable set of health services; many different sets can be just (Emanuel, 1991, 1996). Their justice inheres in fulfilling the over-arching ideals in a way consistent with the procedural principles. Thus, one population-based health system might adopt Eddy's utilitarian view. We might call it the economists' population-based health system. Other systems might reject a strict cost-effectiveness approach, endorsing less effective interventions for reasons of equity or compassion.

Fifth, and related, part of the process required by the procedural principles will include giving reasons for decisions and policies. A core set of substantive principles that are widely endorsed can offer such reasons. More importantly, they can offer guidance to decision makers in how to make decisions and develop policies. This indicates how the substantive and procedural principles are mutually supportive. The substantive principles provide guidance to decision makers in formulating decisions and policies and in providing reasons that can be invoked to justify the decisions and policies. For instance, these principles would suggest coverage of smoking cessation programs. In most of these programs, 20% to 30% of the participants remain tobacco-free after one year. And cessation significantly reduces the risk of lung cancer; for light smokers, the risk can approximate the risk of nonsmokers after several years. And, while former heavy smokers always have elevated risks compared to those of nonsmokers, they do significantly reduce their lung cancer risk. The effectiveness of the cessation programs and the significant reduced risk of lung cancer suggest smoking cessation treatments should be covered.

Nonetheless, the indeterminacy of the substantive principles means that the procedures are necessary to supplement the principles and to ensure that the elaborations and refinements are deemed legitimate because they were achieved through fair procedures. These substantive principles can provide practical guidance in fundamental decisions.

CONCLUSIONS

One of the key health policy challenges for the next decade will be to resolve the ethical dilemmas posed by shifting to a population-based health system. Most of the attention surrounding this challenge has been focused on physician resistance to population-based health care, but the real ethical dilemma, and probably the more serious problem, arises from the public's resistance. The public's suspicions and hostility towards utilitarian approaches to many public policy issues easily translate to Eddy's version of population-based health care. The alternative approach is to consider the kinds of procedural and substantive principles a reasonable person would require to be cared for in a population-based health-care system. I have argued that the key requirements can be captured in four ideals: (*1*) improving health, (*2*) fair sacrifice, (*3*) trust, and (*4*) self-determination. These ideals are best realized when decision making in a population-based health-care system adheres to five procedural principles: (*1*) fair consideration, (*2*) publicity, (*3*) empowerment, (*4*) appeals, and (*5*) impartiality.

These would be accompanied by substantive principles outlining what treatments, services, medications and so on were to be covered. Together, these ideals and principles suggest important practical changes if a population-based health system is to be ethically justifiable.

REFERENCES

Anders G (1996) *Health Against Wealth: HMOs and the Breakdown of Medical Trust.* New York: N Houghton Mifflin.

Brock DW and Daniels N (1994) Ethical foundations of the Clinton administration's proposed health care system. *Journal of the American Medical Association* 271:1189–96.

Council on Ethical and Judicial Affairs, American Medical Association. Ethical issues in health care system reform: The provision of adequate health care. *Journal of the American Medical Association* 272:1056–62.

Crowley W (1996) *To Serve the Greatest Number: A History of Group Health Cooperative of Puget Sound.* Seattle: University of Washington Press.

Daniels N and Sabin J (1997) Limits to health care: Fair procedures, democratic deliberation, and the legitimacy problem for insurers. *Philosophy and Public Affairs* 16: 303–50.

Daniels N and Sabin J (1998a) Last chance therapies and managed care: Pluralism, fair procedures, and legitimacy. *Hastings Center Report* 28:27–41.

Daniels N and Sabin J (1998b) The ethics of accountability in managed care reform. *Health Affairs* 17:50–64.

Davis K and Schoen C (1978) *Health and the War on Poverty: A Ten-Year Appraisal.* Washington, D.C.: The Brookings Institution.

Dougherty CJ (1992) Ethical values at stake in health care reform. *Journal of the American Medical Association* 268:2409–12.

Eddy DM (1990) Connecting value and costs: Whom do we ask, and what do we ask them? *Journal of the American Medical Association* 264:1737–9.

Eddy DM (1991a) The individual vs society: Is there a conflict? *Journal of the American Medical Association* 265:1446–50.

Eddy DM (1991b) The individual vs society: Resolving the conflict. *Journal of the American Medical Association* 265:2399–406.

Eddy DM (1991c) What care is "essential"? What services are "basic"? *Journal of the American Medical Association* 265: 782–8.

Eddy DM (1994) Principles for making difficult decisions in difficult times. *Journal of the American Medical Association* 271:1792–8.

Emanuel EJ (1991) *The Ends of Human Life: Medical Ethics in a Liberal Polity.* Cambridge, MA: Harvard University Press.

Emanuel EJ (1996) Where civic republicanism and deliberative democracy meet. *Hastings Center Report* 26:12–4.

Emanuel EJ and Emanuel LL (1996) What is accountability in health care? *Annals of Internal Medicine* 124:229–39.

Epstein A (1996) Performance reports on quality-prototypes, problems, and prospects. *New England Journal of Medicine* 333:57–61.

Flexner A (1910) *Medical Education in the United States and Canada.* New York: Carnegie Foundation for the Adancement of Teaching.

Geiger HJ (1984) Community health centers: Health care as an instrument of social change. In: Sidel VW and Sidel R (eds) *Reforming Medicine: Lessons of the Last Quarter Century.* New York: Pantheon Books.

Greenlick MR (1992) Educating physicians for population-based clinical care. *Journal of the American Medical Association* 267:1645–8.

Gold MR, Siegel J, Russell LB, Weinstein M (1996) *Cost-Effectiveness in Health and Medicine*. New York: Oxford University Press.

Gutmann A and Thompson D (1996) *Democracy and Disagreement*. Cambridge, MA: Harvard University Press.

Hall MA and Berenson RA (1998) Ethical practice in managed care: A dose of realism. *Annals of Internal Medicine* 128:395–402.

Hobbes T (1962) *Leviathan* [1651] New York: Collier Books.

Kymlicka W (1990) *Contemporary Political Philosophy: An Introduction*. New York: Oxford University Press.

Levinsky N (1984) The doctor's master. *New England Journal of Medicine* 311:1573–5.

Menzel P (1990) *Strong Medicine: The Ethical Rationing of Health Care*. New York: Oxford University Press.

Menzel P, Gold MR, Nord E, Pinto-Prades JL, Richardson J, Ubel P (1999) Toward a boarder view of values in cost-effectiveness analysis of health. *Hastings Center Report* 29:7–15.

Nuland S (1989) *Doctors: The Biography of Medicine*. New York: Vintage Books.

Rawls J (1971) *A Theory of Justice*. Cambridge, MA: Harvard University Press.

Rodwin MA (1996) Consumer protection and managed care: The need for organized consumers. *Health Affairs* 15:110–23.

Sardell A (1988) *The U.S. Experiment in Social Medicine: The Community Health Center Program, 1965–86*. Pittsburgh, PA: University of Pittsburgh Press.

Shortell SM, Gillies RR, Anderson DA, Erickson KM, Mitchell JB (1986) *Remaking Health Care in America: Building Organized Delivery Systems*. San Fransisco: Jossey-Bass.

Starr P (1982) *The Social Transformation of American Medicine*. New York: Basic Books.

Ubel PA (2000) *Pricing Life: Why It's Time for Health Care Rationing*. Cambridge, MA: MIT Press.

Accountability

13

Accountability: regulating health care as a public good

CHRISTINE K. CASSEL AND ELAINE MCPARLAND

A new ethic for health professionals, including a new understanding of accountability, is required by the reality of today's medical marketplace. We do not have a well-developed notion of accountability for the current health care environment, where the physician–patient relationship occurs in the context of more complex systems, where the physician has less control, and where the patient is also seen as a "consumer." Traditional models of accountability are no longer adequate as the dyadic nature of the relationship between physicians and patients has changed. Accountability is a central notion in a modern approach to quality and to the ethical relationships required by transformations in health care. This chapter will first describe the traditional accountability structure and its evolution and then examine the construction and potential advantages and disadvantages of a new accountability structure more consistent with the realities of current clinical practice. A newly articulated ethic for health-care professionals, which recognizes the centrality of the patient as an individual but is more consistent with social priorities such as cost containment and population health, is warranted in today's medical marketplace.

INTRODUCTION

Accountability is a multilayered and multifaceted component of the ethical relationship of health care providers and institutions to patients and consumers. It derives from ancient concepts of medical ethics and professionalism but has become much more complex because of evolving concepts regarding the responsibilities of the health-care professional. Along with concerns about accountability of a physician to his or her patients, questions are being raised about physicians' accountability in the contemporary world to health-care management systems and employers, to governance bodies such as trustees, to the government as payer and as regulator, to the patient as consumer, and to the public or society at large.

Each of these has dimensions that are not clear in any existing code of ethics and has incontrovertible effects on the traditional ethos of the doctor–patient relationship. These newer accountability relationships are often assumed in discussions about setting priorities for health policy and research. Yet the evolving nature of health-care delivery necessitates questioning these assumptions and clarifying the ethical frameworks for the physician's emerging relationships.

TRADITIONAL ACCOUNTABILITY STRUCTURE

Centering the concept of accountability in the context of a discussion on connecting ethics and health policy sheds light on the inherent moral components within the concept of accountability and requires articulation of the relationships encompassed by this term. Webster's definition of *accountable* is twofold: (*1*) subject to giving an account, that is, answerable ("every sane man is accountable to his conscience for his behavior") and (*2*) capable of being accounted for, that is, explainable ("their apparently strange customs are now accountable"). The use of the term in contemporary health policy and ethics focuses on the first of these meanings: accountable means answerable. It implies a relationship, expectations, and duties commensurate with those expectations. However, as the practice of medicine has become increasingly complex, both in terms of its management and its ability to affect and be affected by larger groups, the relationships and corresponding extent of a physician's responsibilities to parties other than his or her patients has remained unclear.

The notion of the social contract, born in the Enlightenment, is a primary source of the demand for accountability, both for the individual and society. Once leaving behind the idea of the divine right of kings or other tyrannical approaches to governing, forms of democracy emerged. While there are various articulations of it, the fundamental concept of the social contract is that people bind together because it benefits them all to be enjoined in a social arrangement where each foregoes some aspect of his freedom or resources in order to gain benefits that can best be gained by common effort. It is the extent to which the individual benefits from a specific cohesion brought together by the social contract that the foregoing of absolute freedom, including the paying of taxes and other levies and the restraints or standards imposed by governmental and regulatory bodies, are justified. This idea is so inherent in our society that we rarely question it, but it needs to be stated clearly as a presumption in exploring how accountability in health care has and continues to evolve in our society. Stated more directly, the individual physician–patient relationship is not the only context of accountability, but it is a central one. The others all derive from the societal mechanisms for regulating professions such as licensure, complex approaches to spreading financial risk, such as insurance, and the reality that illnesses of individuals may affect others, as in epidemics. In addition to the social contract, there are social values—less direct but just as influential—that affect accountability. Examples of these values are the care of the suffering (compassion) and the value of a healthy and productive population.

The professions, of which medicine is one, exemplify a microcosm of the larger social contract. In the professions, sociologists have described a social arrangement whereby elevated status is accorded an occupational group in return for the provision of an essential and specialized benefit (Sharpe, 2000). The sociology of professions has characterized autonomy and self-regulation as essential attributes of professions. However, limitations are imposed on the professional's autonomy to the extent that the professional must meet democratically established normative criteria grounded in concepts of the public good (Sharpe, 2000). The standards to which professionals are held are comparatively high, and professionals are expected to find ways to regulate themselves in accordance with those standards or else be subject to sanctions for misbehavior.

In the traditional model of medicine, on which other health professions also base their ethical codes, the provider is held to be, first and foremost, responsible for (and therefore, for the purposes of our discussion, accountable to) the patient. The patient is defined as the individual seeking care. It is largely a voluntary relationship. Once entered, the physician is expected to act in the best interest of the patient (Shortell et al, 1998). In the words of Plato's *Republic*, "no physician, insofar as he is a physician, considers his own good in what he prescribes, but the good of his patient . . ." (Plato, Book I, 342-D). The physician in the Hippocratic tradition is responsible and therefore accountable to the patient to act professionally. This ethic derives from ancient precepts and has been examined by philosophers throughout the ages. Its justification is based primarily on the observation of the differential power between the patient and the physician. The inequality has two components. First, one party has knowledge that the other party needs but does not have. Second, one party is healthy and in control and the other party is sick and in an inherently vulnerable state asking for help. That is, the patient is sick, or is at least worried or concerned about her health and does not have the knowledge or the skills the physician possesses. Thus, this relationship is inherently unequal at its core and could embody a potential for exploitation. It is because of this inequality that ethicists through the ages have so strongly asserted the importance of the primary responsibility of the physician to the patient (Shortell et al, 1998).

In this context the physician is accountable to the patient for aspects of his professionalism, that is, to have the knowledge he professes to have, to be competent in methods of diagnosis and treatment, and to be respectful toward the patient. Anything that falls short of the first two responsibilities is considered fraudulent or unethical behavior, for which the physician is justly held accountable by statutory and regulatory entities. Similarly, in the full definition of accountability, respect and compassion are behavioral characteristics that, if missing, do not constitute fraud but can be said to constitute unprofessional behavior. Society holds the physician responsible for meeting quality-of-care standards and accountable if these standards are not appropriately respected.

In the traditional structure of health-care delivery, the prospective model of accountability includes the accreditation process of medical schools and training programs, the process of licensure at the state level, and the process of specialty certification and credentialing, which provides peer evaluation by attestation or actual testing throughout a physician's practice life. These intrusions on professional autonomy have been justified by the state's responsibility to protect the public, especially its most vulnerable members (Mechanic, 1996).

The retrospective way in which accountability has been exerted in the traditional doctor–patient relationship is through the medical negligence malpractice system (Emanuel and Emanuel, 1996). As has been well documented, much negligence appears to occur that is never called to account through the malpractice system. It is probably also fair to say that a good deal of malpractice suits may not be related to negligence. Nonetheless, the system has functioned, in a very individualized, piecemeal way, to hold physicians accountable for their actions (Gosfield, 1997). What has emerged from this method of physician regulation and oversight is not so much improved quality of care, but a significant increase in administrative responsibilities and risk management in the practice of medicine. Currently there are requirements for scrupulous documentation by the physician of both actions and justifications for those actions so that an interaction that occurred some time ago may be examined in the future. Standards of care are retroactively reviewed so that damages are theoretically appropriately redressed. The physician is thus accountable for his or her activities in a court of law, and the findings in this forum often inform professional censure for breach of standards of care.

In addition to these traditional methods of regulating professionalism and accountability, there have been additional attempts to formalize the nature of a physician's accountability to his or her patients (Sharpe, 2000). Physicians are often regarded as fiduciaries, or agents, for their patients. In any profession where an imbalance of knowledge and powers exist, the concept of the fiduciary, or agency, can be central. The assumption in these relationships is that some limits are established to the ability to exploit a need or exploit a market because of the inequality of the parties involved. Professional groups have provided guidelines for the individual professional's behavior, and oversight for a fiduciary, or agent, is often by peer or colleague review.

The professional who is fiduciary is both morally and legally liable to those with whom a relationship has been established. Once a relationship is established, the fiduciary owes the principal duties of loyalty, obedience, and care and has the responsibility for ensuring that these duties are fulfilled (Calamari, 1987). A key component, then, of these traditional conceptualizations is that accountability is established only to those with whom a relationship has expressly or implicitly been demonstrated. One of the fundamental attributes of the agency relationship, for example, is the question "Who am I the agent for and on whose behalf am I acting?" A specific relationship must be evidenced before expectations are imposed in the context of these relational definitions. Thus, characterizing the physician as the patient's fiduciary underscores the traditional importance of clearly designating those to whom a duty is owed by the physician. In the traditional medical regime the patient was invariably the recipient of that duty of care.

TRANSFORMATIVE SHIFT

While most people would support the value of accountability between doctor and patient, the context of the relationship has changed in ways that call for a redefining of the relatively straightforward delineation described above (Gray, 1997; Relman, 1988). Some of these factors include the following: (*1*) health care is now often seen as preventive, with an empowered and responsible role for patients in partnership with physicians; (*2*) much of health care is provided by interdisciplinary teams rather than a single doctor;

(*3*) clinicians are part of larger health-care delivery institutions; (*4*) consumers (those who buy insurance and the patients themselves) hold health-care institutions accountable not only for quality of care but also for cost containment; and (*5*) some health care institutions are publicly owned, and the shareholders hold them accountable to produce profit. How do all these new layers of accountability potentially affect physicians' accountability relationships to the patient?

EVOLUTION OF POPULATION HEALTH

In recent years data-processing technology has begun to transform the way health information is acquired and used. Epidemiology, the science of population-based health, has benefited greatly from this technological revolution. Our improved ability to aggregate and synthesize data has enabled scientists to acquire a broader understanding of health-care trends and enhanced their ability to examine population health as an outcome measure of effective health-care policy making (ABIM Forum, 1998).

The focus in epidemiology is on public rather than private health goals. Much of the emphasis in population health is on prevention using a more utilitarian ethic to address preventive needs. Early population-based interventions, patient education, and demographic group screenings are promoted as more cost-effective ways to promote health for the greatest percentage of the population. Decision making in the context of population health is more politically motivated than is that for individual patients because of the finite nature of health-care dollars and resources. Resource constraints and rationing—the explicit process of setting priorities for the allocation of resources—are necessary as a means for distributing population health. The physician's role in setting priorities is indistinct. There are no existing guidelines regarding standard of care because there is no consensus in our society on principles of distributive justice (Bloche, 1999). Decisions regarding expensive but marginally beneficial treatments particularly challenge the physician, as the dual roles of quasi-public servant and provider of individual care conflict.

The concept of population health has taken on even greater significance with the advent of managed care. Managed care plans purport to "manage" populations of patients and thereby support the objective of population health. However, in a managed care organization the goal of population health may be secondary to commercial concerns and the desire for cost control. The ethical basis for decision making is different from that of the traditional provider, with less impetus to defend decisions on behalf of the individual patient (Hiatt, 1975).

Also, in this evolving era of health care in the United States, there is often no stable and identifiable fiduciary relationship between any given provider, health plan, or insurer and a given population of individuals, and, consequently, the definition of *population* in the managed care context may differ. Few health plans have members only in a specified geographic area, and the "community" of their insured members is not the same "community" in which some members live. Rather, people switch from one payer to another, from one health plan to another, and from one provider to another very frequently, as companies are bought and sold, merged, and acquired. Thus, even a good health plan with goals in population health has objectives that may conflict because, as patient demographics change, so might health-care priorities.

Whether the definition of *population* is inclusive or exclusive, it is clear that the ethical ethos shifts when the goal is population health (Mechanic, 1996). A focus on population health inherently suggests that the primary goal of benefits (as evinced in the social contract) has shifted from the individual to the larger community. The accountability of health-care providers, when faced with the needs of the community, changes and may even directly conflict with that of the individual patient. There are situations in which the physician's responsibility to public health may override what the individual patient and family believe is best.

The tensions between public health and individual patient goals translate to complex realities that are framed by underlying ethical dilemmas. Privacy, for example, is an area that exemplifies the ethical tension generated by the clinician faced with conflicting loyalties. In the traditional physician–patient relationship, the physician is accountable to the patient for quality of care, completeness of information about personal health status, explanation of options available, and respect for privacy. However, in a context concerned with public health, the physician's ethical responsibilities to the individual patient may conflict with the socially desirable end of improved health for the community at large. The question arises whether the physician's relative ethical responsibilities to the patient are greater than those to population-based interests seeking aggregate data. For example, it may be necessary to divulge the presence of sexually transmitted or infectious diseases to public health officials or to notify motor vehicle licensing bureaus of the presence of certain neurological disorders in one's patients. Compromise solutions can offer an approach of procedural fairness in aiming for resolution. For example, a process of appeal and exception for individuals could be established, thereby acknowledging the risk that certain kinds of information (such as that pertaining to sexually transmitted diseases or mental illness) might be so incomplete that quality-of-care data is inaccurate. Patient identities can be erased from grouped data, but not everyone is equally confident that electronically processed data will not somehow be used to identify individuals with specific health risks. More importantly, the procedural solutions do not resolve the ethical questions covering the accountability relationship. If population health is examined as the outcome measure for the effectiveness of health-care systems, individual patients need involvement in and perhaps even consent to the priorities established by the population health focus (ABIM Forum, 1998).

MEDICAL MARKETPLACE

A second transformative shift that strongly affects traditional ethical paradigms has been in the economics of health-care delivery. The financing of health care has gradually become more institutionally based, developing from a private fee-for-service structure to government and employer-sponsored insurance and then to for-profit managed care organizations and multispecialty practice groups. The financial structures of our health-care delivery systems have become increasingly complex, and care management practices are shaped by a myriad of commercial and public health considerations (Bloche, 1999).

We have discussed how public health considerations affect the traditional accountability structure. Contemporary management systems in the commercial sector, such as managed care organizations and physician practice groups, also generate considerable conflict with the conventional paradigms. Many of them relate to how money flows within these systems and cost-control measures to maximize profits. The clinical ramifications of decisions made and positions taken in for-profit organizations are more than monetary but are subject to little public or governmental oversight or control. Clinical decisions may be questioned and restrictions on physicians imposed; however, accountability and consequences for questionable practices are often attributed to the individual physician.

For example, an employer or oversight body may not agree with what a physician feels is necessary for a patient. The physician may then find herself in a conflict of accountability. While the physician maintains the moral obligation to make decisions in the best interests of her patient, the decision-making process to ensure quality care for the patient is not straightforward. The consequences of a physician not meeting her organizational responsibilities can significantly affect the patient. For example, if the physician loses her position because she remains inflexible in her opinions, she is no longer in a position to help that patient. Continuity of care is compromised and the patient's interests have not been served. Another level of complexity arises when the physician is part of a multispecialty practice group in which the group sets quality-of-care standards (Lundberg, 1997). Although ideally such a situation should lead to quality improvement as physicians are accountable to peers and colleagues for clinical decisions that should be increasingly evidence-based, it is also a situation that can lead to a conflict of loyalties.

A more clear-cut conflict arises in the case of publicly held, for-profit health-care systems in institutions. In this case there is a legal responsibility of the managers of the systems to the investors to maximize profits. This structure does not allow for the Platonic rule. This is not simply a disagreement about the best approach to a certain clinical problem in which the dispute can be based on a discussion of the evidence among peers, but rather is a situation in which a physician executive could be held legally accountable to shareholders for protecting their investment and, at the same time, be held morally and legally accountable to a patient for acting in the patient's best interests.

As the nature of the business transaction between patient and provider has changed, so has the nature of their professional interaction. The unprecedented access of patients and their families to medical information and alternative treatment options has increased patient desire for input into their care and informed consent about that care. Distrust regarding the financial structures and incentives under which physicians operate has prompted calls for increasingly sophisticated measures to assess physician performance and protect patient well-being. This has been most evident in the growing crescendo of concern about quality of care—its measurement, reporting, and ongoing improvement and the increasing number of constraints on physician autonomy (Relman, 1988). Newly emerging entities such as the National Forum for Healthcare Quality Measurement and Reporting are implementing new initiatives to ensure physician accountability and increase patients' roles in health-care decision making.

As patients began to take a more active role in health care, they began to demand more as a unified group and became more sophisticated about presenting those demands. Demands have evolved into expectations, and the patient has become a health-care "consumer" with stronger abilities to advocate for health-care services. The ongoing debate, about the Consumer Bill of Rights and Responsibilities signifies this new status in a very literal sense, as they specifically delineate a number of rights to which the health-care consumer is entitled. This reflects a new standard in medicine, giving the patient responsibilities as a consumer and explicitly making the relationship more of a commercial one. The "consumer" language empowers the patient but leads to less protection of the vulnerable if caveat emptor rules apply. Consumers also include employers who buy health insurance plans for their workers and, indeed, the government itself in its role as purchaser through Medicare and Medicaid. These larger consumers obviously have much more power than the individual consumer, who may change physicians if dissatisfied but may have to stay within a certain network or hospital system depending on the insurance arrangements. One thing is clear: To call a patient a consumer is not itself sufficient to create an equal relationship with the physician, especially at a time when the patient is sick and in need of care. It does, however, put additional claims on the physician to respond to the patient's needs and to do so in a cost-effective manner. These claims can, of course, be conflicting—the patient may want affordable insurance premiums and co-payments but may also reject any limits when in need of personal services. Conflict arises over which role of the physician most clearly defines his or her accountability and how both claims of the patient can be effectively served.

The effectiveness of the consumer voice has been demonstrated in recent years in the backlash against managed care (Gray, 1997). Successful lobbying efforts on the part of consumers have led to legislatively imposed restrictions on the decisions made by managed care companies regarding some clinical practices. However, accountability has not been well delineated for these corporate entities, and, for the most part, individual providers have borne a large part of the responsibility for questionable decision making. Although managed care companies are increasingly being held responsible for adverse outcomes through tort law and legislative fiat, an ethical framework that more appropriately allocates the legal and moral responsibility for quality care is necessary.

NEW ACCOUNTABILITY STRUCTURE

The recent changes in the economics of health care and patients' roles in the delivery of health care services, as well as the growing awareness of the importance of the social obligations of physicians in addressing the population's health needs, herald a new ethic in medicine (Lundberg, 1997). The fundamental shifts that have occurred in our perceptions of health care should be exhibited in new health-care policies that reflect the movement toward more organizational responsibility and help achieve the objective of reasonable access to quality health care for the greatest percentage of the population (Cassel, 1999).

We currently have a significant segment of our population who are underinsured or who have no insurance at all and a large number who are handled by managed care companies with little or no accountability structures in place. Another segment of the population is served by governmental programs such as Medicare and Medicaid, but quality controls have been implemented only sporadically under these systems. Since no broad regulatory authority is authorized to establish comprehensive controls over any of these populations or corporate entities, accountability in the system remains physician centered. This does not reflect the realities of health-care delivery as it has evolved, nor does it apportion responsibility for decision making to the appropriate parties or groups. As influences on medical decision making expand, the expectations of the individual medical professional must be extended to the larger society of medical providers, with a shift in emphasis from personal accountability to collective responsibility and resolution (Rodwin).

The organizational sources of accountability will, in large part, depend on how the economics of health-care delivery is prioritized in our culture. Currently, government (federal, state, regional, and local) provides forums for decision making, communication, security, and certain services deemed essential to the conduct of contemporary life, such as police, roads, electricity, and sewers. Ensuring the provision of these "public goods and services" is largely the province of government, and restraints and regulations are justified by the need to maintain standards of quality for the good of society. Protection of these essential services is justified as being in the public interest and is generally governed by an administrative or regulatory agency authorized at the state or federal level. Generally, this form of governance is designed to ensure uniformity, veracity, and quality in the provision of these services. An example is the securities industry, which was once unregulated and susceptible to fraudulent practices. The industry is now comprehensively regulated, and issues regarding disclosure, duty, and accountability are addressed explicitly by statute. Furthermore, controls are in place to monitor questionable transactions and provide early intervention and investigation into potential problems. This type of model may be useful in the health-care field.

Transformations in medicine and the health-care delivery system have resulted in a health-care structure in which it is both appropriate and necessary to characterize health care as analogous to a public good or utility. The most important reason for this is protection of the individuals who use these essential services. As the social purposes of medicine have evolved, the recognition that it is both economically sound and socially desirable to strive for the goal of population health has resulted in fundamental changes in our health-care environment. Promotion of various protocols, therapies, and standards of care affect a far greater number of individuals than ever before, and the ramifications of care decisions are more widespread. As the onus of personal rights and responsibilities in the context of a clinical relationship has shifted away from the individual physician and patient, so, too, has the need for coordinated regulation of the various institutions influencing the state of the art of medical care. Thus, it has become crucial that there be an oversight system to ensure quality and uniformity in the provision of health-care services.

Also, the ethical and economic realities of today's medical marketplace, in which health care is considered a valued and concrete resource, are not reflected in the traditional model of market competition. Our accountability structures have become so diversified and our delivery systems so complex that coordinated directives and regulations would help to ensure that cost concerns are disassociated as much as possible from issues of quality of health-care delivery and decisions regarding access.

Characterizing health care as a "public good" would result in an accountability structure by which many aspects of cost, quality, and access to health services would be regulated by the government on behalf of the public. The government, in this case, would and should engage in setting these standards in its role as purchaser, especially on behalf of particularly vulnerable populations. Incentives to balance individual and societal care would be managed by administrative oversight, and that management system would be required to answer to those who are paying for the care (i.e., the taxpayers).

Administrative oversight of health care would serve the interests of patients more effectively, with many advantages over the current system. A more population-based approach to medicine would be facilitated, and this would allow the disciplines of medicine and public health to become more closely aligned. This would also promote improved health-care planning, as strategies for managing care could be more systematically developed and implemented rather than having, as is current practice, reactive legislation address singular issues. Preventive care would be encouraged as a more cost-effective way to achieve the goal of population health and would encourage use of population statistics to promote the most effective interventions.

Public input, in a professionally driven context, would have a greater role in such a system and would thus be more responsive to the current climate of consumerism in health care. Clinical interventions with marginal utility would be evaluated and scrutinized to a greater degree as usage became increasingly value-driven, and quality-of-life issues would be analyzed and used more concretely.

Although cost containment would be an essential reality, administrators would know they were accountable to the public for providing access to quality services. A regulatory agency could operate independently of profit incentives and be less influenced by special interest groups. Rationing would become a public debate, and discussions of different constituencies, a "basic minimum" of services, and "cost-effectiveness" of various approaches would occur in a forum that allowed input from the recipients of care.

Although a publicly regulated health-care system would provide a number of advantages over the current system, it is important to note potential problems with such an arrangement. Administrative burdens associated with the regulatory model potentially could lead to an increase in external requirements without quality improvement. It would be important to implement such a system in a manner that would decrease, not increase, administrative requirements that interfere with physicians' clinical responsibilities. Privacy issues could also be cause for concern. Controls would have to be in place to ensure that the information collected from individuals for health care data systems would not be misused or misappropriated. Finally, new ethical problems would be raised by such a system, which would require attention. For example, public preferences in prioritizing resources would raise moral and ethical dilemmas. Choices regarding experimental interventions or those with marginal utility would have to be balanced against the need for cost-effective care. Safeguards would have to be implemented to ensure that vulnerable populations, such as the elderly and the poor, were adequately represented in decision-making processes. Anticipating these problems will go a long way toward avoiding their generation.

CONCLUSION

It may be the case that the physician is the subject of a good part of the ethical discourse regarding competing responsibilities in health care because, in our society, physicians are the most identifiable sources for accountability. However, the simple and moral relationship between the physician and patient and the clear social purpose of the healing professions will never again be as simple as they once were purported to be. Overall, however, it is clear that we must move beyond the Hippocratic tradition and embrace a new accountability structure more aligned with population needs and the goal of universal access to health care. The real value of ethics in relation to health policy can be understood in its ability to reconceptualize these complex issues in a broader context and thereby clarify directives for moral principles to be reconciled with the realities of our health-care delivery system.

REFERENCES

American Board of Internal Medicine (ABIM) (August 3–5, 1998) *Forum for the Future: New Science, New Markets and New Ethics*. Sun Valley, ID.

Bloche MG (1999) Clinical loyalties and the social purposes of medicine. *Journal of the American Medical Association* 281(3): 268–74.

Calamari JD (1987) *The Law of Contracts*. 3d ed. St. Paul, MN: West Publishing.

Cassel CK (1999) The challenge of serving both patient and populace. *The American Medical Ethics Revolution*. Baltimore, MD: Johns Hopkins University Press.

Emanuel EJ and Emanuel LL (1996) What is accountability in health care? *Annals of Internal Medecine* 124:229–39.

Gosfield AG (1997) Who is holding whom accountable for quality? *Health Affairs* 16(3): 26–40.

Gray BH (1997) Trust and trustworthy care in the managed care era. *Health Affairs* 16(1): 34–49.

Hiatt HH (1975) Protecting the medical commons: Who is responsible? *New England Journal of Medicine* 293(5): 235–41.

Lundberg GD (1997) The business and profession of medicine. *Journal of the American Medical Association* 276(20): 1703–4.

Mechanic D (1996) Changing medical organization and the erosion of trust. *Milbank Quarterly* 74(2): 171–89.

Relman AS (1988) Assessment and accountability: the third revolution in medical care. *New England Journal of Medicine* 319(18): 1220–1222.

Rodwin MA (1998) Conflicts of interest and accountability in managed care: The aging of medical ethics. *Journal of the American Geriatrric Society* 46:338–41.

Sharpe VA (2000) Behind closed doors: accountability and responsibility in patient care. *Journal of Medicine and Philosophy* 25(1):28–47.

Shortell SM, Waters TM, Clarke KWB, Budetti PP (1998) Physicians as double agents: Maintaining trust in an era of multiple accountabilities. *Journal of the American Medical Association* 280(12):1102–8.

14

Perspectives on accountability: past, present, and future

RUTH E. MALONE AND HAROLD S. LUFT

Beginning in the early 1990s and continuing to the present, multiple structural changes within health care have contributed to a sense of instability and increased concern about ensuring accountability for health services. These changes include the economic incentives arising from new financial relationships among patients, clinicians, insurers, and payers; new organizational settings for the delivery of care; and new decision-making roles for patients. Changes of such magnitude and pervasiveness engender debate and resistance, and an unfortunate amount of finger-pointing has characterized much of the discussion to date.

Those advocating stronger organizational and payer controls over medical decision making point to deficiencies in clinical accountability under fee-for-service arrangements and see evidence-based decision rules and economically efficient use of resources as increasing accountability. Physicians, in turn, resent growing intrusions into what was once a self-contained sphere of professional control and peer evaluation, often feeling they are being held accountable for care but denied the autonomy and authority to control the necessary resources (Pont, 2000). Other clinicians, such as nurses, who have traditionally held "in-between" (Bishop and Scudder, 1990) positions in which they served as the interpreters of and negotiators among the interests and wishes of patients, families, physicians, and hospitals or other institutions, complain of having less control over the conditions in which they practice even as they are expected to assume more responsibility for supervising the work of less-educated staff. Patients are increasingly suspicious of all parties and are bombarded by information about the promises of new technological advances. They are offered increased opportunities to make decisions about health practices while finding their options to control their health care increasingly constrained.

These issues raise important questions about how we conceive of accountability and what is at stake in how we address issues of accountability from a policy perspective. We speculate here on how these concerns are likely to manifest themselves in the next decades, what obstacles may be encountered in enhancing accountability, and how we might recognize "good" accountability. In this chapter, we focus primarily on accountability issues involved in the clinician–patient treatment relationship, although we readily acknowledge that there exist equally important accountability issues regarding many other aspects of health services that call for further discussion.

ACCOUNTABILITY DEFINED

To be accountable is, according to the *Oxford English Dictionary*, to be "liable to be called to account, or to answer for responsibilities and conduct" and, secondly, "to be counted or reckoned on" (Simpson and Weiner, 1989) At bottom, accountability rests on the foundation of moral obligation to the other. However, in the current context, the nature of that obligation is complex, contested, and often somewhat diffused. At issue are understandings of what it means to be a person who is accountable and what it means to be a person to whom a duty to provide an accounting is owed. These, in turn, are mediated through the institutions within which individuals act (or do not act) and the social values these institutions embody.

Emanuel and Emanuel (1996) identify three components of accountability: the loci of accountability, or the parties involved; the domains or subject matter for which the parties are to be accountable; and the procedures for assessing or ensuring such accountability. They posit a stratified model of accountability in which competing constructions of accountability drawing on professional, economic, and political conceptions are operative within different health-related spheres. Thus, for example, the clinician–patient relationship would remain under a professional accountability model, while the political model of accountability would guide relations between managed care plans and other institutional networks.

Daniels and Sabin (1998) and Daniels (1985) emphasize that ethical accountability requires a process characterized by fairness and openness. In their emphasis on public accountability, which they posit as requiring both market accountability and "accountability for reasonableness," they suggest a distinction between public accountability, or the kind of issues with which policy is concerned, and private accountability, which would involve commitments to obligations between private individuals that are not mediated through institutional or professional relations. This distinction is an important one to bear in mind because it reminds us to attend not only to the loci, nature, and assessment of accountability, but also to the institutions that mediate all these. For example, hospitals have traditionally served as community benefit institutions, last-resort social service providers, and sources of public pride, embodying community values of mutual aid, charitableness toward the less fortunate, and provision of rest and respite. Under increasing competitive pressures, however, these institutions' values have shifted in many instances away from these community values and toward economic survival in a cutthroat business climate (Noble et al, 1998). As the institutions through which accountabilities are mediated change, the possibilities for accountability likewise change.

It is not always possible to separate public and private accountability, because so many public policies structure the contexts within which individuals interact and thus shape the nature of their private accountability. As a simple example, what we now call spousal abuse was once regarded as private (if regrettable) behavior, and accountability for spousal violence (short of severe assault or murder) was regarded as a private issue, something to be worked out by the unhappy couple. The reframing of this behavior as a public concern, including policy making that set requirements for protection of victims of abuse, expanded the locus of accountability to include police, social workers, and clinicians, and consequently, in these instances, restructured the nature of the relations between spouses. Thus, perceived lack of private accountability may lead to pressure for public policy intervention and regulation.

ACCOUNTABILITY IN THE PAST: FROM MARCUS WELBY TO MANAGED CARE

In the recent past accountability in health services in this country was lodged chiefly within the professions, particularly professional medicine, and was presumed to be assured through a system of peer review. It should be noted here that public health services have operated under somewhat different structures of accountability, which we will not address here except to the degree that medical services are part of public health services. We also acknowledge that medical care does not equal health or even health care

(McKeown, 1979); however, medical care is central to contemporary discussions of health care because it is on medical care that the great majority of health-related dollars are currently spent.

In the idealized version of the traditional relationship, as exemplified by Doctor Marcus Welby, lead character of a popular television show that aired from 1969 to 1976, the physician acted selflessly to do his or her best for the patient. Dr. Welby, like many real-life doctors of his time, was accountable to the profession for upholding its standards, even though these were, in many instances, quite general expectations rather than explicitly agreed-upon standards. Dr. Welby was also accountable to the patient for acting in such a way as to benefit him or her. The patient was understood to be in need of expert knowledge and guidance and was portrayed as relatively helpless and ignorant, while the physician was the unchallenged expert in medical matters. Accountability under this arrangement was embedded within a relatively closed system that was integrated within the larger community.

A few decades before Dr. Welby, accountability was even more direct because, in the absence of health insurance, the patient was directly responsible for the costs incurred. Physicians often would discount their fees or waive them entirely, but it is probably the case that in situations in which ability to pay was limited, some care would not be offered. The spread of health insurance in the middle of the century made it possible for hospitals and clinicians to be paid for their services without the patient bearing the full burden. Cost was spread to other insured individuals, employers, or the public. In this halcyon era, however, no one was being held accountable for the overall costs.

As many have commented (Mechanic, 1998), this arrangement perpetuated paternalistic relations between doctors and their patients, since patients had little basis on which to judge whether a physician was truly acting for the patient's benefit. In addition, the profession's peer review system worked poorly in ensuring quality and minimizing the use of unnecessary or questionable procedures by the unscrupulous or overzealous practitioner (Leape, 1992; Wennberg et al, 1980). While the insurer paid physicians on a fee-for-service basis, with relatively little cost to the patient, one would expect a bias on the part of the physician toward "doing more" for his or her patient. It is unlikely that "doing more" reflected a crude income maximization effort; rather, it probably arose from a true desire to help the patient and reduce one's own clinical uncertainty by gaining more information. Physicians and other practitioners were at least theoretically liable to be called to account for their practices, but this was rarely done by peer organizations and by patients generally only in the case of a lawsuit or by use of the exit option through choosing another physician (Hirschman, 1970).

During the late 1960s and 1970s, social protests against the Vietnam War, the movement to win equal rights for women, the scandals of Watergate, the disability rights movement, and other social struggles provided a backdrop for a general questioning of established authority. Simultaneously, the United States witnessed the emergence of an increasingly vocal "consumer" movement led by the publication in 1965 of Ralph Nader's book on the automobile industry, *Unsafe at Any Speed* (Nader, 1965). In addition, the revelation of abuses in medical research (Caplan, 1992; Jones, 1981) also resulted in widespread discussion and policies to ensure informed consent.

These and other social changes brought about challenges to physicians' traditional authority. Patients began to question doctors and to demand a greater role in decision making about their care, exerting pressure on physicians to be more accountable for the process and content of care they provided. Hospitals were likewise questioned, for example, about restrictive policies that excluded fathers from being present for the births of their children.

At the same time, pressures mounted for physicians and other clinicians to be more accountable for the costs of care. Under traditional fee-for-service arrangements, clinicians and hospitals had covered the costs of caring for the poor and uninsured by adjusting the prices they charged those with insurance, an arrangement known as cost-shifting. However, as the overall costs of care continued to increase, payers, including government and private insurance programs, began to demand that physicians consider cost when choosing among alternative courses of treatment and to search for alternative financing structures that would promote cost containment. Cost pressures in the Medicare program led to the Prospective Payment System, which gave hospitals a fixed number of dollars based on the illness of each patient. No longer could one speak of reimbursement (for legitimate costs incurred); instead hospitals were paid fixed amounts and thus needed to ask their physicians to alter practices, especially the lengths of stay they prescribed. While capitation, under which a clinician or group of clinicians agrees to care for a patient or group of patients for a preset amount regardless of what the care needed actually costs, had been used by HMOs and their predecessors for decades, other forms of managed care,[1] such as preferred provider organizations (PPOs), were primarily a result of these cost-containment pressures.

ACCOUNTABILITY IN THE PRESENT: FROM COST SHIFTING TO BLAME SHIFTING

The widespread implementation of these various managed care arrangements has raised concerns on the part of clinicians and patients. In some instances a health plan must approve in advance whether it will pay for specific services for its enrollees. In 1999 United Health Care, a major HMO, received national attention when it announced it would abandon that policy (Freudenheim, 1999). In other cases, plans pay clinicians so little on a fee-for-service basis that they feel they have no time to adequately care for the patient and, in other instances, capitation payments make clinicians feel they must withhold care in order to stay within their budgets. Patient and consumer advocates charge that payers are not being held accountable for real or potential harms suffered by patients as a result of their external decisions to limit access, minimize costs, and/or control use. (In many instances managed care plans claim they are merely implementing coverage policies required by the employers and government agencies that pay for the coverage.)

Payers, in turn, argue that scientific evidence of a treatment's efficacy must be the standard by which medical decisions be judged rather than merely traditional professional judgment. In some instances payers go beyond efficacy to substitute one service or drug for another because it is markedly less expensive and perhaps only a little less efficacious—an efficiency argument. In this context the lack of rigorous scientific studies to support the use of many treatment options has had the double effect of contributing to patient mistrust (Mechanic, 1998) and creating a small industry in outcomes research. Accountability, once lodged primarily in the patient–doctor dyad, now is diffused by economic, structural, and institutional arrangements that did not previously exist, and the transition has led to considerable finger-pointing and blaming, a sure sign that moral values are at issue.

Several aspects of the current situation are worth noting in relation to the issue of accountability. The increased capability for surveillance of the clinician–patient encounter, which has come about as a result of improved information technology, has multiple implications. Data originally developed by payers to process payments began to be used for research on what interventions worked best. Other studies demonstrated that not all hospitals and clinicians achieved the same success with specific procedures and treatments. Increasingly, then, not only cost, but also clinical aspects of practice are monitored by payers and by others concerned with assessing standards of care, raising new questions about privacy for both patients and clinicians.

Clinical care has also become much more complex than it was in the days of the mythical Dr. Welby. Staying abreast of new developments is increasingly difficult given the demands on clinicians' time. To the degree that clinicians are able and willing to make use of them, new systems of information sharing can potentially aid their decision making. The substantial resistance by many physicians to the use of guidelines (Tanenbaum, 1994) may reflect a resistance to change or to "outside" recommendations. However, the social and moral complexity involved in diagnosis and treatment encounters (Bliton and Finder, 1996) points to the limitations of even the most elegant averages-based science when applied to particular patients.

Finally, the reconstitution of "patients" as "consumers" has been based on certain assumptions associated with individualism in general and with market individualism in particular, each of which is consonant with prevailing U.S. political ideology, but each of which has potential conflicts with earlier understandings of personal and professional accountabilities. For example, the ability of health care "consumers" to influence health services markets through their purchasing behaviors is dependent upon a model of information access and processing that currently does not exist. In addition, referring to patients as "consumers" obscures power inequities, since the actual purchasers of care are in most instances employers or government agencies, not individuals.

ACCOUNTABILITY IN THE FUTURE: CREATING "GOOD" ACCOUNTABILITY

Where could we go from here? What would constitute "good" accountability, and how could a system be structured to best encourage it? In the remainder of this chapter, we propose a working set of criteria that might be useful to consider in evaluating whether a model of health-care services encourages accountability to and from patients, clinicians, and payers. We then provide a rough outline of a model we believe might come close to meeting the criteria we have identified. We conclude with some observations about aspects not addressed here but that call for a thoughtful dialogue about what kind of world our health systems will help sustain.

"Good" accountability, by any measure, would include ways to assess whether treatment decisions are (*1*) reasonably consistent with scientific evidence and practice guidelines, (*2*) reasonably flexible in acknowledging that other kinds of knowledge besides scientific knowledge are relevant to clinical decision making at all stages, (*3*) reasonably consistent with the values of patients and their families, (*4*) reasonably fair in terms of the distribution of health care goods, and (*5*) procedurally reasonable in terms of minimizing the burdens of assessment and evaluation they place on clinicians and patients. In repeatedly using the term "reasonable," we draw on Daniels and Sabin's (1998) discussion of "accountability for reasonableness." Reasonableness, in this view, requires some public explicitness as to the reasoning behind choices, reasoning that makes sense under a "prudent layperson" conception. Furthermore, reasonableness allows for some flexibility in the application of these criteria in specific situations. We will address each of these in turn.

Consistency with Scientific Evidence and Practice Guidelines

The twin issues of limited information and information overload are relevant here. To the extent that well-done scientific studies provide guidance as to the probability of a positive outcome, a "good" accountability would require that information to be considered. However, the overwhelming (and increasing) quantities of information available make "keeping current" a daunting task for any practitioner, no matter how dedicated. Rather than viewing this criterion as one of retrospective surveillance or mandatory "enforcement," we would assess it by considering whether access to current scientific studies is made readily available to clinicians in their practice settings, whether clinicians use it regularly, and whether they are paid for their time in accessing and considering such information. A "good" accountability would also require disclosure of mistakes and of corrective measures taken to prevent their reoccurrence. The focus should be on whether the clinicians generally consider the relevant evidence and whether the organizational settings in which they work facilitate the appropriate and timely use of such information in practice.

Flexibility in Incorporating Types of Evidence

Research-based evidence is not the only kind of knowledge relevant to clinical practice (Benner et al, 1996; Schon, 1988; Tanenbaum, 1994). In theory, one could identify all the relevant variables that determine the best treatment for each patient. In practice, however, in order to undertake studies of the effectiveness of various interventions, researchers have to collect information from various sources, including a wide variety of patients and settings. The result is an assessment of which strategy is best on average, but it may not be best for a particular patient. We have an expectation that our clinicians will act on our behalf, and the ability to recognize what is likely to be best in our particular instance is dependent upon our clinician's knowing us and perceiving our situation in all its moral complexity (Vetlesen, 1994). While, on average, we might expect a clinician's practice to be consistent with evidence-based guidelines, "good" accountability would allow occasional nonadherence to the guidelines based upon a clinical assessment of why this patient is not average. "Bad" accountability, by contrast, might rigidly control such exceptions or make them so procedurally burdensome that they were, for the most part, unavailable. For example, the practice of some health plans of dropping or threatening to drop physicians from plan provider lists if some of their patients are too high-cost, thereby forcing patients to seek new doctors (who would presumably care for them more cheaply), would not meet this criterion, because such practices result in unnecessary disruptions of clinical relationships and do nothing to identify and address better or worse clinical practices.

Treatment Decision Making Consistent with the Values of Patients and Families

It seems self-evident that it is morally harmful to make treatment decisions that are at odds with the values of patients. However, how a system structures the clinical encounter and the decision-making process affects whether those values are communicated, understood, and respected. "Good" accountability is facilitated by a system that provides clinicians with ample time to talk with patients and families, educates and rewards them for sensitivity to the whole range of patients' concerns and values, provides patients and families with clear and accessible information about options, and evidences high rates of patient–clinician continuity and low rates of complaints. For example, this means that the system of accountability should include mechanisms for regular feedback from clinicians and patients into procedures for scheduling appointments, accommodating language or cultural differences, and making arrangements for smooth transitions to new places or providers when necessary. Even though guidelines based on science may recommend against a therapy for cancer on the basis that it will not provide a cure for a patient with late-stage cancer, on balance we would want a system of "good" accountability to be flexible enough to allow or even encourage the clinician to occasionally make exceptions, for example, in the case of therapy that will not cure or significantly extend life but might allow a patient to live just a bit longer to see his first grandchild graduate from college.

Fair in Terms of Distribution of Health-Care Goods

A system for medical treatment must be accountable to its members and/or to the public for distributing the medical goods it has available fairly; for example, it cannot arbitrarily decide to provide treatments to some patients with a given condition and not to others with the same condition. This is not to say that some plans may not set limits on the types of treatments they will provide, but "good" accountability requires that those limits be publicly disclosed in advance in a form patient–consumers and families can understand. A "good" accountability would also involve some form of public discussion and input into decision making regarding both the limits imposed and the adding of new benefits. The Oregon health plan (Jacobs et al, 1999; Leichter, 1999), while imperfect in its technical execution and questioned because it focused only on rationing decisions for the care of Medicaid-eligible individuals, was an important first attempt at implementing just this sort of public conversation about how to set priorities for health-care goods. This plan offers an example of the kinds of processes that might be used, whether for a single program of universal coverage or for one of many individual health plans in determining what services should be offered within the context of a global budget, even one whose overall magnitude is socially determined.

Procedurally Reasonable in Terms of Assessment Burdens

A "good" accountability uses evaluation procedures that cause the least possible disruption to the relationships between clinicians and patients or their families and that respect patient privacy. "Bad" accountability consists of coercive or intrusive demands for information that go beyond quality assurance to punitive surveillance. Similarly, "bad" accountability might overemphasize some features, such as outcomes, that can be objectively measured at the expense of others and thereby skew performance. For example, a focus on mortality reduction may ignore much more important improvements in the quality of life.

A POSSIBLE MODEL OF "GOOD" ACCOUNTABILITY

At the risk of being found guilty of ignoring the elephant in the living room in favor of elaborating on the gnats buzzing around its nether quarters, we have chosen for the purposes of this discussion to assume that access to care is not at issue. The problem of injustice in health-care access looms large over all health policy discourse in the United States and must be addressed in order for any reasonable system of ensuring accountability to succeed. This injustice, in addition to its moral repugnance, creates perverse incentives and contributes to increased costs when care is delayed and conditions thereby worsen or spread to others. However, even if we assume equitable and universal access, there are still major issues of accountability in terms of treatment style and decision making, and we hope to address some of those here.

Assuming, therefore, that everyone has access to health care, our model proposes that health-care services be centered around units of clinicians who self-selectively group together according to their shared philosophies of practice. Even if the body of research evidence about various treatments continues to expand at an enormous rate, there will remain large "gray areas" in which the evidence is either lacking or inconclusive. We would assume that, other factors being equal, all clinicians would treat patients similarly when the evidence is very strong that a treatment does or does not work for a particular condition.

However, within the gray areas that probably constitute the majority of clinical decision making, we suggest that clinicians may fall along a continuum in their approaches to treatment. At one end of the continuum of practice groups, for example, would be those clinicians who generally favor more aggressive treatment. These clinical groups (which could include physicians, nurses, nurse practitioners, pharmacists, and others, possibly including practitioners of various forms of "alternative" medicine) would tend overall to have a greater predilection to pursue every avenue of treatment and undertake every test to rule out any possible uncertainty. They would be those most inclined to try new and potentially risky therapies and procedures and to use new technologies that seemed promising but were not yet proven superior. These clinicians would try any possible therapy, even in cases in which the therapy might be little better than doing nothing. In a best-case scenario, many patients would feel that everything was being done to provide a cure, and some patients might be saved; in a worst-case scenario, patients might suffer unnecessary harm or death as a result of the treatment itself.

At the other end of the gray area continuum would be groups of conservative clinicians who generally recommend only those new treatments that have high levels of certainty as to effectiveness and potential effects. These clinicians would rely on the "tried and true" and on their skills as healers and comforters. Patients who were dying would be treated with compassionate palliative care. In a best-case scenario the patient feels "cared for," and the standard and recommended treatment is effective and in line with patient expectations; in a worst-case scenario the clinician does not adequately treat a condition, the patient suffers unnecessary harm or death due to lack of treatment, and the family feels that potentially helpful treatment was withheld. These are extremes along a continuum, and many groups will be in more moderate positions, perhaps distinguishing themselves by philosophies with respect to aggressiveness in testing vs. treatment.

Within each group along the continuum, clinicians would develop and periodically review and update guidelines for treatment. As much as possible, these guidelines would be based on the most currently available scientific evidence considered in conjunction with the group's general philosophy of treatment. A patient advisory group would review and provide input into the guidelines.

An annual peer review within the clinician group, in which a random sample of a clinician's patient charts was reviewed, would provide opportunities for discussion and learning and for elucidation of the kinds of circumstances under which departures from treatment guidelines would be advisable. This arrangement could provide a formal pedagogical setting in which probabilistic knowledge of the aggregate and narrative knowledge of particular patients could be compared and contrasted, thus addressing criteria (*1*) and (*2*) in our list.

There would be open access to all groups, and consumer–patients could choose a group whose treatment philosophy most closely matched their own. One can imagine consumers being able to review and compare responses to a series of patient scenarios or narratives that would describe how each group would envision good care for patients with particular conditions. For example, cases could range from what would happen with an infant spiking a fever, to a 30-year-old woman with no risk factors asking for annual mammograms, to a 78-year-old man with multiple chronic conditions and a positive prostate exam. In each instance the clinicians' response would allow them to indicate not only what they would do, but why. Some might focus primarily or even entirely on the biomedical aspects of a case; others might be drawn to comment on important emotional or social factors that might lead to an unexpected conclusion. While this may be a difficult undertaking to conceive in a print-based world, it is fairly easy to imagine both how different clinicians would extract different information from the same underlying scenario available on a Website and how their responses could be made easily accessible in video format. While such an approach has obvious limitations, including the disjuncture between what people say they would do in the abstract and what they actually do in particular situations, it might offer a way for consumers to assess and appreciate differences in groups' general philosophies of practice. As is the case now, some consumer–patients would rely solely on advice from friends and relatives in making decisions about which group of practitioners might best suit them, but others could use information technology to research and compare groups.

Patients could also change groups, perhaps at a specific time each year. Allowing patients to switch among groups means there might be differential selection by health risk. High-risk patients might preferentially choose one style of treatment while low-risk people choose another. This would require that sophisticated forms of risk adjustment be implemented so the clinical groups would be paid fairly for the mix of patients they attract (Giacomini et al, 1995; Kahn, Luft, & Smith, 1995; Luft, Romano, & Remy, 1996; Luft, 1995; Rosenkranz and Luft, 1997). There would need to be a socially determined level of how much care should be covered in this risk-adjusted amount. This could be derived from public decisions regarding how much money we as a society want to spend or by determining how much and what types of care are desired by, say, 80% of the population. Alternatively, we could choose to pay for all the services that, on average, meet some criteria of efficacy and, perhaps, efficiency. Our key point is that the "basic package" be socially determined.

However, we would anticipate that the aggressive treatment group might require that additional costs be borne by patients if, in concert with their clinicians, they wanted to try unproven, risky therapies or therapies shown to be of minimal therapeutic value. (It is possible, but less likely, that the less aggressive treatment pattern would actually be more expensive because it chooses to use a far wider range of supportive services or involves more time-intensive care. It is also important to consider the economic costs of informal and family caregiving that are not currently included in most cost calculations.) Some treatments might simply be denied by clinicians as inappropriate, regardless of whether a patient was willing to pay for them. For example, it would not be ethically reasonable to expect that a surgeon would amputate a patient's limb simply because the patient felt that his or her condition would be improved thereby, in the absence of any other evidence to support that notion. Subsidies could be devised to help address the equity problem of lower-income people unable to pay for the more aggressive, unproven therapies, even if these were consistent with their values. For example, the extra premiums needed above and beyond the base plan would be based not on a fixed amount but instead on a percent of income after allowing for basic living expenses.

Similarly, the model for medical decision making might vary among groups. Some groups (and the patients who selected them) would emphasize a shared model of decision making in which all options were thoroughly explained to the patient and decisions were undertaken mutually. Other patients might prefer not to be burdened with details and choices and would choose a group that emphasized a more paternalistic style of practice. Treatment *availability* would be consistent across all patients within a group (although actual delivery of treatments might vary to reflect patients' individual needs and preferences, even within the group). Group performance would be assessed through monitoring of patient complaints, rates at which patients switched from one group to another, and random chart audits.

Patients and families would self-select to a group most consistent with their values, perhaps with the aid of improved mechanisms for presenting choices, such as interactive shared medical decision-making programs and publicly available information about group treatment coverage, practice styles, and decision-making protocols. The availability of information on groups' practice styles, decision-making models, and clinical guidelines and the ability of patients/families to select their group meet our criterion (*3*).

In conjunction with a regulatory authority and a consumer advisory panel, uniform complaint reporting and response mechanisms would be part of all plans. This would enable collection and public dissemination of aggregate complaint data and of groups' responses to the types of problems identified in complaints, which would be a move toward ensuring that all our accountability criteria were being addressed. Our example, however, shows that such an accountability system would not be trivial to design. One might well expect that patients attracted to a "try everything" plan might be more likely to complain than those attracted to a "let's talk about how to make you comfortable" plan. While this expectation may or may not hold, the nature of the complaints would almost certainly differ, and accountability systems would have to be sensitive to such differences.

LIMITATIONS OF THE MODEL AND ISSUES FOR THE FUTURE

The model relies on a "market" mechanism, namely individualized patient–consumer choice among clinician groups in a context of scarce resources that may carry its own baggage. We assume a collective commitment to providing universal coverage and thus a strong implicit acceptance of shared social needs. However, the language of consumer choice sets up our view of the issues in particular ways (Malone, 1998; Malone, 1999) and may limit our ability to talk about health care in terms of broader social goods. For example, we are pragmatic in recognizing that American individualism establishes the discourse about health services differently than occurs in countries in which social solidarity is a primary value. Individualism suggests that differences in patient–consumer preferences should matter and that it is acceptable for different people to have different clinical services as long as pricing does not hinder low-income people from exercising choice. It is possible that, even given the American tradition of individualism, a unitary system would be preferable or even necessary to maintain quality. However, it is also possible that a system that encourages variety in approaches to clinical decisions would lead more rapidly to understanding which techniques work better.

If, as our model suggests, there is to be a "basic package" of services to which members of any plan would have access, the focus on individual choice may shift from public discussion of what that package should entail to discussions about individual preferences or those of organized groups. It may be that, prior to the development of effective models of accountability, another more important public conversation must occur concerning the vastly disproportionate funding of tertiary treatment and new technologies over preventive and health promotion efforts. On the other hand, given the U.S. political structure, it may be better to focus national policy discussion on broad structural issues and leave trade-offs to the local level. Special interest groups, from device manufacturers to antiabortion campaigners, are more likely to be able to influence national than local decisions, for a number of sociopolitical reasons. (For example, President Reagan, supported by anti-abortion groups, forced HMOs to remove abortion coverage from their benefit package for federal employees, even if they did not charge the government for this.) Focusing public discussions at the local level may reduce the influence of special interest lobbyists and engage the public to a greater degree.

Our model is also limited by our capacity to be explicit about values, practice styles, and the clinical contexts in which diagnosis and treatment decisions occur. As human beings, we are constantly interpreting our situations and those of others. Human situations cannot be treated as mere physical states (Dreyfus, 1992), and values are not properties or independent characteristics of objects (Dreyfus, 1992) but are embedded within social worlds and individual situations. Much of the knowledge we use to navigate clinical worlds is implicit, embodied, and largely unconscious, as philosopher Hubert Dreyfus has illustrated using the example of distance standing practices:

> We have all learned to stand the appropriate distance from strangers, intimates, and colleagues for conversation. Each culture has a different "feel" for the appropriate distances. . . . These practices are not taught by the parents. They do not know that there is any pattern to what they are doing, or even that they are doing anything. Rather, the children . . . simply pick up the pattern. There is no reason to think there are any rules involved; rather, we have a skilled understanding of our culture. Indeed, if one tried to state the rules for distance-standing, one would require further rules, such as stand closer if there is noise in the background, or further away if the other person has the flu, and the application of these rules would in turn require further rules, and so on, always leading us back to further everyday, taken-for-granted practices.
>
> (Dreyfus, 1991, 18–19)

In the same way, there are taken-for-granted understandings about what it means to be a patient or to be a good clinician that resist articulation or measurement yet profoundly influence the kinds of choices we are able to see and to see as reasonable. While some strategies (such as peer review groups that use narratives to learn about actual cases) may help practitioners partially articulate their understanding and reasoning in clinical situations, attempts to force clinicians to be entirely explicit about their decision making may inadvertently interfere with their clinical ability to grasp a situation as a whole rather than as a series of disconnected elements (Benner et al, 1992).

We need to make sure that real world implementation of approaches to enhance accountability does not inadvertently degrade what we wish to accomplish. Accountability, under almost any system, has costs of its own, which may become burdensome. We must, as Carolyn Wiener has observed, "decide if we are measuring what is important or expending dollars and energy making important what we can measure" (Wiener, 2000, p. xi). Setting up processes for accountability is not the same thing as preserving and nurturing the growth of moral practices and should not be seen as a substitute.

Another element not yet addressed by the model is how it would equalize accountability to patients whose language and culture may make information about choices have different meanings. It is not sufficient to say that interpreters would be found; a "good" accountability requires that good-faith efforts be made to ensure culturally sensitive care (Tervalon and Murray-García, 1998). For example, discussions of prognoses with Navajo patients may be interpreted as potentially harmful (Carrese and Rhodes, 1995) because of Navajo understandings of the role of language in shaping reality and events.

We have not addressed what would be appropriate and ethically justifiable boundaries to protect patient privacy while preserving the capacity to monitor quality of care. A model based on choice may be difficult in rural settings, where there may be insufficient numbers of clinicians to provide patient–consumers with choices, but the limited availability of providers in such areas is a problem for any approach.

Finally, the model is also limited by our society's lack of clear vision about what kind of society we wish to shape through our rapidly changing technologies and institutions. For example, a "good" accountability should, we would argue, also address accountability to future generations and possibly to other species on our shrinking planet, as "bridge" bioethicists have argued (Donnelly, 1995; Potter, 1999; Whitehouse, 1999). Daniel Callahan (1998) is among those who have urged us to rethink our goals in relation to a "sustainable" model of health progress. To the extent that our aims are muddy, our systems may contribute to a discontinuity between practice and rhetoric that can be demoralizing to clinicians and patients; that is, the expectations vocalized in policy and operationalized in systems may be impossible to achieve in actual practice. If we are to develop new systems of accountability, we must first develop more clarity about what kinds of human relationships we seek to shape through our health-care institutions and policies. Doing it the other way around risks missing the point.

NOTES

1. The term *managed care* is not value-free and may encompass a range of options (Dudley and Luft, 1999; White, 1999).

REFERENCES

Benner P, Tanner C, Chesla C (1992) From beginner to expert: Gaining a differentiated clinical world in critical care nursing practice. *Advances in Nursing Science* 14:13–28.

Benner P, Tanner C, Chesla C (1996) *Expertise in Nursing Practice: Caring, Clinical Judgment, and Ethics*. New York: Springer.

Bishop AH and Scudder JR (1990) *The Practical, Moral, and Personal Sense of Nursing: A Phenomenological Philosophy of Practice*. Albany, NY: State University of New York Press.

Bliton MJ and Finder SG (1996) The eclipse of the individual in policy (Where is the place for justice?) *Cambridge Quarterly of Healthcare Ethics*. 5:519–32.

Callahan D (1998) *False Hopes: Why America's Quest for Perfect Health is a Recipe for Failure*. New York: Simon and Schuster.

Caplan AL (1992) Twenty years after: The legacy of the Tuskegee Syphilis Study: When evil intrudes. *Hastings Center Report* 22:29–32.

Carrese JA and Rhodes LA (1995) Western bioethics on the Navajo reservation. *Journal of the American Medical Association* 274:826–9.

Daniels N (1985) *Just Health Care*. Cambridge: Cambridge University Press.

Daniels N and Sabin J (1998) The ethics of accountability in managed care reform. *Health Affairs* 17:50–64.

Donnelly S (1995) The art of moral ecology. *Ecosystem Health* 1:170–6.

Dreyfus HL (1991) *Being-in-the-World: A Commentary on Heidegger's Being and Time*. Cambridge, MA: Massachusetts Institute of Technology Press.

Dreyfus HL (1992) *What Computers Still Can't Do: A Critique of Artificial Reason*. Cambridge, MA: Massachusetts Institute of Technology Press.

Dudley RA and Luft HS (1999) Goals, targets, and tactics: Making health care policy decisions explicit. *Journal of Health Politics, Policy, and Law* 24:705–13.

Emanuel EJ and Emanuel LL (1996) What is accountability in health care? *Annals of Internal Medicine* 124:229–39.

Freudenheim M (November 9, 1999) Big HMO to give decisions on care back to doctors. *New York Times*.

Giacomini M., Luft H, Robinson J (1995) Risk adjusting community rated health plan premiums: A survey of risk assessment literature and policy applications. *Annual Review of Public Health* 16:401–30.

Hirschman AO (1970) *Exit, Voice, and Loyalty: Responses to Declines in Firms, Organizations, and States*. Cambridge, MA: Harvard University Press.

Jacobs L, Marmor T, Oberlander J (1999) The Oregon health plan and the political paradox of rationing: What advocates and critics have claimed and what Oregon did. *Journal of Health Politics, Policy and Law* 24:161–80.

Jones JH (1981) *Bad Blood: The Tuskegee Syphilis Experiment*. New York: Free Press.

Kahn JG, Luft HS, Smith MD (1995) HIV risk adjustment: Issues and proposed approaches. *Journal of Acquired Immune Deficiency Syndromes and Human Retrovirology* 8:S53–66.

Leape LL (1992) Unnecessary surgery. *Annual Review of Public Health* 13:363–83.

Leichter H (1999) Oregon's bold experiment: Whatever happened to rationing? *Journal of Health Politics, Policy and Law* 24:147–60.

Luft HS (1995) Potential methods to reduce risk selection and its effects. *Inquiry* 32:23–32.

Luft H, Romano P, Remy L (1996) *Second Report of the California Hospital Outcomes Project Volume 1: Study Overview and Results Summary*. Sacramento, CA: California Health and Welfare Agency Office of Statewide Health Planning and Development.

Malone RE (1998) Against "consumers." *Administrative Radiology Journal*, 17 (6 [June]), 17:27–8.

Malone, RE (1999) Policy as product: Morality and metaphor in health policy discourse. *Hastings Center Report* 29:16–22.

McKeown T (1979) *The Role of Medicine: Dream, Mirage, or Nemesis?* Princeton, NJ: Princeton University Press.

Mechanic D (1998) The functions and limitations of trust in the provision of medical care. *Journal of Health Politics, Policy and Law* 23:661–86.

Nader R (1965) *Unsafe at Any Speed: The Designed-in Dangers of the American Automobile*. New York: Grossman.

Noble AA, Hyams AL, Kane NM (1998) Charitable hospital accountability: A review and analysis of legal and policy initiatives. *Journal of Law, Medicine, and Ethics* 26: 116–37.

Pont EA (2000) The culture of physician autonomy: 1900 to the present. *Cambridge Quarterly of Healthcare Ethics* 9:98–119.

Potter VR (1999) Fragmented ethics and "bridge bioethics." *Hastings Center Report* 29: 38–40.

Rosenkranz SL and Luft HS (1997) Expenditure models for prospective risk adjustment: Choosing the measure appropriate for the problem. *Medical Care Research and Review* 54:123–43.

Schon DA (1988). *Educating the Reflective Practitioner*. San Francisco: Jossey-Bass.

Simpson JA and Weiner ESC (1989) *The Oxford English Dictionary*, 2d ed. Oxford: Clarendon Press.

Tanenbaum SJ (1994) Knowing and acting in medical practice: The epistemological politics of outcomes research. *Journal of Health Politics, Policy and Law* 19:27–44.

Tervalon M and Murray-García J (1998) Cultural humility versus cultural competence: A critical distinction in defining physician training outcomes in multicultural education. *Journal of Health Care for the Poor and Underserved* 9:117–25.

Vetlesen AJ (1994) *Perception, Empathy, and Judgment: An Inquiry into the Preconditions of Moral Performance*. University Park, PA: Pennsylvania State University Press.

Wennberg JE, Bunker JP, Barnes B (1980) The need for assessing the outcome of common medical practices. *Annual Review of Public Health* 1:277–95.

White J (1999) Targets and systems of health care cost control. *Journal of Health Politics, Policy, and Law* 24:653–96.

Whitehouse PJ (1999) The ecomedical disconnection syndrome. *Hastings Center Report* 29:41–4.

Wiener CL (2000) *The Elusive Quest: Accountability in Hospitals*. New York: De Gruyter.

Vulnerable populations

15

Health resource allocation for vulnerable populations

DAN W. BROCK

Should vulnerable populations receive special moral concern in the prioritization and allocation of health care and other resources and programs that affect health? The meaning of this question is not clear on its face. By "vulnerable populations" I shall follow both the Agency for Healthcare Research and Quality (AHRQ) account as populations with special needs for or barriers to care from a variety of conditions or circumstances and less able than others to safeguard their own needs and interests and Lu Ann Aday's account of at-risk populations as populations or groups at high relative risk of suffering poor physical, psychological, and/or social health (AHRQ, 1999; Aday, 1993). In asking whether these vulnerable populations should receive special moral concern, I mean should an account of justice or equity in health and health care distinguish vulnerable populations from other groups or the population at large, or can just treatment of vulnerable populations simply be derived from an account of just treatment of other groups or the population at large?

The chapter is organized as follows. First, I will discuss why this question has received relatively little attention to date in bioethics. Then I will explore some of the complexities in defining vulnerable populations and some differences in AHRQ's and Aday's accounts of them. Next, I distinguish three different moral categories of vulnerable populations—those whose risk of poor health is caused by conditions that are themselves unjust, those whose conditions causing their high health risks are an undeserved misfortune but not themselves a social injustice, and those who are at fault or responsible for their high health risks—and explore the relevance of these differences for prioritization of health resources for vulnerable populations. The remaining pages explore what I believe is the most plausible general ethical framework for determining the special claims of vulnerable populations in health resource prioritization. More specifically, the shared disadvantage of different vulnerable populations of relatively poor expected health suggests that our obligations to them in resource prioritization should be understood within a general ethical framework focusing on what priority worse-off groups should receive. I explore three groups of questions for developing that framework and applying it to vulnerable populations. First, why should improving the condition of the worse-off receive priority? Second, who are the worse-off for the purposes of health resource priorities—for example, are they the sickest or those with worse overall well-being, the sickest now or those with worse lifetime health? Third, since giving the worse off absolute priority in health resource prioritization is not plausible, how much priority should they receive? Relatively little systematic work has been done on these issues, and my discussion of them will raise far more questions than it will answer; much remains to be done in developing and applying this ethical framework to resource prioritization for vulnerable populations.

WHY BIOETHICS HAS FAILED TO ADDRESS THE CLAIMS OF VULNERABLE POPULATIONS IN HEALTH RESOURCE PRIORITIZATION[1]

In most work in bioethics, the answer to whether vulnerable populations should receive special concern in health resource prioritization would appear to be no—vulnerable populations seem not to be regarded as raising distinct issues that require special treatment in an account of justice in health and health care since they in fact rarely receive such separate treatment. (Of course, it is possible that bioethicists believe they do require special treatment, although they haven't bothered to provide it, but I do not think this a plausible inference.) Why is that? One reason is that most work in bioethics has been done from the perspective of medical ethics, which is concerned with the ethical problems that arise between medical professionals and patients in the course of the delivery of medical care to patients. These microproblems have been addressed with the principles of personal and professional morality applied to issues like treatment decision making, paternalism and autonomy, truth telling, and confidentiality. Until recently, macroissues of justice and equity in health and health care have received far less attention from bioethicists.

Even bioethics work specifically addressing macroissues of justice and equity, however, has focused on health care, not health, and, as I will suggest, this has had consequences for the treatment of vulnerable populations. There are several reasons for the focus on health care. It is possible to determine the distribution of health care by how we organize and structure the health-care system, but the distribution of health is not entirely under social control. At the present time at least, the genetic contribution to health and illness is largely beyond our control, as are many of the effects of the vicissitudes of life, such as accidents, contact with contagions, and so forth. Philosophical theories of justice largely presuppose that justice concerns actions, institutions, and outcomes that are within human control; unfortunate health outcomes that are beyond anyone's control, such as the effects of being hit by lightening, are just that, unfortunate but not something to which principles of justice directly apply or could regulate.

Related to this point is the fact that much work in justice in health care focuses on elucidating individuals' moral rights to health care, and, on standard views, rights must be possible to secure or to avoid violating; this follows from the fact that a right entails obligations on the part of others not to do what would violate the right and to secure what the person has a right to. Now, it would be possible to secure for all Americans, for example, at least a basic level of health care, even if we now shamefully fail to do so, but it would not be possible to secure for all Americans even a basic level of health; because of genetic differences and other unfortunate circumstances and events in part beyond anyone's control, some individuals suffer poor health that cannot be prevented or substantially improved. So it has been natural to think that rights must be rights to health care, not to health.

Moreover, most philosophical work on justice in recent years has been "resourcist" rather than "welfarist" (Marchand et al, 1998). In the enormously influential work of John Rawls, for example, fundamental principles of justice concern the distribution of primary goods, which are roughly all-purpose resources or means useful in carrying out nearly any plan of life, not the distribution of well-being or happiness that individuals achieve with them (Rawls, 1971). Other influential work departing from Rawls's view, such as that of Amartya Sen on capabilities and various theories appealing to principles of equality of opportunity, remain focused at the most fundamental level on resources (Sen, 1985). Of course, utilitarians remain focused on individual welfare or well-being, but their position on distributive justice is widely thought to be unsatisfactory.

When resourcist theories are applied in the health sector, they naturally focus on the distribution of health care, a resource, instead of health, a component of welfare or well-being. The most sophisticated and influential extension of general theories of justice to the area of health is Norman Daniels's book *Just Health Care*, whose title alone betrays its primary focus on the distribution of health care, though Daniels does address other nonhealth-care causes and interventions affecting health (Daniels, 1985).

Why does a focus on health care instead of health usually result in ignoring the special problem of vulnerable populations? When theorists focus on health care and then defend some general moral right to health care, the principal injustice in the health-care system seems to them to be lack of access to health care, as evidenced in particular in the United States by the 44 million Americans without health insurance. And it is often assumed as well that the principal controllable differences in individuals' or groups' health status are caused by differential access to health care. But public health professionals and many bioethicists know better—the principal differences in individuals' or groups' health are not the result of differential access to health care, but other factors (Wilkinson, 1996) Some of these other factors, such as genetic determinants, are not now under our control to any significant extent. Others, such as good or bad luck in avoiding injury, contagious diseases, and so forth, are likely always to remain significantly beyond social control. But many other social determinants of health such as poverty, economic and educational inequality, and homelessness as well as unhealthy behaviors like smoking, alcohol and substance abuse, high fat diets, and sedentary lifestyles are within our control to alter, at least to a substantial degree, if we have the will to do so.

So when work on justice focuses principally on access to health care, it misses most of the causes of inequality in the health of individuals or groups. To be sure, bioethicists are increasingly clear about the important contribution of social and behavioral factors to ill health and health inequalities, but their work on justice remains focused largely on health care, not health and its social and behavioral determinants. This focus on health care to the exclusion of other factors that have a greater impact on health and health inequalities has led to generally impoverished accounts of justice and equity in the health sector. And more to the point regarding vulnerable populations, it has led to the assumption that the principal vulnerable population consists of persons without health care insurance and a regular source of access to health care. But many empirical studies identify other social, medical, and behavioral factors that put people at high risk of poor health and so define them as members of a vulnerable population (Aday, 1993; Wilkinson, 1996). This focus on health care largely to the exclusion of health in work on justice in the health sector has had a number of bad consequences, and one of them is an overly narrow view of who are vulnerable populations at high relative risk for poor health.

Another reason work in bioethics on justice has had little to say about vulnerable populations is that the work has largely, certainly until recently, focused on establishing a right to health care from some more general moral perspective or theory. That right is what philosophers call a general right, or sometimes a human right, which individuals have just by virtue of being persons, unlike special rights, which arise out of specific actions or roles, such as a promisee's right to have a promise kept or a child's right to be cared for by its parents. As a human right, its existence should not depend on or vary with social circumstances. A general right holding against a person's society and its government as the agent securing persons' rights in the society is also possessed equally by all members of the society. From this perspective, there is no need for a special account of the rights of specific groups, such as vulnerable populations—the fundamental moral right to health care that the health-care system should be organized to secure is the same for all citizens. This is consistent, of course, with recognizing the different health-care needs of different individuals or groups, since the right to health care is virtually always defined, at least in part, in terms of meeting some level of health-care needs and so will be sensitive to their variation. But the greater health-care needs of vulnerable populations will be accommodated by the responsiveness to differential needs of the general right to health care, without requiring any separate account of the just treatment of vulnerable populations. Of course, in the application of general and universal moral principles establishing a right of all persons to have their basic health-care needs met, empirical evidence will be needed of the differential needs of particular vulnerable populations, but no special treatment of vulnerable populations will be needed at the level of basic moral principles in a theory of just health care.

Thus, there are a number of explanations of why work in medical ethics and even in justice in health care has had little to say specifically about at-risk or vulnerable populations. These populations have been recognized as suffering most from our failure in the United States to secure a right to health care for all, but they have not been recognized as requiring separate treatment at the level of fundamental principles of justice in health care. Nonetheless, an explanation is not a justification of inattention to vulnerable populations. As already noted, I will argue that the most plausible ethical framework for considering the claims of vulnerable populations in health resource prioritization is that of priority for worse-off groups. While this subsumes vulnerable populations under the category of worse-off groups, it does not simply assimilate their claims within a general right to health care.

CONCEPTIONS OF VULNERABLE OR AT-RISK POPULATIONS

A particular population will be at high relative risk for poor health when the condition(s) that defines that population causes or is associated with poor health. Aday's list of nine high-risk groups illustrates this (Aday, 1993).

1. high risk mothers and infants;
2. chronically ill and disabled persons;
3. mentally ill and disabled persons;
4. persons with AIDS;
5. alcohol and substance abusers;
6. suicide or homicide prone persons;
7. abusing families;
8. homeless persons;
9. immigrants and refugees.

Likewise, AHRQ defined vulnerable populations as those populations "made vulnerable by their financial circumstances or place of residence; health, age or functional or developmental status; ability to communicate effectively; presence of chronic or terminal illness or disability; or personal characteristics." It went on to add: "These populations may be less able than others to safeguard their own needs and interests adequately during this period of rapid health system change. These populations may incur different health outcomes traceable to unwarranted disparities in their care or stemming from special needs for care or barriers to care."

Besides their special needs for and/or barriers to care, the feature that on AHRQ's formulation creates groups' vulnerability to poor health is their "being less able than others to safeguard their own needs and interests adequately." In other contexts, young children are probably the most familiar example of a group similarly vulnerable, in their case to not having all their basic needs and interests safeguarded. Once they have grown to adulthood, we expect that, for the most part, they will be responsible for safeguarding their own basic needs and interests, but until then others must have this responsibility. As primary caretakers, parents have this responsibility for their children, with the state having the responsibility to intervene when parents fail in their responsibility. What is important is that this responsibility be clearly and effectively assigned. It is not morally optional whether children's basic needs for shelter, nutrition, and health care are met—morality and justice require it—and so it is society's responsibility to ensure that the responsibility for doing so is clearly assigned in a manner that will ensure that they are met.

A variety of other, usually nondevelopmental, factors are responsible for the vulnerability of the groups of concern here, but since their having effective access to adequate health care is as much a requirement of justice as it is for children, others bear a responsibility to protect them from the effects of their vulnerability as well. How that responsibility is most effectively assigned is an empirical matter and may vary depending on the particular vulnerable group, but it is a social responsibility to ensure that it is effectively assigned and met, and government is society's primary agent for carrying out that responsibility.

Both Aday's and AHRQ's lists of conditions defining at-risk or vulnerable populations are diverse in interesting ways. Some conditions are themselves conditions that constitute poor health, such as being chronically ill or terminally ill or disabled, mentally ill and disabled, and having AIDS; these conditions do not put individuals who have them at risk of poor health. Instead, they are conditions that *define* these individuals as having poor health. If these groups are *at risk* of poor health or vulnerable to poor health, it must be because these conditions, themselves constitutive of poor health, put them at further risk for other health problems. For example, persons with AIDS are subject to a variety of opportunistic infections. These groups may also be at further risk either because their conditions create special needs for and/or barriers to care and so make them less likely than others to get appropriate health care for their condition. For example, mental illness is less adequately covered in most health insurance plans than is physical illness. Care for conditions that are less able to be effectively treated, such as chronic illness, which can be ameliorated but not cured, may also be underfunded.

In other of Aday's and AHRQ's categories, the condition is causally related, sometimes in indirect ways, to a high relative risk of illness and/or of not getting, or being able to get appropriate treatment for illness. For example, the condition of homelessness is associated with a high relative risk of being subject to violence, to conditions causing physical harm such as exposure to extreme weather conditions, and to some infectious diseases as well as to not having access to regular sources of care to treat one's health needs. People's financial circumstances and place of residence also often create barriers to securing adequate care. Of course, and as Aday emphasizes, often these conditions interact or are cross-cutting, such as the high rate of mental illness and of alcohol and substance abuse among the homeless, thereby exacerbating their vulnerability to poor health. The complex heterogeneity of these conditions that define at-risk or vulnerable populations is of obvious policy importance in designing programs to reduce their vulnerability and risk of poor health. For example, reducing some of the high health risks of homeless persons requires, among other things, decreasing their vulnerability to violence as well as improving their access to regular sources of health care.

THREE MORAL CATEGORIES OF VULNERABLE POPULATIONS

Aday's and AHRQ's groups are heterogeneous as well in the nature of their moral claims on others to reduce their high relative risks of or vulnerability to poor health, and this heterogeneity will be even more apparent if we expand their lists, as I will do shortly. I want to distinguish at least three distinct moral categories of vulnerable or at-risk groups. The significance of these differences for health policy depends both on features of our general account of justice in health care and on pragmatic policy considerations. The first category consists of groups who are vulnerable or at high relative risk of poor health because of conditions that themselves constitute an injustice independent of their also putting the group at high risk of poor health. Extreme poverty and low levels of training due to lack of access to jobs or adequate education constitute an injustice on most theories of justice, and certainly would do so in a rich, developed country like the United States. Theories of justice differ on the degree and kinds of inequality in income and wealth that they permit, but few sanction extreme economic deprivation. The federal poverty level is one practical definition of the point below which individuals' incomes should not fall, and some theories of justice would place the level higher, others lower; only libertarian accounts, among major alternative theories, deny that justice requires any income floor below which individuals should not fall. Some commitment to equality of opportunity also has a deep place in American moral and political culture, and access to adequate education is typically considered a fundamental component of equality of opportunity because of its pervasive effects on individuals' access to jobs, careers, and the more general opportunities that are part of the normal range of opportunities available to most members of society.

Extreme poverty and lack of access to adequate basic education are both unjust, independent of their effects on individuals' health. But we also know that they result, in a variety of ways, in poorer levels of health as well. Thus, the poorer than average health caused by poverty and lack of education only compounds the injustices of poverty and lack of educational opportunity themselves. Our country's social structure causes these two injustices, and our society has a moral responsibility to remove them. Doing so would in turn remove the further injustice of poor health that the very poor and uneducated suffer. It is important to see that the moral responsibility to remove these two injustices that result in poor health for some vulnerable populations need not depend on any particular account of justice in health and health care because it need be grounded in no such account, but rather in the independent injustice of the conditions causing the disadvantage of poor health. In many particular accounts of justice in health and health care, this disadvantage in health may be unjust independent of the fact that it was caused by these further injustices, and that will be a further moral reason to remove this health disadvantage.

The second category of at-risk or vulnerable populations consists of groups whose defining conditions that result in poor health are morally undeserved but not themselves a social injustice. For example, many disabilities are a result of genetically inherited diseases; inheriting the genes for those diseases is an undeserved misfortune and disadvantage, but typically a result of bad luck in the "genetic lottery" and beyond anyone's control. Likewise, being a child of a young high-risk mother or having a mental illness are not risk factors that the child or mentally ill person deserves or for which he or she is in any sense responsible. These and many other risk factors or vulnerabilities for poor health are undeserved disadvantages that some individuals or groups suffer. Nonetheless, they are not themselves the result of any social injustice.

Of course, that these conditions do not result from any social injustice does not entail that there is nothing unjust about them. There is a sense of justice, and more particularly of fairness, in which it is common to claim that suffering a misfortune like a serious chronic disease or disability that one acquires through no fault of one's own is unfair. What this means is that one has suffered an undeserved misfortune that others have not suffered, and this comparative disadvantage makes the notion of fairness appropriate; this is the sense of fairness people invoke when they say that "life is unfair"—individuals do not always get what they deserve, and they often get what they do not deserve. However, this is morally different from having been treated unfairly or unjustly by other persons or social institutions, the condition present in the first category of vulnerable populations I distinguished above.

On a few moral views, no instance of this second category of undeserved harm or disadvantage for which no one is responsible grounds any moral claim or requirement that society or any other individual attempt to rectify or compensate individuals for the harm they have suffered (Engelhardt, 1986). We might, out of compassion or concern for those who have suffered such undeserved harms, attempt to help in some way, but there is no moral requirement on this view to do so and, in particular, no injustice or unfairness that morally must be made right. If we help out of general charity or beneficence, that will reflect our generous and compassionate character, but no one can make any moral claim that we must do so. This position is most often found among libertarians. However, most people and most moral theories reject libertarians' position that there is no moral obligation to aid or prevent harm to another, no matter how great the harm prevented or benefit that could be conferred, and no matter how little the cost or sacrifice to one in doing so, in favor of some moral obligation of mutual aid, although there is much disagreement about the extent of this obligation.

Persons whose misfortune or disadvantage has been unfairly or unjustly caused by other persons or social institutions have a specific moral claim against those persons or institutions for remedy of or compensation for the harm suffered. This is a different moral claim than that of persons who suffer an undeserved misfortune or disadvantage for which no other person or social institution is responsible. At the least, in the latter case, who is responsible to do anything, and if so what, about the undeserved harm the individual has suffered is often unclear or indeterminate. Moreover, few people believe and few theories of justice hold that all morally undeserved disadvantages that people suffer morally require rectification or compensation from others, either other individuals or from the society at large through its social and political institutions. Being physically unattractive or short or being of somewhat below-average intelligence are both morally undeserved disadvantages, but few people believe that all disadvantages such as these morally require rectification or compensation. Likewise, few theories of justice require that we attempt to equalize people's overall happiness or in turn all the factors that contribute to people's overall happiness.

The most plausible moral position, I believe, is neither that all or no undeserved disadvantages morally require rectification, but rather that whether they do depends on their nature, seriousness, and relation to specific requirements of justice. This means that we must examine those disadvantages one by one to determine what response, if any, morality and justice require. What of the undeserved disadvantage suffered by this second category of vulnerable populations of being at high relative risk of poor health? On Norman Daniels' theory of just health care, for example, preserving or restoring people's health is a matter of justice because of the way disease and ill health limit their function and in turn their opportunities (Daniels, 1985). Many Americans and many theories of justice share a commitment to equality of opportunity, even if there is much disagreement about just what equality of opportunity requires. When the poor health of this second category of vulnerable populations adversely affects their opportunity, justice and, in particular, equality of opportunity do require action to reduce their health risks and to preserve or restore their health. This moral claim of the second category of vulnerable populations, unlike that of the first category, will be grounded in a particular theory of just health care. However, even if their claims have different moral sources, the members of both of these first two categories of vulnerable populations suffer from an undeserved disadvantage of poor expected health that justice requires removing or remedying.

The third moral category of vulnerable populations at high relative risk for poor health consists of those individuals or groups who are believed at fault or responsible for that risk. It might be thought a confusion to distinguish a category of at-risk or vulnerable populations who are responsible for their risk or vulnerability. None of Aday's or AHRQ's categories of at-risk or vulnerable populations in any obvious way consist of persons responsible for being at risk. Alcohol and substance abuse once were thought to be behaviors for which individuals were responsible, and so responsible in turn for the predictable consequences of those behaviors, including the health consequences. Today, however, these are more commonly characterized as diseases, and in particular as addictive behaviors over which alcoholics and substance abusers lack normal degrees of control. Lacking such control, they cannot reasonably be held responsible for their behavior, or in turn for its health consequences. Homelessness may be the free choice of a few individuals, but for the vast majority it results from mental illness, alcohol and substance abuse, or economic adversity and is thus not their freely chosen lifestyle.

However, the implicit criteria for inclusion on Aday's list of at-risk populations, despite her definition of at-risk populations, must be more complex than merely whether the group is at high relative risk of poor health. Otherwise, as we shall see shortly, important additional groups would be on the list. Likewise, some of the conditions enumerated by AHRQ in its list of vulnerable populations are largely beyond individuals' control, such as financial circumstances, age, functional or developmental status, and presence of chronic or terminal illness or disability. Other conditions that are under individuals' control, such as personal characteristics or place of residence, presumably should not affect one's health status and access to health care, and so individuals should not have to alter them in order to protect their health or access to health care. But here, too, the criteria for inclusion are more than simply whether one is vulnerable to being in poor health. Rather, these are groups at high relative risk for poor health *because* "of unwarranted disparities in their care stemming from special needs for care or barriers to care" and *because* they "may be less able than others to safeguard their own needs and interests adequately during this period of rapid health system change." In other words, these are essentially groups vulnerable to poor health because of conditions that should not affect their health and who lack a reasonable ability to prevent those adverse effects on their health. Accordingly, the criteria defining vulnerable populations are not just empirical—

groups at high relative risk of poor health—but normative as well—groups whose health is at risk because of conditions that should not put it at risk and who cannot reasonably prevent or avoid the conditions.

If the definitions of at-risk or vulnerable groups are solely empirical—simply those at high relative risk of poor health—then other examples of at-risk or vulnerable groups include persons with sedentary lifestyles, persons with high fat diets, and persons who engage in high-risk activities such as mountain climbing or auto racing or who freely choose high-risk jobs. These risk factors for poor health are behaviors usually, at least in significant part, under the control of the individuals who engage in them, and so for which those individuals can reasonably be held responsible, at least in significant part. Part of what it means to hold them responsible in this sense is that they and not others bear the responsibility for the predictable consequences of the behavior. Nonetheless, this is not to deny that these behaviors can and should be reduced by public health interventions, such as efforts to increase seat belt use, reduce dangerous workplace conditions, and encourage healthy diets.

Determining which behaviors or conditions properly place an at-risk group in this third category is more complex and problematic than is often supposed. Smoking-related health risks are often thought to belong in this third category, and they illustrate some of the complexity. In this case, to determine whether smokers legitimately constitute an at-risk group of this category, we need to consider, first, how much the additional health risks are due to individuals' behavior and how much they are due to other factors beyond their control. For example, many smokers do not develop smoking related diseases such as lung cancer and heart disease, suggesting important genetic and/or environmental, as well as behavioral, contributions to the development of these diseases. Second, the behaviors need to be substantially voluntary and so reasonably under individuals' control; the early age at which smoking typically begins and its addictive nature undermine its voluntariness. Third, persons must know that the behavior causes the additional disease risks. Fourth, individuals must know before engaging in the behavior that doing so will reduce their priority for treatment in comparison with individuals not responsible for their own health needs. Determining whether, or the extent to which, these conditions are satisfied for various at-risk groups will often be complex and controversial in practice. As such, typical attributions of personal responsibility for the health consequences of individual behavior are far more problematic than is often supposed.

If persons in this third category of vulnerable populations have put themselves at a risk that others have chosen to avoid, they do not have the same moral claim as do members of the first category of vulnerable populations, whose vulnerable condition is caused by other social injustices. Moreover, an argument can be made that it is unfair to expect others who have chosen to avoid these risks to bear the costs of relieving persons of the health consequences of their risky behavior. Even when substantial responsibility is established, however, there may be persuasive reasons not to have the health-care system distinguish individuals' claims to health care by whether they are responsible for their health care needs. One reason is that the complexities noted above in determining whether individuals are truly responsible for their health needs would make doing so administratively complex and expensive. More importantly, this strategy would involve serious invasions of individuals' privacy to obtain the necessary information. Furthermore, we all may benefit from being able to engage in behaviors that carry some health risks without fear that doing so will later deny us access to needed health care. This can be an important aspect of ensuring peoples' autonomy in constructing and pursuing their own plans of life (Fried, 1971).

There may be other reasons in some policy contexts to ignore one or more of the differences between these three categories of at-risk populations in the nature of their moral claims on others for social resources and action to reduce their health risks. For example, we might adopt the goal of increasing the health of the population, whatever the different moral claims of its members on our efforts, or we might want to reduce the social and economic costs of poor health in the population, and so forth. But at the least, we should be clear about the differences in the nature of the moral claims of these different categories of at-risk or vulnerable populations and clear in turn about our policy reasons for ignoring them when in specific contexts we do so. And the definition of vulnerable populations employed by AHRQ seems not entirely to ignore them: its definition and enumeration of vulnerable populations includes the first two categories, even while it essentially excludes the third one. What this may show is a significant difference between Aday's account of at-risk populations and AHRQ's account of vulnerable populations. AHRQ's account is normative in the sense I noted above; it picks out conditions that should not put individuals at risk of poor health and whose health effects they are largely unable to prevent or avoid. It is this latter feature of the groups in question that makes the characterization of these populations as vulnerable especially apt. As AHRQ put it, they are "less able than others to safeguard their own needs and interests adequately" (AHRQ, 1999).

I will largely follow AHRQ in what follows in ignoring the third category of at-risk populations because it is problematic whether they have comparable moral claims on social resources grounded in justice to meet their special health needs or to lower their special health risks. Both Aday's and AHRQ's accounts of at-risk or vulnerable populations, however, include populations that fit the first and the second categories, and these categories share the condition of being subject to a serious, morally unjustified disadvantage; their relatively high risk of poor health makes them worse off than others and supports a claim grounded in justice for special concern in health policy. What should that special concern be? As we will see, this question is far more complex and relatively unexplored in work both in general moral and political philosophy and in justice and health policy than one might expect.

First, however, it is important to emphasize that the most pressing ethical issue in response to the increased risk of poor health of at-risk or vulnerable populations is not ethically complex or controversial and is addressed by traditional work on justice in health care. That work, as already noted, is centrally focused on establishing a moral right of all persons to health care. That right is acknowledged to be a limited right, not a right to any beneficial care whatsoever no matter how small the benefit and how high the cost. The limit is typically defined by the health care necessary to meet a reasonable level of health care needs under resource constraints. Sometimes this definition is expressed in very general terms, such as an adequate level of health care, sometimes in broad categories of services, and sometimes in a more detailed list of covered services, such as that developed by Oregon for its Medicaid program. However, none of the conditions making a group at risk or vulnerable on Aday's or AHRQ's list could plausibly be offered as a ground morally justifying the group to deserve either a lower level of health care or a lower level of health.

If some groups have special or greater health-care needs than others, those additional needs serve as a ground for their receiving the additional health care necessary to reasonably meet them; virtually all accounts of a right to health care accept that the health care individuals or groups receive should vary with differences in their health-care needs. Moreover, if some groups face special barriers to obtaining adequate health care, for example from poverty, geographical location, or communication problems, these are standardly understood to require efforts to overcome them in order to ensure that the groups can secure the same level of health care available to others, rather than being offered as a justification for their getting fewer needed health-care services. When groups such as some racial or ethnic minorities receive lower quality care than others, this, too, requires efforts to eliminate the difference as part of securing their right to health care. And when particular groups are less able than others to safeguard their own interests or to secure their health-care needs, this, too, requires special efforts by others to ensure their right to health care is made a reality.

All this is required by standard accounts of justice and the moral right to health care. It is all a part of removing the disadvantages in health and health care of vulnerable populations and putting them in an equal position with others. The general point is that the special at-risk or vulnerable status of those groups is an injustice, nearly as straightforwardly as is the fact that 44 million Americans are without health-care insurance, because it denies members of vulnerable groups full realization of their right to health care. No special moral principles are required to identify these injustices. What specific health policies and programs would best reduce or remove these various disadvantages is an empirical matter, not a matter for ethical analysis. I will address below what special moral claims, beyond the general claim of all to a right to health care, vulnerable or at-risk groups have because and so long as their vulnerable or at-risk conditions have not been removed and they remain disadvantaged by their relatively high risk for poor health.

PRIORITY TO THE WORSE-OFF

A concern for the worse-off members of society has long been central to many views of social justice. This is seen in familiar popular aphorisms such as "the justice of a society can be seen in how it treats its least-fortunate members." Many otherwise different religious traditions also share this concern for the worse-off and most vulnerable in their teachings and work on social justice. Concern for the worse-off has a long tradition in political philosophy as well and, in more recent decades, was a central focus of the work of John Rawls and the many others he influenced (Rawls, 1971). Rawls's difference principle requires the basic social and economic institutions of society to be arranged so as to maximize the expectations of the worst-off representative group, although the absolute priority it gives to the worst-off is extremely controversial. However, this principle has a specific and qualified application in Rawls's work, and he did not apply it to health care. An important theme in more recent political philosophy has been the so-called equality of what debate whose participants include many of the most prominent contemporary academic political philosophers. They share a commitment to equality and thus to the priority of improving the condition of the worse-off but disagree about whether the proper focus of egalitarians should be on individuals' well being, resources, opportunities, capabilities, and so forth (Sen, 1980; Dworkin, 1981; Arneson, 1989; Cohen, 1990) Thus, while the condition of the worse-off members of society has been a central concern of recent political philosophy, the proper degree and focus of that concern remains highly controversial.

Moreover, in resource prioritization, specifically that of health care, additional controversies and uncertainties surface about how a concern for the worse-off should be reflected in those priorities. Norman Daniels has characterized this as one of several important unsolved rationing problems (Daniels, 1993). Viewed from the perspective of giving priority to the worse-off, there are at least two alternative ways of thinking about vulnerable populations. One is to think of the different vulnerable populations as homogeneous in their status as among the worse-off with regard to health and health care. The rationale for this can be seen in both Aday's and AHRQ's conceptions of at-risk and vulnerable populations. If at-risk populations are defined by their sharing a high relative risk for poor health, then they are all among the worse-off with regard to their expected health status in the absence of special interventions to reduce their high relative risk. Likewise, AHRQ's conception of vulnerable populations as having special needs for care and/or barriers to care while being less able than others to safeguard their own needs and interests makes these populations also among the worse-off with regard to their expected health status in the absence of special interventions to reduce their vulnerable status. In each case the shared feature of all at-risk or vulnerable populations is being among the worse-off groups in society in terms of their expected health status.

The second way of thinking about different at-risk or vulnerable populations within a framework of priority to the worse-off is to differentiate the various groups to the extent that they have different moral claims as worse-off groups to health-care resources. For example, we might distinguish them according to the three categories of at-risk groups I delineated above—that is, whether their worse-off status is due to independently unjust conditions to which they are subject, to undeserved disadvantages not the result of any social injustice, or to conditions for which they bear responsibility. Yet vulnerable groups are different in other potentially relevant respects. For example, some are already among the worse-off with regard to health status, such as those with a chronic or terminal illness or disability (AHRQ) or with mental illness or AIDS (Aday), while others may not now suffer impaired health but be at risk of it in the future, for example those who face barriers to getting care if and when they need it because of financial circumstances or place of residence (AHRQ) or because they are immigrants or refugees (Aday).

I will pursue the simpler alternative of understanding at-risk and vulnerable populations as homogeneous in sharing the condition of being among the worse-off members of society with regard to their expected health status. What priority, if any, should these populations have in resource prioritization and interventions to reduce their high relative risk for poor health? On what I believe is a common, though by no means universal, view in public health and health economics, the answer is none. In this view, since health resources are inevitably scarce, they should be used in whatever way will maximize the health benefits derived from them and thereby the overall or aggregate health of the population served. Cost-effectiveness analysis (CEA) is the natural and standard analytic tool for pursuing this goal since it enables policy makers to determine how to allocate a given sum of money or resources to different health programs and interventions or to different patients in order to produce the greatest health gains (Gold et al, 1997). Measures like quality adjusted life years (QALYs) and disability adjusted life years (DALYs), which combine into a single unit the two main benefits from health interventions of preserving or extending life and protecting or improving health-related quality of life, are commonly used in CEA for quantitative assessment of the benefits of health interventions. CEA is indifferent to the distribution of health benefits to different individuals or groups except insofar as it affects aggregate health benefits; it does not matter who receives how much health benefit so long as overall benefits are maximized.

From this perspective, when effective health interventions exist to meet the health needs of individuals with worse health status, they will receive more resources whenever their worse initial health status makes possible greater health gains at a given cost. But they receive more health resources because they can be benefited more cost-effectively, not because of their worse health status. And when their conditions cannot be treated as cost-effectively as the conditions of persons whose health status is better and from whom greater health gains will be obtained, then resource priority should go to the better-off, not the worse-off. The cost-effectiveness standard of using limited resources to maximize health benefits is a utilitarian, or consequentialist, standard of distributive justice, and this account of distributive justice is widely considered one of consequentialism's most problematic features. It gives no direct weight to the degree of inequality in different distributions, and in particular to bettering the condition of those who are worse-off.

If the cost-effectiveness standard for prioritizing health resources is rejected in part in order to give priority to the worse-off, then we face three main sets of issues. First, for what reason should the worse-off receive priority for health resources? Second, who are the worse-off for the purposes of health resource prioritization? Third, how much priority should the worse-off receive? These issues are complex, controversial, and unsettled in general theories of distributive justice, as they are here, too, in theories of just or equitable health resource prioritization and allocation. If anything, the problem is worse in the health-care context because the issues have received less sustained attention and so, I believe, are less well understood. This means that it will not be possible to provide anything like a precise and definitive account of what priority vulnerable populations should receive in resource prioritization because they are among the worse-off, but we can explore some the issues that must be resolved to develop that account.

MORAL JUSTIFICATIONS OF PRIORITY TO THE WORSE-OFF

Why does justice require some priority to the worse-off in health resource prioritization and allocation? I will set aside cases in which individuals are responsible for their own disadvantage, cases that fall into the third category of at-risk populations I distinguished above, since, in those cases, many would say that the worse-off should not have the same special priority or, if they should, it will not be for the same reasons as when individuals are not responsible for their own disadvantage. Perhaps the most natural reason for giving priority to the worse-off is a concern for equality. When disadvantages are undeserved, then the moral baseline would appear to be one of equality, since it eliminates those undeserved disadvantages. As I have already noted, some commitment to equality is a central feature of most, and perhaps all, theories of justice, with most of the dispute being in what respects people should be equal. However, whatever the relevant respects, there are good reasons to reject a fundamental commitment to equality in outcomes or conditions, both in general and as the basis of a concern for the worse-off. The goal of equality in outcomes is different than the goal of improving the condition of the worse-off, and so equality in outcomes will not always support improving the position of the worse-off. Moreover, equality in outcomes or conditions is an implausible goal in its own right, even for egalitarians and even if achievable. The central difficulty is what Derek Parfit has called the leveling down objection. If it is a morally desirable, even if not always, all things considered, decisive, feature of states of affairs that individuals are equal in some relevant respect, then, to take Parfit's example,

> it would in one way be better if we removed the eyes of the sighted, not to give them to the blind, but simply to make the sighted blind. That would be in one way better even if it was in *no* way better for the blind. This we may find impossible to believe. . . . [I]t is not enough to claim it would be wrong to produce equality by leveling down. . . . Our objection must be that, if we achieve equality by leveling down, there is *nothing* good about what we have done.
>
> Parfit, 1991

An alternative egalitarian view looks not to whether outcomes are unequal, but rather to whether inequality is brought about by unjust treatment or action. In this view, while some of the conditions that make particular groups at-risk or vulnerable are the result of unjust treatment, such as discrimination against minority groups, other conditions need not be, such as chronic illness or disability. Consequently, this form of egalitarianism would not support giving priority to all the worse-off or to all vulnerable groups.

A more promising egalitarian appeal is to equality of opportunity. The most well-developed theory of justice in health care, that of Norman Daniels, focuses on the impact disease has in limiting function and, in turn, limiting people's opportunity (Daniels, 1985). Since some principle of equality of opportunity is common to most theories of justice, providing health care that prevents or restores loss of function would be required by these accounts of justice to protect equality of opportunity. In order to avoid the leveling down objection, the focus must be on bringing people up to the normal opportunity range for their society, not strictly on equality of opportunity. In general, the greater the loss of function caused by illness, the further persons will be from enjoying that normal opportunity range and so, in that respect, the worse-off they will be.

How this view of equality of opportunity applies to the worse-off depends on how it is interpreted. The greater the loss of function that health care can prevent or restore, the greater the increase in opportunity it will produce. If equality of opportunity is given a maximizing interpretation as requiring eliminating as much as possible the aggregate reduction in opportunity from the normal range suffered by the members of society, then providing health care that prevents or restores a greater loss of function and opportunity should have priority over preventing or restoring a lesser loss. This is not the same as maximizing opportunity, since raising people above the normal opportunity range does not have the same moral importance as bringing people up to it. Maximizing opportunity will not give priority to the worse-off when a greater loss of function and reduction of opportunity can be prevented or restored for better-off persons than can be achieved for the worse-off. The issue of priority for the worse-off, however, concerns whether and to what extent we should give priority to the needs of the worse-off when we could provide greater overall improvement in function and opportunity by directing resources to better-off groups; that is, whether and how much we should depart from cost-effectiveness applied to opportunity and accept a lower level of aggregate gain in health and opportunity in order to respond to the needs of worse-off groups. To support this priority for the worse-off, an equality of opportunity account must be interpreted as holding that the lower a person's level of opportunity is, the greater the moral importance of, or the greater priority should be given to, raising it. Most accounts of equality of opportunity are not clear on how they are to be interpreted in this regard, so let us pursue further how this priority for the worse-off might be justified.

Whether in the context of equality of opportunity or more generally, we need an account of why the worse-off should receive priority *because they are worse off*, not because we can often produce greater benefits by treating their greater needs. Here is how Derek Parfit states "The Priority View:

Benefiting people matters more the worse-off these people are." How might one justify this priority view? While I cannot fully explore this large issue here, I will at least suggest two potentially promising responses. First, the worse-off that persons are, the greater the relative benefit a given size of benefit will provide them, and so the more the benefit may matter to them. To illustrate, suppose that on a scale of a health-related quality-of-life index like the Health Utilities Index (HUI), on which death equals 0 and full unimpaired function equals 1, person A is very seriously disabled and at level .20, while person B, who is less seriously ill and impaired, is at level .60; if we could use a given amount of health-care resources to move either of them up the HUI scale by .20, that is, produce the same size health gain for each, doing so would provide A with a 100% increase in health-related quality of life but only a 33% increase for B. (Many will find precise quantification of health status problematic, but I use it only for ease of explication; it is not essential to my argument.)

This may be what people had in mind in empirical studies in which they were offered choices between using limited resources for a treatment program that would serve a group like A or a group like B, but where those same resources would produce a larger health gain for B than for A (Nord, 1993). Most people preferred to treat the worse-off group A, even when doing so would produce substantially less aggregate health benefits than would have been achieved by treating group B instead. The reason many offered for this preference was that they believed it would be more important to the more seriously ill to get treatment, even though they would receive less benefit from treatment. Their thinking may have been that it would be more important because the worse-off's relative, although not absolute, benefit would be greater. This is one way of taking account not just of objective health gains but also of the subjective perspective of individuals, which in one form or another many nonconsequentialist moral theories do (Kamm, 1993). Of course, giving priority to the greater relative benefit will not always result in priority to the worse-off, for example, if A can only be raised from .20 to .25, while B could be raised from .60 to .90. But if relative benefit is the morally important consideration, this may only reflect that the worse-off should not get absolute priority no matter how large the sacrifice to better-off groups.

A different line of justification for the priority view focuses on the degree of undeserved or unjust deprivation A and B suffer from their substantially different degrees of undeserved poor health relative to their being in full health. Because worse-off A's undeserved deprivation is greater, it could ground a stronger moral claim than B's to have that deprivation reduced or eliminated. It is morally more important or urgent to reduce A's greater deprivation than B's just because it is the greater undeserved reduction in health-related quality of life from full health.

WHO ARE THE WORSE OFF FOR HEALTH RESOURCE PRIORITIZATION?

Suppose that one of these or some other line of reasoning, suitably elaborated, succeeds in establishing that it is more important to benefit people the worse-off they are or, more specifically, that it is more important to improve people's health the worse-off they are. We then face the second question: Who is worse-off for the purposes of health-care resource prioritization and allocation? The answer we give to this question will determine whether and how priority to the worse-off applies to at-risk or vulnerable populations with worse expected health. There are several parts to this question. The first is whether, for purposes of health resource prioritization, the worse-off should be understood as those who are sicker, that is, those with worse health, or as those with worse overall well-being. In a general theory of distributive justice that gives some priority to the worse-off, it is overall or global well being that is important; for example, Rawls's statement of the general form of his principles of justice does not distinguish any particular aspect of well-being, although his difference principle requiring maximization of the expectations of the worst-off representative group applies to the basic institutions that determine the distribution of income and wealth (Rawls, 1971). One alternative would then be to treat health care as one among other goods whose distribution should be arranged to give priority to improving the overall condition of those who are overall worse-off. However, this would have what for many are highly counterintuitive implications. For example, we would have to give lower priority to treating the rich than the poor, even when the rich are much sicker than the poor, since the overall well-being of the rich may be higher despite their much worse health. If the worse-off are defined by their level of overall well-being, there would also be no tight correlation between worse-off groups and at-risk or vulnerable populations as Aday and AHRQ define them, since these groups are worse-off only in respect of their lower expected health, independent of their level of overall well-being.

The most common support for restricting the definition of the worse-off in health resource prioritization to those who have worse health is some form of separate spheres argument (Walzer, 1983; Kamm, 1993; Buchanan et al, 2000; Brock, unpublished). The idea is that there are different spheres of goods to whose distribution a theory of justice will apply, and those spheres should be treated separately or independently. Thus, a concern for the worse-off, for purposes of prioritizing educational resources, should look to those who are worse-off with regard to education and educational opportunities. Likewise, a concern for the worse-off for purposes of prioritizing health-care resources should look to those with the worse health. This fits common practices of giving the sickest patients priority for treatment when resources are explicitly scarce, for example, who is treated first in hospital emergency rooms or who gets scarce intensive care unit beds. A separate spheres view might be justified on pragmatic policy grounds—it would be too difficult, costly, and controversial, as well as too subject to mistake and abuse, for health professionals to evaluate people's different levels of overall well-being; health professionals are experts in the evaluation of people's health, not of their overall well-being. Alternatively, some have argued on principled grounds for the autonomy of different spheres of distribution—income and wealth, health care, votes, and so forth—with different moral principles applying to different spheres, although these arguments are controversial.

Even if there is good reason to restrict the concern for the worse-off to the sickest in the prioritization and allocation of health-care resources, additional issues remain. One is how to determine who are the sickest. This may seem obvious and straightforward, even if there will be disagreement about close cases, but it is not. One question is whether the sickest are those with the worse overall health or those with the most serious disease in need of treatment? For example, suppose A has a serious disability that leaves her overall health-related quality of life as measured on the HUI at .5, while B's is much better, at .9; A and B each contract the same disease, but B's case is more serious and will reduce her health-related quality of life to .7 without treatment, while A's less serious case will reduce hers to .4 without treatment. Should a special concern or priority for the sickest favor A or B? A's overall health is worse and will be worse than B's even if she, and not B, is treated, but B has the more serious illness now in need of treatment because her illness will have a greater adverse impact on her health-related quality of life than will A's on her. A natural description would be that B is the sicker now, but A's overall health is worse. It is questionable whether a separate spheres argument implies that in our concern for the worse-off we should ignore large background differences in current health or health-related quality of life and attend only to the seriousness of the illness for which each patient now needs treatment. Treating B would produce the most health benefits but would only increase the degree to which A's health is worse than B's. This question has obvious importance for the priority that some at-risk or vulnerable populations should receive, since many of them are defined by poor background health conditions such as chronic illness or disability.

Another aspect of the question of who is worse-off, again assuming the assessment is restricted to health, is whether only individuals' present health, or instead their health over time, including past and perhaps also expected future health, is relevant. Suppose 65-year-old A developed an infectious disease as an infant that has left him paralyzed in one leg, and 65-year-old B has also just contracted this disease, but his case is more serious and has left him with both legs paralyzed. A new treatment of the condition is developed that would restore the full use of their limbs to each patient, but we can only treat one of them and no future treatment of the other will be possible. Who should be considered the worse-off? B's illness is more serious and results in a greater loss of function than A's, but A has suffered his lesser loss of function his entire life, while B has been healthy all his life and has only now suffered his more serious loss of function. There is a plausible case that A is the worse-off with regard to health because he has had the condition for so long, even though his condition now is less serious than B's. People's lives extend continuously over time, and a concern for the worse-off should reflect this and not ignore the duration of people's poor health. The relevance of past health states for determining who is worse-off will also be important for assessing how badly-off different vulnerable groups are, for example persons with chronic illness or disability. Differences in the duration of expected future health impairments seem relevant as well for who is worse-off. For example, if both A and B contract the disease now at age 65, but A will suffer his lesser impairment for the rest of his life, while B will suffer his greater impairment only for a few years and then will regain use of his limbs, the worse-off is A, not B.

Who will be worse off in the future is sometimes treated as urgency, but that concept is, in fact, more complex. Urgency is a function at least of how great a harm a patient will suffer if not treated, how soon a patient must be treated to prevent the harm, and how soon the patient will suffer the harm without treatment. It is a major factor in selecting patients for transplantation of scarce organs as well as for triaging patients under emergency conditions. Frances Kamm distinguishes two senses of urgency, to reflect its complexity: urgency_t, which refers to how soon the harm will be suffered, and urgency_q, which refers to how much the patient's quality of life will be reduced (Kamm 1993; 2001). However, since there are two aspects of the temporal component of urgency—how soon it is necessary to treat the patient to prevent a harm and how soon the harm will be suffered if the patient is not treated—they may conflict. For example, it might be necessary to treat A now to prevent her suffering a harm one year from now and necessary to treat B in six months to prevent her suffering a harm at that time; B is more urgent in how soon she will suffer the harm, A in how soon she must be treated to prevent the harm. Notice that the aspect of urgency of how great a harm the patient will suffer without treatment, Kamm's urgency$_q$ suitably amended to take account of effects on length as well as quality of life, is, in fact, a measure of expected benefit from treatment when treatment is intended to prevent the patient from becoming worse-off. It displays how one aspect of potential treatment benefit plays a role in determining which patients are worse-off. Urgency captures the aspect of who is worse-off that is future directed but ignores how well- or badly-off a person has been in the past. I believe that both expected and past health states are relevant to a judgment of how badly-off persons are, although how they should be weighted is unclear.

The justification or reason for giving priority to the worse-off is related in complex ways to how the worse-off should be defined, and I can only give one example here. As already noted, in Erik Nord's empirical studies of the priority people give to the worse-off in the prioritization of health-care resources and programs, a common reason offered for favoring the worse-off was that it would be subjectively more important to the sickest to get treatment, even if they would benefit less from treatment than would others less sick (Nord, 1993). First, this justification applies only to the worse-off as determined by their health state, not a broader determination of well-being. Second, we do not know whether people meant by "the sickest" those with the worse overall health-related quality of life or those with the most serious illness to be treated now, although the latter is more likely. And third, this justification ignores how badly-off people may have been in the past in its focus on how sick patients are now. If there are conflicts between the justification(s) for giving priority to the worse-off and how the worse-off are most plausibly defined or determined, then the justification(s), or the definition, or both will have to be revised to reach a consistent and coherent overall position on priority to the worse-off in health care. This is the process that Rawls characterized in another context as attaining reflective equilibrium between our moral principles and our consideed moral judgments (Rawls, 1971).

HOW MUCH PRIORITY SHOULD THE WORSE-OFF RECEIVE IN HEALTH RESOURCE PRIORITIZATION?

The third issue in developing a moral framework for determining what priority the worse-off should receive in health-care resource prioritization is how much priority they should receive. Giving the worse-off absolute priority over others better-off is not plausible because it encounters what has been called the "bottomless pit" problem (Daniels, 1985). If the worse-off are understood as the very severely cognitively and/or physically disabled who have an extremely low health-related quality of life, health interventions in the form of health care and other supportive services may provide them with only very small benefits, but at very great cost. If improving their condition is given absolute priority, there may be almost no end to what could be done to provide them with minimal marginal gains consuming near limitless resources. Greatly expanded medical research on their conditions, even if very unpromising and at very great cost, would also have some very small expected benefit for them. If we give absolute priority to the worse-off, not just the worst-off, and maximize the health-related quality of life of each next most worse-off group after doing everything possible for those worse-off than them, few resources would remain for the important health needs of most of the population who enjoy a higher health-related quality of life.

Some balance is clearly required between giving special priority or weight to the needs of the worse-off and other relevant moral considerations, such as using limited resources to maximize overall health benefits and to meet the needs of those better-off. Ideally, we want a principled basis or reason(s) for determining how much priority to give the worse-off, but it is not clear what that principled basis would be. Rather, it seems that most people have independent moral concerns that must be balanced, but no clear or precise means for doing so and no weighting of different concerns. The balancing required will be more complex still because other moral concerns that bear on overall health-care resource prioritization and allocation, but not on my focus here, must be taken account of as well. Lacking any principled basis for how much priority to give to the worse-off, we could simply ask people, using various hypothetical choice scenarios, how much benefit to others they are prepared to sacrifice in order to treat the worse-off. Empirical research of this sort by Eric Nord and others has begun, but the data are very limited at this point (Nord et al, 1995). Alternatively, we could turn to fair procedures, either political procedures or procedures within private health plans, to make these trade-offs, perhaps informed by the research on how ordinary citizens make them (Daniels and Sabin, 1997).

CONCLUSION

I hope it is abundantly clear by now that if questions about what priority at-risk or vulnerable groups should receive in resource prioritization and allocation are best understood as one aspect of the general issue of priority to the worse-off, there is a large agenda of normative work that needs to be done and that has received far too little systematic attention to date. That work includes systematically exploring the full details and complexities in the context of health-care resource prioritization of the three questions I have briefly discussed: What is the moral justification for giving priority to the worse-off? Who are the worse-off for health-care resource prioritization? How much priority should the worse-off receive in health-care resource prioritization? Moreover, in applying a moral framework for priority to the worse-off in health-care resource prioritization, it will likely be necessary to distinguish different at-risk or vulnerable groups as relevantly different in their moral claims on health-care resources, as well as in the policy responses needed to meet those claims. Finally, the priority to the worse-off is only one of a number of prioritization and rationing problems that a full account of justice in health-care resource prioritization and allocation must confront (Daniels, 1993; Kamm, 1993; Brock, 2000). Especially in my discussion of the priority to the worse-off framework, I have raised many questions and issues without providing and defending solutions to them. In part, this is no doubt my own failing, but I believe it reflects, as well, the quite undeveloped state of serious work on the issues of health-care resource prioritization and allocation. Bioethicists and others of a normative bent should get to work.

Acknowledgments

I am grateful to Norman Daniels and Marion Danis for helpful comments on an earlier version of this chapter.

NOTES

1. This section draws on my paper (2000) Broadening the bioethics agenda. *Kennedy Institute of Ethics Journal* 10:21–38.

REFERENCES

Aday L (1993) *At Risk in America: The Health and Health Care Needs of Vulnerable Populations*. San Francisco: Jossey-Bass Publishers.

Agency for Healthcare Research and Quality (1999) Request for applications on measures of quality of care for vulnerable populations. 25.

Arneson R (1989) Equality of opportunity for welfare. *Philosophical Studies*. 56:77–93.

Brock DW (2001) Ethical issues in the use of cost-effectiveness analysis for the prioritization of health care resources. In: Anand S and Sen A (eds) *Ethical Foundations of Health Equity*. Oxford: Oxford University Press.

Brock DW (unpublished) Separate spheres and indirect benefits.

Buchanan A, Brock D, Daniels N, Wikler D (2000) *From Choice to Chance: Genetics and Justice*. Cambridge: Cambridge University Press.

Cohan GA (1992) Equality of what? On welfare, goods and capabilities. In: Nussbaum M and Sen AK (eds) *The Quality of Life*. Oxford: Clarendon Press.

Daniels N (1985) *Just Health Care*. Cambridge: Cambridge University Press.

Daniels N (1993) Rationing fairly: Programmatic considerations. *Bioethics* 7:224–33.

Daniels N and Sabin J (1997) Limits to health care: Fair procedures, democratic deliberation, and the legitimacy problem for insurers. *Philosophy and Public Affairs* 26: 303–50.

Dworkin R (1981) What is equality? Part 1: Equality of welfare. *Philosophy & Public Affairs* 10:185–246

Dworkin R (1981) What is equality? Part 2: Equality of resources. *Philosophy & Public Affairs* 10: 283–345.

Engelhardt HT Jr (1986) *The Foundations of Bioethics*. New York: Oxford University Press.

Fried C (1971) *An Anatomy of Values*. Cambridge, MA: Harvard University Press.

Gold MR, Siegel JE, Russell LB, Weinstein MC (1997) *Cost-effectiveness in Health and Medicine*. New York: Oxford University Press.

Kamm FM (1993) *Morality-Mortality Volume I: Death and Whom to Save From It*. Oxford: Oxford University Press.

Kamm FM (2001) Deciding whom to help, the principle of irrelevant good and health-adjusted life years. In: Anand S and Sen A (eds) *Ethical Foundations of Health Equity*. Oxford: Oxford University Press.

Marchand S, Wikler D, Landesman B (1998) Class, health and justice. *Milbank Memorial Quarterly* 76:1–19.

Nord E (1993) The trade-off between severity of illness and treatment effect in cost–value analysis of health care. *Health Policy* 24:227–38.

Nord E, Richardson J, Street A, Kuhse H, Singer P (1995) Maximizing health benefits vs. egalitarianism: An australian survey of health issues. *Social Science and Medicine* 41:1429–37.

Parfit D (1991) Equality or priority. The Lindley Lecture. Department of Philosophy, University of Kansas.

Rawls J (1971) *A Theory of Justice* Cambridge, MA: Harvard University Press.

Sen A (1980) Equality of what? In: *Choice, Welfare and Measurement*. Oxford: Blackwell.

Sen A (1985) *Commodities and Capabilities*. Amsterdam: Elsevier Science Publishers.

Ubel P, Scanlon D, Lowenstein G, Kamlet M (1996) Individual utilities are inconsistent with rationing choices: A partial explanation of why Oregon's cost-effectiveness list failed. *Medical Decision Making* 16: 108–19.

Walzer M (1983) *Spheres of Justice*. New York: Basic Books.

Wilkinson R (1996) *Unhealthy Societies: The Afflictions of Inequality*. London: Routledge.

16

Health policy, vulnerability, and vulnerable populations

MARION DANIS AND DONALD L. PATRICK

Health policy consists of a diverse set of legal, legislative, administrative, and social decisions that are enforced to different degrees and operate in different sectors. These decisions shape, intentionally or unintentionally, the ways in which resources are distributed to competing programs and therefore to competing populations (Patrick and Erickson, 1993, 12). In so doing, these decisions reflect how communities make social choices among their members about who receives particular types and quantities of benefits or services. An examination of resource distribution necessarily involves attention both to where the monetary and nonmonetary resources come from, the actors and processes involved in deciding who and which programs receive the resources, and the outcomes of these distribution processes.

Resources that promote health and well-being are not distributed equally. Such resources, which are both intrinsic and extrinsic to persons, range from genetic susceptibility to disease to level of economic prosperity in a particular nation or social group (Evans et al, 1994). Inequalities in the distribution of wealth and material resources (Young, 1990) as well as inequalities in health and well-being (Wilkinson, 1997) have been examined repeatedly. Inequality has also been viewed from the standpoint of risk theory, which has been used by actuaries and economists to calculate the costs of spreading risks (Arrow, 1971). Aday has extended the theory of risk to the concept of vulnerable populations, which are populations "at risk of poor physical, psychological, and/or social health" (Aday, 1993, 4) not only because of their fixed or ascribed characteristics but also because of disparities in social and human capital. Some vulnerable populations are likely to receive fewer benefits and experience poorer outcomes than are less-vulnerable populations. These poorer outcomes are often attributed to disparities in a wide variety of determinants outside the health-care system, such as access to education and income, and culturally influenced attitudes and behaviors. Disparities also occur in the availability and access to health services through differences in health insurance and health-care benefits and in the management of specific health conditions.

Risk factors that influence health are so encompassing that any member of a population may, at some point in his or her life course or in some social circumstance, be vulnerable. For example, persons who are self-employed are vulnerable in the United States as insurance is usually obtained through employment. Children and older adults are often thought of as vulnerable populations, since age is often used to define risk. Some persons, however, are more at risk throughout life, such as persons born with severe cognitive impairment or congenital conditions. Thus, any analysis of health policy and risk should focus on the concepts of universal vulnerability, even while acknowledging that there are particularly vulnerable segments of the populations.

This chapter examines the nature of vulnerability and vulnerable populations. It then defines the goals U.S. health policy ought to adopt in order to reduce the risk of vulnerability. Philosophical arguments for fairness in resource allocation justify the provision of health resources in a manner proportionate to vulnerability, with the goal of maximizing each individual's capacity to achieve full potential. These arguments suggest how universal access to health care might be achieved through changes in health policy in the United States.

THE NATURE OF VULNERABILITY AND VULNERABLE POPULATIONS

Vulnerable populations are those at risk at any particular point in time for unequal opportunity to achieve maximum possible health and quality of life because of differences in intrinsic and extrinsic resources that are associated with good health. Vulnerability may be defined by financial circumstances, place of residence, cultural background and ethnicity, age, and health conditions (such as terminal illness or mental illness, impairments, including psychological and cognitive ones, and functional status or disability, such as an inability to communicate effectively). When vulnerable, persons may be less able than others to access opportunities and to safeguard their own needs and interests adequately. These populations may also experience different health outcomes traceable either to unwarranted disparities in access to the goods and services that others receive or to cultural attitudes, special needs for care, or barriers to care.

Characteristics of those segments of the population that are most at risk in the United States have been identified. They include high-risk mothers and infants; persons with chronic illness, disabilities, AIDS, or mental illness; persons with alcohol or substance dependence; those living with domestic violence; persons without homes; and immigrants and refugees (Aday, 1993).

The term *vulnerable populations* suggests that the characteristic of vulnerability is fixed and immutable. During the course of life, however, almost everyone in the population is vulnerable on the basis of one characteristic or another, in particular regarding poor health or disability as part of acquiring chronic conditions or approaching the end of life. That *everyone is at risk* is an important concept for considering health policy and vulnerability. As Irving Zola observed two decades ago,

> By agreeing that there are twenty million disabled, or thirty-six million, or even half the population in some way affected by disability, we delude ourselves into thinking there is some finite (no matter how large) number of people. In this way, both the defining and the measuring, we try to make the reality of disease, disability, and death problematic and in this way make it at least potentially someone else's problem. But this is not and can never be. Any person . . . may be able-bodied for the moment. But everyone . . . will at some point, suffer from at least one or more chronic diseases and can be disabled, temporarily or permanently, for a significant portion of his/her life.
>
> Zola, 1983

In forging health policy that takes into account universal vulnerability, the concept of vulnerability applies to virtually all persons in the population. While recognizing that some people are always more vulnerable than others, we propose in this chapter a shift in the conception of health policy so that attention to specific vulnerable populations will not preclude acknowledging vulnerability as a universal phenomenon.

PHILOSOPHICAL ARGUMENTS

We draw here upon several previously articulated philosophical arguments in order to develop an ethical foundation for a health policy regarding vulnerability. Recently philosophers and social analysts have produced arguments that form a logical progression and a shifting approach to fairness. In doing so, they offer gradual improvements in conceptualizing the dilemma of how to address vulnerability fairly. Along with theoretical arguments, it is useful to take account of empirical evidence about the impact of health care on health outcomes, since we believe an important ingredient in translating theoretical arguments into goals for health policy is an appreciation of the nature of health-care delivery and its limitations.

The social contractarian view of justice, as articulated by Rawls (1971) and adopted by Daniels (1985), is a fruitful place to begin. While Rawls's theory of justice is commonly the starting point for many discussions and likely to be widely familiar, it is important to clearly articulate why this is so. Subsequently, we will argue that problems with this approach warrant further conceptual developments in search of an adequate ethical underpinning for a realistic policy on vulnerability.

The strengths of the social contractarian approach lie in its understanding that any social arrangements we make to address the fair distribution of goods, and, in particular, any conception we have about a guarantee to health care, are the result of a common social agreement. Rawls offers an advance over utilitarian theory since utilitarian strategies generally provide inadequate insights into how to distribute the sum of goods. His solution includes three essential elements: placement of oneself in the hypothetical original position, principles of justice that identify particular considerations as morally relevant, and priority rules for these principles. By creating this scheme, it is possible to treat questions of distribution as a matter of procedural justice.

Rawls assumes that if one adopts the hypothetical original position, where one is as though behind a "veil of ignorance," unaware of any personal proclivities or circumstances, one would choose guiding principles that would not advantage particular individuals over others. From this position he proposes that two principles would be picked. The first requires equal liberty for all. The second principle, as first outlined by Rawls, states that social and economic inequalities are to be arranged so that they are both (*1*) reasonably expected to be to everyone's advantage and (*2*) attached to positions and offices open to all (Rawls, 1971). As Rawls describes it, under conditions of democratic equality "the higher expectations of those better situated are just if and only if they work as part of a scheme which improves the expectations of the least advantaged members of society. The intuitive idea is that the social order is not to establish and secure the more attractive prospects of those better off unless doing so is to the advantage or those less fortunate" (75). One could argue that American health policies are consonant with this Rawlsian approach. The current U.S. policy of guaranteeing health care to the "poorest-off" through the Medicaid program, Medicare (through Social Security Disability Income), and the Child Health Insurance programs, is consistent with Rawls's second principle. To the extent that Rawls's theory of justice is consonant with some existing policy toward vulnerable populations, it is a good example of an ethical framework that meshes with health policy.

While we agree with the social contractarian approach, once we examine the core elements of Rawls's strategy we begin to doubt, as others have (Buchanan, 1989), that it offers the sort of unassailable arbiter of disputes about allocation that we are hoping to achieve. Rawls's theory of justice leaves room for improvement. Likewise, the current system of health-care delivery needs improvement. Having offered a modicum of guaranteed health care to a fraction of the population that is worst-off, and having no mutually agreeable logic about what to do with the rest of the population or about how to divide the pot for those vulnerable individuals the U.S. has agreed to cover, we are lost at sea. We need only remember the heroic and controversial effort to find a fair allocation scheme for distributing Medicaid dollars in Oregon to provide universal access alongside private insurance to realize how far we are from having a workable approach to distributing resources to vulnerable populations.

The approach that Rawls proposes falls short as a distribution process for at least two major reasons. One is the fact that the arrangement of negotiating under the veil of ignorance, which offers the crucial advantage of bringing stakeholders to the bargaining table in a suitably compromising frame of mind, does not provide sufficient information or traffic rules to identify solutions once we are there. As Buchanan states, "Nothing in Rawls conception of rational decision suggests that once the relevant, concrete information is available, rational persons will agree on a single assignment of weight to primary goods," of which healthcare is one (Buchanan, 1989, 314).

Even Daniels has come to this regrettable conclusion (1996). Having built his arguments for just health care on Rawls's theory of justice, Daniels faces the same difficulty. Arguing for the right to health care because it is the only way to guarantee fair equality of opportunity—an argument that is immensely powerful in justifying some guarantee to health care—does not appear to provide guidance as to how we are to make priority decisions in efforts to achieve fair equality of opportunity. As Daniels writes:

> This point was driven home to me by the way in which my "fair equality of opportunity" account of just health care (Daniels, 1985, 1988) fails to yield specific solutions to the rationing problems. . . . Even the best work in the general theory of justice has not squarely faced the problems raised by the indeterminacy of distributive principles. Rawls (1971), for example, suggests that the problem of fleshing out the content of principles of distributive justice is ultimately procedural,

> falling to the legislature. Perhaps, but the claim that we must in general turn to fair democratic procedure should not be an assumption, but the conclusion, either of a general argument or of a failed search for appropriate moral constraints on rationing. If, however, there are substantive principles governing rationing, then the theory of justice is incomplete in a way we have not noticed.
>
> Daniels, 1996, 318

Among the reasons the Rawlsian approach does not get us all the way home is that it assumes, in suggesting the use of a "veil of ignorance," that it is possible for rational individuals to shed their unique stances and thereby arrive at a common viewpoint that would permit a fair approach to distributing societal goods. In reality, individuals do not all have the same wishes or aspire to common goals, and hence the choices they would make about the distribution of primary goods such as medical care will not be the same. With regard to vulnerable populations this means, for example, that some individuals with disabilities will view their disability as no disadvantage at all and may not wish to alter it. They consider society, with its attitudes and its distribution of goods, as the problem. At the same time, others with the same disability may view it as undesirable and wish to prevent or eliminate it at any cost. Some deaf adults, for example, view deafness as the basis of a unique culture and wish to have deaf children. As Dolnick writes, "So strong is the feeling of cultural solidarity that many deaf parents cheer on discovering that their baby is deaf" (Dolnick, 1993). At the same time, pregnant women with hearing might wish to be tested for a genetic mutation associated with deafness with the aim of preventing deafness. Any policy must take this sort of diversity of views into account and accommodate them.

The importance of different views is considered particularly compelling by people with disabilities. As a case in point, Pfieffer argues against the International Classification of Impairments, Disabilities and Handicaps (ICIDH) that has been published by the World Health Organization and is undergoing a revision. Pfeiffer writes:

> Its conceptual basis is the medical model, which leads to the medicalization of disability. From this point it is a short step to eugenics and a class-based evaluation of people with disabilities using the concept of "normal." People with disabilities are found to be lacking and a burden. The language and the logic of the ICIDH are faulty. It is replete with biased, handicapist language. In its present form and even in its proposed revised form (ICIDH-2) it is a threat to the disability community worldwide.
>
> Pfeiffer, 1998

Needless to say, this view is difficult to reconcile with that of others who would argue with equal fervor that the medical model addressing disabilities is ethically sound and humane. The recognition that a shared view is not achievable, nor even desirable, because it would require the devaluation of different legitimate and irreconcilable perspectives in a diverse world, has made the resolution of distributive questions through a common lens a less plausible and attractive solution. As Young writes, the tendency of modern political theory "to reduce political subjects to a unity and to value commonness or sameness over specificity and difference" cannot serve as an approach to distributive justice because it ignores social groups and differences (Young, 1990, 3). Young argues that "where social group differences exist and some groups are privileged while others are oppressed, social justice requires explicitly acknowledging and attending to those group differences in order to undermine oppression" (Young, 1990, 3).

This recognition of the implausibility of arriving at a common view about what goals to aim for is an important advance simply because it is more reflective of the reality that diversity exists, politically and personally. In acknowledging this reality about human diversity, we revisit, however, the difficulty of possibly overwhelming divisiveness in achieving the goal of a health policy that provides protection for all persons who are vulnerable. The difficulty with this attempt to correct injustices by recognizing irreducible differences and calling for elimination of oppression of minority groups is that it is an argument that inevitably leads to partisanship—a reaction that simply fuels divisiveness and is thus bound to create further divisions, rather than overcome them.

How shall we recognize difference without fueling partisanship? Here it is useful to examine the arguments of several philosophers who provide grounds for us to attend to the needs of one another, including Scanlon (1998), Habermas (1990), and Churchill (1994). Scanlon takes the view that when we articulate what we owe each other, we must be able to defend our position to others. We must be prepared to give convincing arguments that could not be rejected by others (Scanlon, 1998). Habermas argues that the case one makes on one's own behalf must be acceptable to all (Habermas, 1990). Churchill suggests that we would do well to adopt a type of social contract envisioned by Hume, who believed that just institutions derive from self-interest (Churchill, 1994; Hume, 1998). Since we are all vulnerable, it is in the self-interest of each to provide security for everyone. We need not put ourselves in a hypothetical position because each of us, in the course of our common experience, recognizes the need for a mutual commitment out of self-interest (Churchill, 1994). The Humean contract is thus based on prudent self-regard.

Once we have mustered the arguments for motivating us to attend to each others' needs without necessarily having a common view offered by the veil of ignorance, society must deal with the mechanisms for just allocations even while there is no common view about the dividing lines. Here we turn to the economic philosophy of Sen (1992). Sen makes us aware of the diabolically difficult task entailed in attempting to divide resources equally. He provides the invaluable insight that in equalizing one domain, by dint of human differences, other domains will be made unequal. The pursuit of equality is thus always followed by the creation of other inequalities. Providing equal education and job training may, for example, yield unequal job performance and income because of the diversity of human talents. Sen is not denigrating the pursuit of equality. In fact, he argues:

> Every normative theory of social arrangement that has at all stood the test of time seems to demand equality of *something*—something that is regarded as particularly important in that theory. The theories involved are diverse and frequently at war with each other, but they seem to have that common feature. In the contemporary disputes in political philosophy, equality does, of course, figure prominently in the contribution of John Rawls (equal liberty and equality in the distribution of "primary goods"), Ronald Dworkin ("treatment as equals," "equality of resources"), Thomas Nagel ("economic equality"), Thomas Scanlon ("equality"), and others generally associated with a "pro equality" view. But equality in some space seems to be demanded even by those who are typically seen as having disputed the "case for equality" or for "distributive justice." For example, Robert Nozick may not demand equality of utility or equality of holdings or primary goods, but he does demand equality of libertarian rights—no one has any more right to liberty than anyone else. James Buchanan builds equal legal and political treatment—indeed a great deal more—into his view of a good society. In each theory, equality is sought in some space—a space that is seen as having a central role in that theory.
>
> Sen, 1992, 12–13

Sen argues that even utilitarianism values equality in the form of equal treatment of human beings in the space of gains and losses of utilities. There is an insistence on equal weighting of everyone's utility gains in the utilitarian objective function.

In short, Sen maintains that human diversity necessitates that the search for equality with regard to one variable tends to clash both in fact and in theory with equality in terms of other variables. Diversity in age, gender, general abilities, talents, and illnesses as well as social backgrounds, environment, and ownership of assets makes insistence on egalitarianism, in the sense of equality across multiple or all domains, impossible. Yet while recognizing the impossibility of seeking equality in more than one domain, Sen goes on to propose that the domain worthy of concern is the domain of functioning and capability. Living involves "beings" and "doings" that may be labeled "functionings." The various functionings that a person can achieve may be called that individual's "capability" to function.

The relevance of a person's capability to his well-being arises from two distinct but interrelated considerations. First, if the achieved functionings constitute a person's well-being, then the capability to achieve functionings (i.e., all the alternative combinations of functionings a person can choose to have) will constitute the person's freedom—the real opportunities—to have well-being. The second connection between well-being and capability takes the direct form of making achieved well-being itself depend on the capability to function. The first consideration—choosing—may itself be a valuable part of living, and a life of genuine choice with serious options may be seen to be, for that reason, richer (Sen, 1992, 40–1).

Sen traces the roots of this approach to the Aristotelian view of "the good of man" in the sense of activity. In this approach, "well-being" is synonymous with "human flourishing" (Sen, 1992, 38):

> (T)he capability approach differs from utilitarian evaluation (more generally "welfarist" evaluation) in making room for a variety of doings and beings as important in themselves (not just *because* they may yield utility, nor just to the extent that they yield utility). In this sense, the perspective of capabilities provides a fuller recognition of the variety of ways in which lives can be enriched or impoverished. It also differs from those approaches that base the evaluation on objects that are not, in any sense, personal functionings or capabilities, e.g. judging well-being by real income, wealth, opulence, resources, liberties, or primary goods.
>
> Sen, 1992, 43–4

Sen translates these concepts into a proposal to judge individual advantage by the freedom to achieve, incorporating actual achievements (Sen, 1992).

Both his recognition of the impossibility of equalizing multiple domains, and the selection of capability to function as the domain to equalize when a domain must be chosen, pose useful strategies for developing health policies that deal with vulnerability. To the extent that the distribution of health-care resources takes place at two separate levels—at the level of the individual through individualized health insurance policies and at the level of appropriation of funds to communities for community services—Sen's insights can be marshaled to address these distributive tasks separately. Where funds are apportioned to individuals, an opportunity exists to let individual visions of what matters dictate how funds are spent. Needless to say, the *amount* apportioned to each is where negotiations will take place. Where community services are being determined, the domain of capability and the goal of maximizing potential should be selected.

Young's philosophical perspective brings an additional important insight for health policy. She argues that justice is not merely a matter of distribution of resources.

> Distributive theorists of justice agree that justice is the primary normative concept for evaluating all aspects of social institutions, but at the same time they identify

> the scope of justice with distribution. This entails applying a logic of distribution to social goods which are not material things or measurable quantities. Applying a logic of distribution to such goods produces a misleading conception of the issues of justice involved. It reifies aspects of social life that are better understood as a function of rules and relations than as things. And it conceptualizes social justice primarily in terms of end state patterns, rather than focusing on social processes. . . . Rights are not fruitfully conceived as possessions. Rights are relationships, not things: they are institutionally defined rules specifying what people can do in relation to one another. Rights refer to doing more than having.
>
> Young, 1990, 24–5

James Nickel defines opportunities as "states of affairs that combine the absence of insuperable obstacles with the presences of means—internal or external—that give one a chance of overcoming the obstacles that remain." As Young writes, "Opportunity in this sense is a condition of enablement, which usually involves a configuration of social rules and social relations, as well as an individual's self-conception and skills" (1990, 26).

The claim that justice is not merely a matter of distribution of resources rings true when we recognize the numerous influences on health care and health outcomes. Health policy is a complex array of layered arrangements involving the allocation of funds to individuals for their personal medical expenditures as well as funding at numerous levels of government and nongovernmental agencies, both public and private. Influences upon policy derive from various sources, including court decisions, legislative regulations, administrative rules, and community decisions. What would matter in Young's view, in this process of making health policy, is not merely the distribution of funds to programs but the participation of all stakeholders, and the selection of programs that lead to the inclusion of and respect for vulnerable individuals within communities.

For example, parents of children with severe impairments that require one-on-one personal assistance have argued for inclusion of their children in regular schools that would provide these children with respirators or other forms of assistance. Many schools do not want to pay for the extraordinary services of attendant care and want parents to pay for the benefit of attending regular classes. In a recent Supreme Court case (*Cedar Rapids v Garrett F*, No. 96–1793, 7–2), access to community participation or school inclusion was argued, and the Court ruled that students with disabilities who require special care during the school day are entitled to the care at public expense as long as a doctor is not required to deliver the necessary services. This case clearly is a question of justice and resource distribution, involving the community through local taxes supporting the schools. But it is also a question of justice as a matter of inclusion and respect. Although the child may receive health coverage either privately or through Supplemental Security Income, this "health" issue was decided as an educational issue, with the judgment that such children are capable of benefiting from, and indeed can maximize their potential by, attending regular school. These deliberations illustrate Young's insight that rules, relations, and opportunities for participation are as much a part of the full picture of justice as is attention to the distribution of financial resources.

In summary, we have argued that we must synthesize various and sometimes disparate approaches in order to think adequately about just policies regarding health care and vulnerable populations. The vision of a social contract provides a foundation that prepares for negotiation, yet it does not contain the right ingredients given our differing assets, liabilities, and aspirations. For the social contractarian approach fails to take into account differences through any workable mechanism. At the same time, an approach that seeks to acknowledge multiple views but casts only *some* as vulnerable is insufficient—it ignores the fact that vulnerability is universal and that the failure to acknowledge this universality is divisive. Labeling individuals as "vulnerable" risks viewing vulnerable individuals as "others" worthy of pity, a view rarely appreciated.

Moreover, the vulnerable are not "others," for no one is invulnerable. To see the vulnerable as other always risks doing less than the best by them, because decisions affecting them are made by those who often see themselves as invulnerable. Finally, to isolate and champion vulnerable individuals risks alienating those who see themselves as invulnerable. For, given that they conceive of the vulnerable as a minority group, they may protest the advantage or special treatment this group receives.

A combination of arguments converges to suggest that nearly all current arguments regarding justice value equality of some sort. Yet no argument for the importance of equality in a particular domain permits maintenance of equality in other domains. Thus one might argue for allowing individuals to hold and exercise their own view whenever and to the greatest extent possible. We come then to the suggestion that we ought to find ways to allow individuals to maximize their capability as they aspire to do. When allocation decisions must be made at the group or community level, a negotiating process should aim to maximize capability through equal opportunity for participation in the decision process.

The theoretical line of arguments we have developed serves to shift our approach to thinking about medical insurance and vulnerability. It should serve to persuade us to consider medical insurance not as a matter of debatable obligation to citizens but rather as a matter of mutual interest and benefit to the society and its citizens as a whole because we are all vulnerable. Furthermore, given the lack of consensus about what matters to each of us, we must find an approach to insurance that permits and respects our different visions.

LIMITING ASSUMPTIONS

The reasoning developed above provides the basis for claiming that the aim of a policy on vulnerability and vulnerable populations should be to provide resources to all individuals and populations in proportion to their vulnerability with the goal of allowing individuals choices to maximize their capacity to achieve. Several limiting features of health care and the societal milieu must be recognized in translating this goal into practice.

First, health care is not the major determinant of health of a community. A corollary of this reality is that disparities in health that have been created by social forces are not entirely erased by health care (Evans et al, 1994). Thus, while it is an ethical and plausible aim of medical care to minimize disparities in health for vulnerable individuals, it is unrealistic to aim to equalize opportunities for individuals through medical care alone.

Second, in a society with a market-based economy, there is debate about the role of government and the balance of responsibilities between the public and private sectors. The vociferousness of this debate should not dissuade us from recognizing that universal vulnerability warrants a universal guarantee of health insurance.

Third, rationing of health care is necessary to provide universal coverage. By rationing we simply mean that some strategy is necessary for distributing limited resources (Hiatt, 1987; Daniels, 1996). The rationale given for the need to ration varies (Patrick and Erickson, 1993). Some argue that the ceiling on expenditures for health care is an arbitrary one and that we could spend more but simply choose not to. Others may believe that the ceiling is less optional because other legitimate expenses pose competing demands. Regardless of how elective and elastic the limit is seen to be, resources are finite and must be distributed by some means.

TOWARD A STRATEGY FOR A POLICY ON VULNERABILITY

Building on these philosophical arguments for recognizing and addressing universal vulnerability and acknowledging the existing limitations, how should health policy aim to provide resources to individuals and populations in proportion to their vulnerability with the goal of maximizing individuals' capacity to achieve? A policy ought to have the following features:

First, for personal health services, an insurance scheme should be designed based on a tailored package of benefits. Although there are core coverage benefits that all persons would do well to have, some flexibility in the remainder of the package must exist, thereby providing choice within constraints in a manner consistent with respect for diversity. By constraints we mean both constraint on choices and constraint on resource use. Choices should be constrained, first, in that individuals could not opt out of some modicum of benefits covering health care at the beginning and end of life, given the near universal need for care at these times and, second, in that individuals could not have every conceivable benefit.

Second, the size of the benefit package and its cost to the individual should vary. The size of the health-care benefit package under this principle should be determined by age and health status. The cost to the individual of premiums for the benefit package and/or co-payments should be based on income. This would be similar to any means-tested federal program, except that there would be no income level at which individuals would be excluded.

Third, the opportunity to maximize achievable potential must be translated into the opportunity to actually exercise choices about health care within constraints whenever possible. Services must be available in the community that allow individuals who are particularly vulnerable or have disabilities to meet their needs. Provision of insurance without availability of services will not really yield the opportunity to achieve potential.

Fourth, the burden of rationing should fall on everyone. One might call this an argument for equal rationing. Specifically, the burden of rationing should fall equally on individuals' shoulders, and the benefits of receiving a portion should be experienced equally as well.

Fifth, all persons are vulnerable, and thus all persons must participate in protection for vulnerability through health insurance coverage. No one should be able to opt out of insurance, just as all people who drive must have automobile insurance.

Most proposals to date have focused on provision of a minimum benefit package provided to all persons covered under the insurance plan. We suggest that a *uniform* service or procedure-based benefit package across the entire U.S. population will *not* be the most effective and accommodating approach to achieving universal coverage and that we must diversify and base entitlement on age, health status, and income eligibility criteria. This proposal would include a core of benefits that would apply to all, such as preventive services, hospital stays, and maternity benefits. In addition, however, the total individual benefit package would be calculated based on age and health status. Contributions to this package, including any deductibles or co-payments, would be based on income.

An individual's total benefit package would contain considerable options to choose from, including degree of comprehensiveness and flexibility of inpatient and outpatient benefit levels, mental health benefits, choice of providers, and other current features of managed care. These different packages are currently available to consumers through employer-provided health insurance and publicly funded insurance.

Consistent with the logic argued so far, it is possible to imagine a health insurance proposal that has some of the following assumptions and features. Individuals would be required to have health insurance coverage. We assume that ultimately the source of funding would come from the public; whether it would be paid for through taxation or premiums is irrelevant, but the amount derived from each individual would be related to individual or family income.

Responsibility for administration of the sort of program we describe is irrelevant to the merits of the proposal and a matter for public debate. However, we suggest that implementation of the proposal through expansion of the Medicare program would likely be the most feasible option. The availability of an existing administrative structure offers an advantage. As the population gets older, the percentage of the population that will be insured through Medicare will be expanding, in any case. While the Medicare program is currently funded partly through direct taxation of income and partly by general revenues, this tax base need not be altered. Those in the population who are employed and insured through a combination of contributions by employee and employer could channel these funds through Medicare. Those who are employed but uninsured would have the opportunity to participate through taxation of their incomes. Strategies to avoid any financial disadvantage to individuals who do not work for contributing employers would need to be developed. Those who are unemployed would be able to participate since means testing would permit them to do so at minimal personal cost.

When individuals signed up for their health insurance, they or their representative would pick a package tailored to their goals and designed to maximize their capability. The cost would vary with their income either by varying premiums, varying deductibles and co-payments, or both. The selection process would involve picking among a variety of benefits and among more or less tightly managed options for these benefits, similar to the sort of tailored benefit selection process that has begun to be explored (Biddle, 1998; Danis, 1997; Danis, 2002; Goold, 2000). Individuals with extremely poor health status or cognitive impairment would have a case manager or counselor with whom they, their family, or someone else designated on their behalf might consult to pick their package.

The administration of this proposal would be facilitated by advances in computerized insurance claim processing. Such processing would be expected to minimize the administrative burden of varied benefit packages and reimbursement for utilization of services.

Where community resources must be pooled to provide health care (for example, public health or school health), communities would choose how to allocate available public resources. These choices would be made with the aim of maximizing potential to function and participate in the community.

ILLUSTRATIVE CASES

Hypothetical cases serve to illustrate how the imagined policy might function in relation to individuals who are variously vulnerable.

Genetic Disorder

A family has a father who has developed Huntington's chorea. The adult children have seen him develop a dementing illness and are aware that they are at risk for this disease. One daughter has chosen to be tested and tests positively for Huntington's chorea. She would like to have children through assisted reproduction using an egg donor in order to avoid transmitting the disease. When she picks her benefit package, she selects infertility coverage and chooses to forgo eye and dental benefits, which she instead plans to pay for out of her own pocket.

Her brother chooses not to be tested. Several years later he develops Huntington's chorea. His new diagnosis relegates him to a new health status, so the total dollar figure for his benefit package increases. When selecting his health benefits he chooses a package that includes long-term care in anticipation of the need for nursing home placement at some point. He picks the most basic primary care and pharmacy benefit packages in order to select the highest long-term care benefit.

Mental Illness

A young woman in her 30s has schizophrenia. With the help of her case manager, she picks a package that includes long-term care and payment for living in a half-way house, since this will help her avoid the periods of homelessness she experienced previously. To make this choice, she picks the most basic, tightly managed primary care services, hospitalization coverage, and mental health services. Her psychiatrist agrees with this coverage choice, particularly the trade-off of higher mental health benefits for long-term care, believing that she would not benefit from frequent psychiatric visits as much as she would from a supportive residential arrangement.

Another schizophrenic patient, who is able to function more independently and work at his job in a library, decides on advice from his case manager to pick the mental health services and pharmacy benefit so he can pay for both his visits to his psychiatric social worker as well as his antipsychotic medications.

Severe Impairment

The parents of a child with cerebral palsy pick a package that has the most comprehensive and flexible option for durable medical equipment and other medical services since they have extremely large bills for specialized equipment and physical therapy. They do not select coverage for long-term care since they feel committed to taking care of their child at home and have made arrangements with their extended family to help with this plan.

A young adult had meningitis at age 3 and now has mild cognitive impairment and hearing deficits. His parents have debated about how to educate him and would like to send him to the local school. They are hoping to get some expensive equipment to aid him in hearing in the classroom. They opt to select the highest coverage for medical equipment as well.

Chronic Disease

A woman in her 40s has had multiple sclerosis for the last eight years. She had previously picked a benefit package that had the highest hospitalization benefit because she had several hospitalizations when she first developed the disease. In the last few years she has been receiving immunotherapy and has required fewer hospitalizations. She therefore decides with her case manager that she will change from selecting the highest hospitalization benefit to the highest pharmacy benefit so her co-payments for immunotherapy will be less. She has been able to work more effectively since she has been taking the medication, she has had a promotion at work, and her health insurance premiums have gone up.

An HIV-infected man has been taking highly effective antiretroviral therapy for the last two years. In past years he had selected the most restrictive pharmacy benefit package, which required a 20% co-payment on his pharmacy bills. This year, after a discussion with his primary care provider, who now works closely with a comprehensive HIV treatment team, he selected the pharmacy benefit option that only requires him to pay a 10% co-payment and a more restrictive primary care option that requires more restricted referrals to specialists.

Substance Abuse

A 35-year-old man has had a problem with alcohol abuse for the last nine years. He lost his job as an accountant three years ago because of his unreliability at work. For the last several years he has had the maximum mental health benefit because his case manager and primary care physician advised him that he ought to work with a counselor and a support group. But he has continued to drink heavily and lately has developed signs of cirrhosis. This year his primary care physician suggests to him that he drop his mental health coverage and get the highest hospitalization benefit because he has begun to require hospitalizations for bleeding esophageal varices.

A 31-year-old woman who has been an intravenous drug abuser is ready to try giving up the habit. Her mental health counselor sends her to a rehabilitation facility, and she has recently begun taking methadone. When she selects her benefit package this year in consultation with her counselor, he mentions that methadone alone will not help her deal effectively with her recovery and that she might want to think now about what her goals are and about strategies that could help her reach her goals, since she has been on the methadone program for the last year. He refers her to a local community college counselor. Thus, her individual policy is coordinated with community-wide services.

Unexpected Illness

A 47-year-old man was about to begin his own computer software company two years ago when he was informed by the consultant provided by the Small Business Administration that he was required by law to set aside money for health insurance. He was reluctant to do so since he needed as much cash as possible to invest in his business and pay for his son's college tuition. The consultant informed him of one of the legal options, which was to set aside only that amount of funds needed for a basic benefits package. He chose this option and, among the basic options of catastrophic coverage or basic inpatient and hospitalization, he selected catastrophic coverage. One year ago, during a particularly stressful period, he developed a bleeding ulcer. His insurance covered 80% of his hospitalization.

A 27-year-old woman was employed at a small dry-cleaning store. She had an automobile accident on her way home from work one evening and suffered acute spinal cord injury. Her automobile insurance did not pay for all of her medical bills. She has been getting rehabilitation therapy for the last several months that is paid for by the insurance that she receives through work.

These examples serve to illustrate the possibilities offered by a healthcare policy that acknowledges the universality of vulnerability and deals effectively with populations at particularly high risk. It aims to maximize capability and accommodates individual goals. It incorporates rationing through a mechanism that allows room for choice. It acknowledges that health care alone is not expected to bring individuals to their full capability.

The policy illustrated here is based on the assumption that fairness is not merely a matter of just distribution. It recognizes that a policy allowing some degree of individual benefit selection must dovetail with available community resources to work effectively. Individual policies meet individual needs because there are community services, case managers, school counselors, community facilities, primary care providers, and coordination of care that make individual choices feasible.

ADVANTAGES AND DISADVANTAGES OF THE ILLUSTRATED PROPOSAL

A plan that has societally defined parameters that incorporate financial limits, rules about allocation that are based on enrollee characteristics, and choices based on enrollee preferences can afford the following advantages:

- It assumes that all are vulnerable to some extent.
- It accommodates individuals with varying degrees of vulnerability.
- It accounts for the need to ration.
- It strives to be fair and incorporates various views of fairness including liberty and equality.
- It provides a mechanism for arbitrating disagreements since the rules have been chosen both to be even-handed to all enrollees and to accommodate individual preferences in a way that is very specific.
- It avoids some of the vagueness and arbitrariness involved in current disputes about insurance coverage.
- It does not place the physician in the awkward situation of arbitrating decisions about resource use because the ground rules have been set based on individual choice

Despite these advantages, a variety of disadvantages must be addressed regarding this imagined proposal. Efforts to individualize are problematic in designing insurance. In the imagined plan, the benefits of pooled risk, which are inherent in insurance, are arguably lower than when everyone has the same benefit packages. The moral hazard incurred in allowing individuals to tailor their insurance is large. In tailoring a package of one's own the likelihood that selected services will be used increases and the actuarial costs for these services will rise. But while the benefits of pooling risk are lower, they are not nil. Individuals are still insuring for possible health events, not for certain outcomes. One must assume then that the actuarial costs for any given service will rise and, to compensate for this, the total number of packages that an individual could pick from may need to be restricted. It is likely, however, that research would show patterns of choices among groups of individuals, and thus, while it would not be possible to offer an infinite number of package options, it should be possible to offer a few more commonly preferred insurance package options for individuals to select from.

It may be objected that prospective self-denial, which is entailed in forgoing some services in favor of others, will be hard to live with. While this is inevitably the case, one might counter that prospective self-denial is no worse than denial by someone else. It may be objected, as well, that individuals will make imprudent choices. This concern may be addressed by having the most commonly used or needed benefits automatically included in benefit packages. Others might argue that individuals will not want to make choices for themselves. As mentioned above, one might design a default package for such individuals.

Finally, given that we have suggested expansion of the Medicare program as the most feasible approach to implementing the strategy we have proposed, it may be objected that problems of intergenerational equity will arise. But we might argue that, on the contrary, if Medicare were expanded and individuals of all ages were enrolled in the program, a more straightforward calculation of how health-care funds should be distributed as a function of age could be developed. The dollar amount of the benefit package would be a function of age, and we would argue for applying age-appropriate guidelines, as suggested elsewhere in the chapter by Callahan.

FURTHER IMPLICATIONS

While the implications of this proposal are numerous, the major ones relate to shifts in conceptions of vulnerability, the consequences for risk stratification and measurement of preferences, and consideration of feasible implementation of the proposal. The proposal suggested here entails a change from rationing by procedure to rationing on the basis of risk stratification. It requires actuarial estimates for costs as a function of health status to determine the size of the benefit package that individuals will receive.

A focus on maximizing the potential to achieve has major implications for measuring the benefits of health care and technology. The strategy of evaluating benefits on the basis of cost-effectiveness using quality-adjusted life years (QALYs) or some other type of health-adjusted life expectancy, as currently construed, does not incorporate opportunity or potential capability to function, but instead incorporates actual level of function, with conditions that are less susceptible to improved function being given lower priority or fewer QALYs (Gold, 1996). As currently practiced, the QALY approach has severe limitations in incorporating concerns of fairness that are well recognized. (Patrick and Erickson, 1993; Nord et al, 1999; Carr-Hill, 1989; Williams, 1997) Persons who have lesser potential for health improvement than others are disadvantaged by the traditional QALY estimation. Equity weights may be one solution to this problem. For example, one might assign a life year gained for people with disabilities the full value of 1 as long as the person concerned considers the year preferable to death (Nord et al, 1999). Other alternatives seem less satisfying. For instance, it has been suggested that persons with disabilities be left out of the resource allocation schema (Patrick and Erickson, 1993). This does not seem like a viable alternative, however. Alternatively, some have proposed that a weighting system be incorporated that does not systematically place a lower value on persons with lower health potential. A reconfiguration of the QALY estimation procedure would be necessary to implement this suggested policy consistent with the ethical arguments described in this chapter.

One might wonder about the place of evidence-based medical practice if individuals are to have a great deal more say in their health-care coverage, yet the role that evidence plays in medical decision making would not necessarily change substantially. The use of individual procedures would remain a matter of discussion between doctor and patient, with the doctor using an evidence-based rationale for advising procedures and a patient contributing a personal perspective, on the goals of care. We argue here for a more important role of the patient in selecting his or her insurance coverage up front, not for a change in the way treatment decisions are made once illness ensues.

This approach to prioritizing individual health care offers a partial solution to distributing health-care resources, but it does not address the planning of community services required by individuals who have vulnerable conditions. Societal weighting of lower functional status conflicts with the views of individuals with lower functional status. Some strategy for weighing the views of all relevant parties, including people at risk, must thus be developed. Any community weighting must incorporate the views of individuals across the health status spectrum. While some have argued that a useful approach to recognized differences involves creating numerous homogeneous communities that can each develop its unique set of goals, we would suggest, consistent with our earlier discussion, that diversity makes the aspiration for solutions based on homogeneous communities an impossibility.

Some readers may consider the proposal here akin to a proposal for a voucher system. While there are similarities to a voucher system, the intent of the proposal differs from voucher proposals. More specifically, recent proposals for the use of a voucher system as an option for reforming the Medicare program involve offering Medicare enrollees a fixed dollar contribution from the government to purchase health insurance from the private sector (Luft, 1984; Oberlander, 1998). Such vouchers have been intended as an approach to cutting costs and promoting a choice of providers through privatization of Medicare, yet privatization is not the goal of our proposal. The aim of providing choices as described here is to allow health insurance to facilitate the achievement of personal goals and functioning. By offering the strategy suggested here, we introduce the possibility of structuring a mechanism for individuals to make responsible choices for use of publicly or privately funded programs. We acknowledge that the attempt to accommodate choice does entail the difficulties encountered by voucher systems. In particular, the need to rely on risk adjustment in order to determine the size of the benefit package for individuals of differing health status is as pressing as is the need to risk adjust in order to design a voucher system. The administrative and monitoring burden may seem similar to that of a voucher system, given the complexity of the proposal. Of course, if the proposal were to be carried out through a single-payer system, the complexity would be less, but the proposal does not require a single payer.

The proposal may raise concerns about the possibility of pooling risk when individuals select tailored insurance packages. We imagine, however, that the fact that enrollees select to forgo coverage (or accept more restricted coverage) for some benefits for the sake of benefits they would prefer (or would prefer to have available more comprehensively or flexibly) means that the net effect will be a shift in use patterns rather than a net gain in use. If this is the case, then the advantages of pooled risk will not be lost.

A final implication of the proposal is the assumption that cost controls should be an individual responsibility (Danis, 1991). This again is a feature that is similar to voucher systems. Critics have argued that individuals should not have to bear the responsibility for rationing (Marmor, 1998). We suggest that, ultimately, individuals always bear the consequences of rationing. Whether it occurs through global budgeting, at the discretion of the provider, or through individual choice, in the end the consequences are felt by individuals who are subjected to compromises of some sort in delivered services and shared costs. The opportunity to have a say in how rationing will occur is preferable to bearing the burden of rationing without having a say in the matter.

A SUGGESTED RESEARCH AGENDA

While we have focused specifically on arguments for developing a policy on vulnerability, if scholars in ethics, health services research, and health policy are effectively to contribute to addressing vulnerability and the needs of vulnerable populations, a broad array of research and deliberation is warranted. At the conceptual level, there is much room for debate about how to address the universal but uneven vulnerability of the population. Certainly, a critique of what we have proposed as well as proposals for other strategies are warranted, particularly by persons in especially vulnerable populations

Regarding the strategy we have suggested, there is room for experimental research, particularly demonstration evaluations of allocation exercises. If we focus on a capability theory, what capabilities matter to people? When determining how to apportion community resources, how might simulation exercises be developed that allow the public to make choices within resource constraints? If the public is reluctant to ration (Lomas, 1994), can this reluctance be overcome with the development of more easily used decision tools?

The proposal we have suggested warrants some risk adjustment in apportioning benefit packages. Suggestions similar to those proposed (Newhouse et al, 1997) for deciding how to apportion must be developed and justified. The Social Security Administration, for example, is looking at functional capacity and its assessment for eligibility for income maintenance in its National Study of Health and Activity (Social Security Administration). This type of research will provide guidance in health status measurement for risk adjustment. A broader set of questions deserves to be addressed. We enumerate but a few.

As health-care organization and financing change, what are the implications for more vulnerable segments of the population? Evidence suggests that vulnerable segments of the population fare differently than do less vulnerable segments of the population with regard to access to care and medical outcomes (Miller, 1998; Ware, 1996). How should we deal with this differential response?

Those health-care organizations and delivery mechanisms that have had a track record of delivering service to vulnerable populations, such as community clinics and school-based clinics, have had a difficult time remaining financially solvent under current reimbursement arrangements (Schauffler, 1996; Brindis, 1997). How do we rectify this?

If the United States chooses to continue with a multiple payer arrangement, this strategy affects the fulfillment of health-care needs of vulnerable populations (Soman et al, 1996; Ware, 1996). How can this arrangement be coordinated more effectively to address the needs of vulnerable individuals?

Finally, the following issues need to be further explored. Development and testing of innovative strategies for organizing and delivering coordinated services to vulnerable populations need to take place (Chermak, 1990; Bergman, 1997). The training of providers in ways that properly prepare them for treating vulnerable populations has been suggested, and the impact of such training needs to be evaluated (Lurie, 1990). Creative strategies for organizing the care of vulnerable individuals need to be further developed along the lines of those strategies used in home care settings (Feldman et al, 1996). Finally, ongoing collection of data to monitor the impact of policies on vulnerable individuals and populations needs to occur (Bindman, 1993).

CONCLUDING COMMENTS

We have developed arguments for and an outline of a policy regarding vulnerability and vulnerable populations without having fully pursued its practical application. While much practical effort would be required to develop the approach suggested here, it should not be dismissed lightly out of concern about its feasibility. The philosophical arguments, if accepted, should facilitate the debate on how to achieve fair funding of health care for all.

NOTES

1. The opinions expressed here are those of the authors and are not official policy of the National Institutes of health, the Public Health Service, or the Department of Health and Human Services.

REFERENCES

Aday LA (1983) *At Risk in America.* San Francisco: Jossey-Bass.

Arrow KJ (1971) *Essays in the Theory of Risk-bearing.* Chicago: Markham.

Bergman H, Beland F, Lebel P, Contandriopuolos AP, Tousignant P, Brunelle Y, Kaufman T, Leibovich E, Rodriguez R, Clarfield M (1997) Care for Canada's frail elderly population: fragmentation or integration? *Canadian Medical Association Journal* 157: 1116–21.

Biddle AK, DeVellis RF, Henderson G, Fasick SB, Danis M (1998) The health insurance puzzle: A new approach to assessing patient coverage preferences. *Journal of Community Health* 23:181–94.

Bindman AB, Grumbach K, Keane D, Lurie N (1993) Collecting data to evaluate the effects of health policies on vulnerable populations. *Family Medicine* 25:114–9.

Brindis CD (1997) School-based health clinics: Remaining viable in a changing health care delivery system. *Annual Review of Public Health* 18;567–87.

Buchanan A (1989) Health care delivery and resource allocation. In: Veatch R (ed) *Medical Ethics.* Boston: Jones and Bartlett.

Carr-Hill R (1989) Assumptions of the QALY procedure. *Social Science and Medicine* 29;3:469

Chermak GD (1990) A global perspective on disability: A review of efforts to increase access and advance social integration for disabled persons. *International Disability Studies* 12:123–7.

Churchill LR (1994) *Self-Interest and Universal Health Care: Why Well-Insured Americans Should Support Coverage for Everyone.* Cambridge, MA: Harvard University Press.

Daniels N (1985) *Just Health Care.* New York: Cambridge University Press.

Daniels N (1996) *Justice and Justification: Reflective Equilibrium in Theory and Practice.* Cambridge: Cambridge University Press.

Danis M and Churchill LR (1991) Autonomy and the common weal. *Hastings Center Report* 21:25–31.

Danis M, Biddle AK, Henderson G, Garrett JM, DeVellis RF (1997) Elderly Medicare enrollees choices for insured services. *Journal of the American Geriatric Society* 45: 688–94.

Danis M, Biddle A, Goold SD (2002) Insurance benefit preferences of the low-income uninsured. *Journal of General Internal Medecine* (in press).

Dolnick E (1993) Deafness as culture. *The Atlantic Monthly* 272:37–53.

Evans RG, Barer ML, Marmor TR (eds) (1994) *Why Are Some People Healthy and Others Not?* New York: Aldine DeGruyter.

Erickson P, Wilson R, Shannon I (2000) *Healthy People 2000 Statistical Notes, Number 7.* Washington, DC: Centers for Disease Control and Prevention.

Feldan PH, Latimer E, Davidson H (1996) Medicaid-funded home care for the frail elderly and disabled: Evaluating the cost savings and outcomes of a service delivery reform. *Health Services Research* 31:509–13.

Gold MR (1996) *Cost Effectiveness in Health and Medicine.* New York: Oxford University Press.

Goold SD, Biddle A, Klipp G, Danis M (2000) Choosing healthplans all together: a game to assess consumer values and preferences for health insurance. *Journal of General Internal Medicine* 15:68.

Habermas J (1990) *Moral Consciousness and Communicative Action.* Cambridge, MA: MIT Press.

Hiatt HH (1987) *America's Health in the Balance.* New York: Harper and Row.

Hume D (1998) *An Enquiry Concerning the Principles of Morals.* New York: Oxford University Press.

Lomas J (1997) Reluctant rationers: public input to health care priorities. *Journal of Health Services Research and Policy* 2:103–11.

Luft HS (1984) On the use of Medicare vouchers for Medicare. *Milbank Memorial Fund Quarterly* 62:237–250.

Lurie N, Yergan J (1990) Teaching residents to care for vulnerable populations in the outpatient setting. *Journal of General Internal Medecine* 5 (1 Suppl):S26–34.

Marmor T, Oberlander J (1998) Rethinking Medicare reform. *Health Affairs* 17:52–68.

Miller RH (1998) Healthcare organizational change: Implications for access to care and its measurement. *Health Services Research* 33 (3, pt2):653–80.

Newhouse JP, Buntin MB, Chapman JD (1997) Risk adjustment and Medicare: Taking a closer look. *Health Affairs* 16:26–43.

Nickel J (1988) Equal opportunity in a pluralistic society. In: Paul EF, Miller FD, Paul J, and Ahrens J (eds) *Equal Opportunity.* Oxford: Blackwell.

Nord E, Pinto JL, et al (1999) Incorporating societal concerns for fairness in numerical valuations of health programmes. *Health Economics* 8:25–39.

Oberlander J (1998) Remaking Medicare: The voucher myth. *International Journal Health Services* 28:29–46.

Patrick DL and Erickson P (1993) *Health Status and Health Policy*. New York: Oxford University Press.

Pfeiffer D (1998) The ICIDH and the need for its revision. *Disability and Society* 13: 503–23.

Rawls J (1971) *A Theory of Justice*. Cambridge, MA: Belknap Press of Harvard University Press.

Scanlon TM (1998) *What We Owe Each Other*. Cambridge, MA: Harvard University Press.

Schauffler HH (1996) Community health clinics under managed care competition: Navigating uncharted waters. *Journal of Health Politics Policy and Law* 21:461–88.

Sen A (1992) *Inequality Reexamined*. Cambridge, MA: Harvard University Press.

Social Security Administration. National Study of Health and Activity. Available at: www.ssa.gov/nsha/

Soman LA, Brindis C, Dunn-Malhotra E (1996) The interplay of national, state, and local policy in financing care for drug-affected women and children in California. *Journal of Psychoactive Drugs* 28:3–15.

Ware JE, Jr, Bayliss MS, Rogers WH, Kosinski M, Tarlov AR (1996) Differences in 4-year health outcomes for elderly and poor, chronically ill patients treated in HMO and fee-for-service systems. Results of the Medical Outcome Study. *Journal of the American Medical Association* 276:1039–47.

Wilkinson RG (1997) Socioeconomic determinants of health. Health inequalities: Relative or absolute material standards? *British Medical Journal* 314(7080):591–5.

Williams A (1997) Economics, QALYs and medical ethics: A health economist's perspective. *Journal d'Economie Medicale* 1: 49–54.

Young IM (1990) *Justice and the Politics of Difference*. Princeton, NJ: Princeton University Press.

Zola IK (1983) *Sociomedical Inquiries*. Philadelphia: Temple University Press.

Ethical considerations of health services research

17

Values in research: picking research priorities ethically[1]

BERNARD LO

The choice of topics for study, the specification of research questions, and the design of a health services research project all involve a series of value choices. At each decision point the investigator's choices have important implications. Many factors influence the design of a research project, including such external considerations as information available in databases, access to databases, and funding priorities. However, the justification for a research project should never be merely that the data and funding are available to carry out the work. The personal interests of the researcher in a topic or methodology have an important influence in shaping research projects. Indeed, because difficulties and complications always occur in projects, it is easier to sustain a project in which the investigator has a heartfelt personal interest. However, the personal interests of the investigator are also not sufficient justification for a research project. Ultimately, health services research should benefit the public. Arcane "pure" research may eventually have important real-world implications, but a researcher developing a research agenda or protocol should articulate how it will affect clinical care, decisions by health care organizations, or public policies. If the researcher cannot give a plausible account of how the research might have such an impact, the investigator should consider whether different studies should have higher priority.

This chapter will address two issues concerning health services research:

1. What are the ethical implications of how we define health services research?
2. How do our values shape the research agenda and methods?

WHAT ARE THE ETHICAL IMPLICATIONS OF HOW WE DEFINE HEALTH SERVICES RESEARCH?

Research on human subjects is defined by the goal of obtaining generalizable knowledge (Levine, 1986). Research benefits society as a whole because, ultimately, increased medical knowledge will help reduce human suffering. Research is not intended to benefit primarily the subjects of research. As such, ethical concerns arise because subjects undergo risks or inconvenience for the benefits of others. Research subjects may be treated merely as a means to achieve other ends, rather than being respected as ends in themselves. Clinical research has raised the most ethical concerns because research subjects may undergo invasive clinical interventions and physical risks for the sake of others. Health services research generally carries fewer risks than does clinical research because patients undergo no physical interventions as part of the research study. Instead, many of these projects are secondary analyses of data that has already been collected.

Overlap Between Health Services Research and Other Activities

Health services research overlaps with closely related activities such as disease management, quality improvement, and business functions. A project involving the secondary analysis of personal health information in databases could be carried out for different objectives and characterized in different ways. Consider a project to identify high-cost patients. There are numerous ways to categorize such a project. First, the project objective could be to identify such patients in a reliable and valid way in various organizational and clinical settings. The ultimate goal might be to design a system of risk adjustment for provider reimbursement. Such a project would be properly characterized as health services research. Second, the identification of high-cost patients might be carried out as a disease management project whose goal is to identify patients for case management, education in self-care, or to promote prevention and adherence to recommended therapies. In other words, individuals identified as being high-cost patients might be contacted and offered clinical interventions that presumably would benefit them. Thus, the subjects of this sort of project would directly benefit from the analysis of personal health information in the databases. The project could be considered an adjunct to patient care. Third, the objective of identifying high-cost patients might be to design more efficient ways of providing care by examining high-cost cases more closely. Such a project would rightly be considered quality improvement. Fourth, the goal of identifying high-cost patients might be to help a health-care organization negotiate more favorable contracts and reimbursement rates. Such a project would be characterized as a necessary business function of the organization, namely, that of contracting and financial planning. In the third and fourth possibilities, it is the health-care organization that primarily benefits from the analysis of databases containing personal health information.

Ethical Implications of Classifying a Project as Research

What difference does it make whether we label a specific project as health services research, disease management, quality improvement, or a business function? There are several important ethical implications.

Oversight and protections

For research, federal regulations are in force if the project is carried out with federal funding or at an institution that has a multiproject assurance that all research at the site will comply with federal regulations, even if it is not federally funded. Federal regulations protect the subjects of human research (Protection of Human Subjects, 1999). These protections include informed consent from research subjects and review by an institutional review board (IRB) that is independent of the investigators. The rationale for these regulations is that persons need to be protected if they are asked to accept risks as part of a research project. IRBs have recently been criticized for failing to meet the objective of protecting research subjects (U.S. General Accounting Office, 1996; Office of the Inspector General, 1998). However, the requirement of independent review of research protocols by persons not directly involved in the research remains a sound one.

In health services research, the major risk to subjects is usually loss of confidentiality. Breaches of confidentiality harm research subjects by violating their autonomy. These may also lead to tangible harms, such as discrimination and stigmatization. IRBs are charged with ensuring that the risks of research are minimized and proportional to the benefits. With adequate confidentiality safeguards in place, a good deal of health services research that carries out secondary analyses of data that have already been collected qualifies for an exemption from the requirement of informed consent from subjects.

For projects that are considered disease management, quality improvement, or business functions, however, no federal regulations exist to protect subjects whose personal health information is analyzed. Even though the risks may be similar to those in research projects, no one independent of the project team needs to review the protocol to ensure that confidentiality will be appropriately safeguarded. Because these projects are usually undertaken by the organization that also provides health-care services to the persons in the project, no further disclosure of personal health information to other organizations is required.

Proposed federal policies also distinguish between research and these other activities. More specifically, proposed federal regulations do not subject quality improvement, disease management, and business functions to the same oversight or regulation as research (Department of Health and Human Services, 1999). In particular, there is little discussion of how the confidentiality of personal health information needs to be protected in these other types of projects.

State laws or regulations also may apply to research projects but not to the other types of projects. For example, Minnesota requires disclosure to patients about research that examines a person's health records generated after January 1997. If the patient objects, records may not be released (Minn Stat. §§ 144.335.3a [1997]). However, there are no such requirements concerning notification and authorization for disease management or quality improvement projects conducted by the health-care organization.

Reliability of findings

Findings from projects in disease management, quality improvement, and business activities may be less reliable than are findings from research projects. The absence of a peer review process for studies not characterized as research may lead to projects that are less rigorously designed. Furthermore, projects in disease management, quality improvement, and business activities often accept lower standards of evidence than does health services research. Leaders in health care organizations do not need findings that reach statistical significance at the $p < .05$ level. With much less certainty, they can make sound decisions. In addition, the time frame in which business and organizational decisions need to be made is much shorter than the time frame usually required to plan and carry out rigorous scientific studies. To respond to marketplace forces and competitors, health-care organizations cannot defer decisions for years while definitive studies are carried out. Indeed, in the time it would take to conduct a rigorous scientific study, the market may have changed so drastically that the original question is no longer relevant.

Different balance of benefits to risks

The balance of benefit to risk may be less favorable when a project is characterized as disease management, quality improvement, or business activity. The risks may be greater because safeguards for confidentiality may not be as robust as they are in health services research. For example, less stringent standards may be used for coding and linking, disclosure of information within the organization, and disclosure to third parties. One particular concern is that employers may obtain patient-identifiable health information. Increasingly, employers who provide health insurance to employees are self-insured. As parties that pay for or administer health insurance benefits, employers have a legitimate need to have sufficient personal health information to carry out payment, utilization, and other business functions. However, patients are commonly concerned that information from disease management, quality improvement, or business administration projects will be passed on to the personnel department of the employer (Committee on Maintaining Privacy and Security in Health Care Applications of the National Information Infrastructure, 1997) and that health information will be used in hiring and promotions, notwithstanding the provisions of the Americans with Disabilities Act.

The benefits of quality improvement and business functions activities also differ from the benefits of research. One important difference concerns the beneficiaries of these projects. In research the ultimate beneficiaries are society in general and patients whose suffering may be relieved by improved delivery of clinical care. However, in business activities, such as financial planning and contracting, the benefits accrue primarily to the health-care organization. Indeed, the public is concerned that the efficiency achieved by managed care organizations may compromise the quality of care (Blendon et al, 1998).

Another important difference is that the knowledge gained through research has the potential to benefit many more people than does information derived from quality improvement and business activities. The latter projects seek not generalizable knowledge, but rather local knowledge that pertains to a particular health-care organization or restricted population of enrollees. Furthermore, the findings of quality improvement and business projects usually are not disseminated through publication to other organizations that might find them useful. These unpublished findings will not benefit the public. In research findings are published in sufficient detail that the project can be replicated by others. Everyone benefits from publication of research results, including competitors of the investigators who carried out the research. However, in the competitive managed care marketplace, many health-care organizations do not publish findings from quality improvement, disease management, and business projects for fear that publication would assist competitors.

HOW DO VALUES SHAPE RESEARCH AGENDAS AND METHODS?

Value judgments cannot be avoided in the selection of topics for study, the framing of research questions, and the choice of end points for analysis. Acknowledging such value judgments does not necessarily mean that research is biased or merely a rationalization for preconceived conclusions. However, it is important to make explicit the assumptions on which research projects rest so that discussions about the interpretation and policy implications of research findings can be put into context.

This section will analyze the value judgments implicit in formulating research agendas and methods, with emphasis on the types of health services research that deserve more attention.

Outcomes Research

Outcomes research studies the impact of either specific health-care interventions or the organization of health-care services.

Ethical underpinnings of outcomes research

There are compelling ethical reasons to conduct outcomes research. Beneficence is a cardinal principle of medical ethics: Physicians should act in the best interests of patients and try to benefit them. Health-care organizations should also provide and foster interventions that are beneficial to patients. To achieve these ethical objectives, health-care providers need to know which clinical services and ways of organizing care are associated with improved health outcomes and which are not.

Outcomes research follows a consequentialist model of ethics. Outcomes research studies the consequences of clinical interventions, organizational arrangements, and health-care policies. The underlying assumption is that interventions that result in the most favorable overall outcomes should be preferred, yet consequentialist theories generally have been criticized regarding the selection of outcomes for analysis and the distribution of benefits in a population (Beauchamp and Childress, 1994).

Selection of topics for study

Value choices shape the selection of topics for study. As the research question is specified and operationalized, the researcher faces a series of choices. At each decision point choices have important implications for how the study may affect public policy. An example of an important topic for research is a study of outcomes after myocardial infarction, the leading cause of death in the United States. One researcher might study patterns of underuse of effective secondary prevention measures, such as aspirin and beta-blockers. Another researcher might study variation in short-term outcomes, such as mortality. Still another investigator might be interested in long-term outcomes, such as functional status two years after a heart attack. The choice among such broad topics should reflect the investigator's perception of what issues are most important or most likely to lead to interventions that could improve the outcomes of care.

As the investigator develops a project, he or she must make additional value choices. Consider a project on underuse of secondary prevention. The specific research question might be whether not-for-profit plans or accredited plans have lower rates of underuse. Alternatively, the researcher might decide to study how underuse varies by physician characteristics rather than by organization features. Thus, the investigator might determine whether cardiologists have lower rates of underuse, or whether physicians who have been certified or recertified within the past three years have lower rates. Again, the choices should be based on a consideration of what factors are most important or ultimately most amenable to change.

Another important choice is whether additional outcomes research needs to be carried out on a research question, or whether conclusions are sufficiently well established that efforts would be better directed to changes in practice and policy rather than to additional studies of the same topic. People can always disagree over whether findings are generalizable to a new population of patients or organization, or whether the practice has substantially changed since studies were carried out. However, absolute certainty is never possible in health services research, and, at some point, there are diminishing intellectual returns on applying the same methodology to a different database.

Choice of independent variables for study

What interventions are of interest as independent variables in outcomes research? Organization level independent variables are important. For example, various aspects of "managed care" can be specified and their effects clarified. These include

- different types of financial incentives
- gatekeeping and utilization review arrangements
- tiered co-payments in pharmacy benefits
- hospital arrangements for inpatient care

Other important changes in the delivery of health-care have developed independently of managed care. These include the burgeoning availability of medical information and medical advice on the Internet and the direct-to-consumer advertising of drugs.

In addition to organization level variables, physician-level variables and patient-level variables may be of interest. Even if specific variables are not part of the research hypothesis, they are important to consider as covariates or potential confounders. An important issue is that researchers who are limited to studying data already collected and accessible in a database may not be able to obtain information on certain types of variables. For example, when working with a databases containing patient outcomes, a researcher may not be able to take into account physician reimbursement incentives or utilization review. When faced with such limitations on data, investigators need to decide whether the inability to control for important covariates so compromises the findings that the study is not worth carrying out because it does not give valid answers to the research question. The importance of the research question, not the feasibility of answering it, should be the primary consideration.

Which outcomes should be assessed in determining whether an intervention is beneficial? This is a value-laden question. Some outcomes seem obvious, for example, patient-centered clinical outcomes such as mortality and functional status, and organization-level outcomes such as use of services and disenrollment from a plan. Such outcomes are significant from a clinical, business, and public policy perspective. Moreover, these outcomes are relatively easy to measure because information about them is increasingly collected routinely in the course of providing health care.

Other important consequences of health-care interventions and organization of services, however, are indirect, long-term, and difficult to measure. As with any consequentialist analysis, outcomes of this kind tend to be overlooked.

Underuse of beneficial interventions

Underuse is an important outcome because of concerns that financial incentives and utilization review in managed care may lead physicians to withhold interventions that would benefit patients. Such concerns have led to calls for consumer protection legislation and regulation (Miller, 1997). Empirical studies are needed to assess whether and to what extent underuse occurs, and in what contexts. Data on adherence to preventive and screening interventions, such as vaccinations, mammograms, and the use of beta-blockers after myocardial infarction are collected by health-care organizations because of requirements for accreditation. Eligible enrollees for such interventions can readily be identified using administrative databases that contain patient demographics, medications, and inpatient diagnoses.

Outcomes studies of underuse need to be extended in two significant ways. First, the studies need to include interventions that require complex clinical judgments to identify patients who would benefit from them. Such interventions are more pertinent indicators of the quality of physician judgment than are interventions whose indications can be determined from demographic or administrative data. For example, decisions to perform revascularization after myocardial infarction require clinical judgment. Such decisions call for what philosophers call practical wisdom. In contrast, compliance with guidelines for vaccinations or cancer screening depends more on the organization's computer system than on the wisdom of its physicians. Evaluation of the appropriateness of such decisions is challenging. Clinical practice guidelines and databases fail to capture important information that is pertinent to such decisions (Ellrodt et al, 1995).

A second way to extend studies of underuse is to examine variation according to specific organizational and financial arrangements in managed care. For example, in treatment after a myocardial infarction, do levels of underuse of angiography and revascularization vary according to different physician financial incentives, gatekeeping arrangements, or utilization review? It is not sufficient simply to compare "managed care" with traditional insurance. Instead, the different facets of managed care need to be examined.

Patient trust

Many scholars assert that the doctor–patient relationship begins with the patient's illness, need for help, and lack of expertise relative to the physician (Pellegrino and Thomasma, 1988). Because patients are vulnerable and dependent on physicians, they need to trust their physicians to act in their best interests. Patient trust is desirable both for its own sake and because it may have beneficial consequences. Trust is considered to increase patient willingness to seek care, disclose information to physicians, and accept physicians' recommendations (Mechanic and Schlesinger, 1996). Being able to trust that physicians are acting in their best interests may also decrease patients' anxiety and increase hope.

Today, trust is in jeopardy and hence particularly important to measure because of financial and organizational arrangements in managed care. Capitation and bonuses may create conflicts of interest, leading physicians to act in their own self-interest or in the interest of third parties rather than in the best interests of patients. Because of utilization review and practice guidelines, patients may no longer regard physicians as professionals who exercise independent clinical judgment, but rather as bureaucrats carrying out policies set by administrators. Patients are particularly vulnerable if they have few options to change physicians or plans if they are dissatisfied or receive poor care. In light of these concerns, it is important to conduct carefully designed empirical studies to determine the extent to which various managed care arrangements affect patient trust.

A few studies have confirmed that managed care may exacerbate the vulnerability and uncertainty that is inherent in being sick. Capitated patients have lower levels of trust than do fee-for-service patients (Kao et al, 1998). The reduction in trust was associated with a doubling of the odds that patients had considered changing physicians. Patients whose physicians were paid by salary had even lower levels of trust than did capitated patients. Patient trust in their health plan was significantly lower than was their trust of their physicians.

We need to extend this research to identify what independent variables are associated with patient trust or mistrust. Are financial incentives the most important factor, or are other considerations such as the type of utilization review also important?

Research on trust will be difficult because it requires primary data collection. Patient ratings of trust are not routinely collected by health-care organizations as are satisfaction ratings and clinical and use information. As a "soft" variable, trust is difficult to quantify in a precise, accurate, and clinically meaningful way. Thus it will be more difficult to measure than "harder" variables, such as mortality and hospital days.

Doctor–patient communication

Another understudied area of health services research is doctor–patient communication. Changes in the organization of health care, such as gatekeeping requirements and shorter outpatient visits, may complicate doctor–patient interactions. In addition, physicians may face challenging situations when patients request tests or drugs that the doctor does not think are medically indicated (Kravitz et al, 1994; Gallagher al, 1997). The growing availability of medical information to patients on the Internet and through direct-to-consumer advertising has exacerbated this phenomenon.

Communication skills by physicians may well be an important intervening variable in determining whether physicians accede to requests that are not clinically indicated and whether patients are satisfied with the physicians' decisions. It may be difficult for physicians to dissuade patients from such interventions because of patient mistrust. Patients may believe that physicians are withholding interventions because of financial incentives or utilization review rather than because the interventions will provide little benefit (Blendon et al, 1998). Depending on how the physician responds to such requests, the situation may become confrontational or accelerate patient concerns that beneficial interventions are being withheld.

Thus, questions addressed in outcomes research may not be adequately answered unless the nature of doctor–patient interaction is taken into account. To do so, however, may be difficult because the research project will need to collect primary data about doctor–patient communication. Not only is collecting such data logistically difficult, but studying transcripts of doctor–patient interviews is beyond the expertise of most health services researchers. Hence collaborative projects with scientists with complementary expertise will likely be needed.

Communication skills as a means to explain sound clinical decisions need to be distinguished from communication skills as a means to diffuse patient dissatisfaction with inadequate care. Attempts to persuade patients are ethically appropriate only when it is medically appropriate for the physician not to order a test or drug requested by the patient. Physicians may learn how to discuss these requests with patients in ways that increase patient agreement with physicians' recommendations while also maintaining patient trust and satisfaction. However, if, within a health-care organization, a physician is unable to provide services that would provide significant clinical benefits, it would be ethically problematic to use communication techniques to divert the attention of the patient away from this fact.

Research on doctor–patient communication needs to take into account the organizational context of clinical care. How do such organizational characteristics as financial incentives and utilization review affect the nature of physician responses to patient requests for interventions? Furthermore, it would also be important to understand how organizational variables affect both specific communication behaviors and patient outcomes. It may well be that doctor–patient communication is a significant intervening variable between the characteristics of the health–care organization and such outcomes as use, patient acceptance of recommendations, satisfaction, and disenrollment.

Justice and outcomes research

When assessing the consequences of an action or policy, it is important to determine not only the aggregate benefits and harms, but also the distribution of benefits and harms across a population of interest. Consequentialist, or utilitarian, theories commonly are criticized for not adequately considering whether benefits and harms are distributed equitably (Beauchamp and Childress, 1994). In health services research considerations of justice may be particularly important. An organizational or clinical intervention may have beneficial consequences within the entire population, but the benefits and burdens may be spread unevenly across different subgroups. Such discrepancies are ethically disturbing if more vulnerable subgroups have less favorable outcomes. Some groups, such as persons with chronic illness or Medicaid beneficiaries, may have greater needs or less ability to respond to a complex managed care system. Thus, it would be important to ascertain whether certain financial incentives, utilization review, or formulary benefits programs, although neutral in their design, might in practice have less beneficial consequences or produce greater burdens for persons who have chronic illness or are on Medicaid. Similarly, studies of patient trust need to focus on patients with serious illness, who are more vulnerable and dependent and for whom trust may be a more significant issue.

From a policy perspective, we need to know all the consequences of an organizational intervention, both hard and soft, and how they are distributed. Such research can inform policy choices between improving outcomes for the worst-off enrollees in a health-care organization and improving aggregate outcomes for the entire population. Although this is a matter of justice and equity, the solution is not likely to result from an abstract philosophical debate about justice. Instead, issues are likely to be resolved on the level of specific interventions and problems, and political compromises and pragmatic considerations are more likely to be dispositive than are theories of justice. Nonetheless, sound health services research is essential to illuminate the debate.

Analysis of Ethical Issues Raised by New Practices

Many innovations have dramatically changed the delivery and organization of health care. These innovations include financial incentives for physicians, different types of utilization review, tiered formulary co-payments, and clinical practice on the Internet. The evaluation of these new practices is an important but underdeveloped area of research. Much research will fall within familiar types of health services research, such as descriptive epidemiology and outcomes research. On the level of descriptive epidemiology, research questions will include: What is done? Who is doing it? Where is it done? and How is it done? We have already considered outcomes research. In this section I illustrate the analysis of ethical issues raised by such new practices, using examples from the growing phenomenon of practicing medicine on the Internet (Borowitz and Wyatt, 1998; Eysenbach and Diepgen, 1998; Widman and Tong, 1998).

Patients can use the Internet both to seek advice from a physician they have never met and also to contact a physician who is already providing them care. Although Internet practice is growing, ethical issues have only begun to be analyzed (Spielberg, 1998).

Ethical concerns regarding new practices

Researchers can identify ethical concerns regarding new practices and clarify the nature of those concerns in common clinical situations. For example, when clinical care is delivered on the Internet, the familiar ethical issues regarding beneficence, autonomy, confidentiality, and justice arise, but with new variations.

Non-maleficence and beneficence are pertinent to Internet practice because patients may be harmed if advice is incorrect or if Internet medicine is inappropriately risky. Concerns about risk have been raised for several reasons. First, physicians who practice medicine on the Internet need to make decisions and recommendations without information that is ordinarily available to the physician in face-to-face visits. Internet physicians have no opportunity to observe or examine the patient. Furthermore, in some cases pertinent previous medical records may not be available. Second, the quality of care in Internet medicine has not been evaluated extensively. Studies have raised concerns about the poor quality of medical advice on the Internet (Culver et al, 1997; Impicciatore et al, 1997; Patrick et al, 1999). The balance of benefits to harms may vary in different situations. The clinical situation, the goal of the interaction, and the nature of the doctor–patient relationship may be significant. Concerns about benefit and risk may be greater if doctor–patient interactions on the Internet lead to individualized medical advice rather than merely conveying general information or if the interaction initiates a new doctor–patient relationship rather than occurring as part of an ongoing doctor–patient relationship.

Internet medicine also raises concerns about patient autonomy. The philosophy of the Internet is caveat emptor—the user of the information needs to assess its reliability because information is not reviewed. However, in health care such a marketplace approach to information has traditionally not been accepted. Physicians are given role-specific obligations to help patients make decisions, particularly obligations regarding disclosure of information during the informed consent process. How should this traditional obligation to inform patients be adapted to Internet medicine? Do patients who seek care from a new physician on the Internet appreciate the risks of this new mode of communication? What ethical and legal obligations should physicians have to inform patients of these risks? Boilerplate disclaimers on a Website are more likely to be ignored or misunderstood by patients than are discussions of limitations integrated into the doctor–patient interaction.

Confidentiality is another important ethical concern regarding Internet clinical care. Communication between patients and physicians over the Internet may not be secure (Rind et al, 1997). Moreover, patients who have employment-based Internet access may not realize that if they use their work computers to communicate with physicians, the employer has access to their e-mail (Terry, 1999). Patients may not appreciate how Internet medicine raises these confidentiality concerns, which are not present in face-to-face doctor–patient interactions.

Medical practice on the Internet also raises issues regarding equitable access to care. Patients who do not have computers or Internet access will not be able to take advantage of programs to allow patients to communicate with physicians and to obtain refills by e-mail. Hence, these new modes of communication with physicians may increase existing discrepancies in access to health care.

Paradigmatic cases that raise ethical concerns

Health services researchers can analyze paradigmatic cases in order to identify the pertinent considerations in responding to such ethical concerns. One would first identify clear-cut cases in which people agree that Internet medicine is appropriate or inappropriate (Jonsen and Toulmin, 1988; Sunnstein, 1996). The next step would be to identify the features that make a case appropriate or inappropriate for Internet medicine. Features such as the clinical situation, patient characteristics, the doctor–patient relationship, and type of help the patient seeks might be pertinent. These clear-cut cases set anchor points that can guide other cases. Next, one would identify intermediate, gray-zone cases and analyze how these considerations would be weighed and balanced. The issue is whether the cases resemble the paradigmatic cases closely enough that they should be resolved similarly, or whether there are ethically significant differences that change how they should be resolved. This bottom-up approach contrasts with a top-down approach that starts with general principles. It is similar to development of case law, in which guidelines are developed by working through a series of cases.

Ethical issues that need further discussion

Health services research can identify ethical issues about new practices that need further discussion and research. Such analysis provides both a stimulus and a framework for further discussions. With regard to medical practice on the Internet, researchers might identify a number of issues that require attention. Examples might include

- How can physicians practicing on the Internet identify patients for whom a face-to-face visit is desirable?

- Are patients well informed of the risks and benefits of receiving care via the Internet?
- Do patients who establish care with a new physician over the Internet have comparable outcomes to patients who receive conventional care?
- How can the benefits of Internet care be enhanced and the risks minimized?

Evaluation of Health-Care Policies

Concerns over the recent dramatic changes in the delivery of health care have led to laws and regulations intended to prevent abuses, protect patients, and improve care (Miller, 1997). The impact of such policies is an important research question. Posing empirical research questions acknowledges that a health-care policy may not achieve its goals and that a policy may have unintended detrimental consequences. A number of research studies of this nature have been carried out:

- What is the impact of laws mandating that women with breast cancer be told of the option of breast-conserving therapy on the actual frequency of such treatments (Nattinger et al, 1996)?
- What is the impact of restrictions on psychotropic drugs in Medicaid formularies on drug costs, psychiatric hospitalizations, and total expenditures for patients with psychiatric illness (Soumerai et al, 1991; Soumerai et al, 1994)?
- What is the impact of name reporting of patients with HIV infection on the willingness of persons at high risk for HIV infection to be tested (CDC, 1998)?

Many states have passed consumer protection legislation in response to public concerns about various features of managed care. A frequent feature of such legislation is that when disputes over coverage arise between the enrollee and managed care plan, independent expert physicians must render a judgment on the appropriateness of the requested medical intervention (Sage, 1999). Is such consumer protection legislation associated with beneficial outcomes for enrollees? Specifically, does it reduce underuse of beneficial services? Furthermore, does it increase use of services that have little or questionable benefit?

BARRIERS TO OVERLOOKED AREAS OF HEALTH SERVICES RESEARCH

There are many barriers to carrying out these kinds of underdeveloped outcomes research.

Methodological Challenges

Such research may be harder to carry out than is more conventional health services research. First, in outcomes research data on hard outcomes such as mortality, readmissions, and length of stay are routinely collected in delivering health care. However, studying the impact of interventions and arrangements on the doctor–patient relationship and on patient trust requires the collection of additional primary data. Second, new methodologies need to be developed. Instruments to measure trust and methodologies to measure underuse need to be developed. Third, in analyzing the impact of public policies, it may be particularly difficult to identify appropriate control groups and to control for confounding variables, such as secular trends.

Disincentives to Such Research

Health-care organizations have few incentives to examine such outcomes as patient trust and underuse. For a for-profit, market-oriented managed care plan, it might even be irresponsible to stockholders to study such soft outcomes rather than hard outcomes that have direct, short-term financial consequences. Furthermore, health-care organizations may also have little incentive to cooperate with independent researchers who wish to study such outcomes. A managed care organization may fear disclosure of proprietary information or negative publicity when results are published. Organizations not only may fear unflattering findings but also may want to discourage public discussion of such topics as mistrust and underuse of services.

Even in the public sector there may be disincentives to such research. Research on new practices or public policies may be regarded as political and biased. Such research may seem threatening to stakeholders who have a vested interest in certain ways of organizing and delivering health care. Proponents of new heath-care policies may not be interested in evaluations of the policies. As such, policies may be enacted for symbolic reasons or may be defended even if they do not achieve their intended goals. Their defenders may lobby Congress not to use public funds to carry out research on the effect of health policies. However, to the extent that such research is in the public interest and is not supported by the private sector, a strong case for federal support needs to be made.

In conclusion, values affect health services research in several ways. Ethical values and preconceptions shape the research agenda and the design of projects. Accordingly, unexamined value judgments may result in some important types of research receiving less attention than is warranted. More explicit attention to values and ethics can thus strengthen health services research and make it more relevant to health policy.

NOTES

1. Supported in part by the Robert Wood Johnson Foundation and Center Grant MH42459 from the National Institute of Mental Health.

REFERENCES

Beauchamp TL and Childress JF (1994) *Principles of Biomedical Ethics*. New York; Oxford University Press.

Blendon RJ, Brodie M, Benson JM, Altman DE, Levitt L, Hoff T, et al. (1998) Understanding the managed care backlash. *Health Affairs* 17(4): 80–94.

Borowitz SM and Wyatt JC (1998) The origin, content, and workload of e-mail consultations. *Journal of the American Medical Association* 280: 1321–24.

CDC (1998) HIV tesing among populations at risk for HIV infection—nine states, November 1995–December 1996. *Morbidity and Mortality Weekly Report* 47: 1086–91.

Committee on Maintaining Privacy and Security in Health Care Applications of the National Information Infrastructure (1997) *For the Record: Protecting Electronic Health Information*. Washington, DC: National Academy Press.

Culver JD, Gerr F, Frumkin H (1997) Medical information on the Internet: A study of an electronic bulletin board. *Journal of General Internal Medicine* 12: 466–70.

Department of Health and Human Services (1999) 45 CFR §160–164. Standards of privacy of individually identifiable health information; proposed rule. *Federal Register* 64: 55918–60065.

Ellrodt AG, Conner L, Riedinger M, Weingarten S (1995) Measuring and improving physician compliance with clinical practice guidelines. *Ann Intern Mec* 122: 277–82.

Eysenbach G and Diepgen TL (1998) Responses to unsolicited patient e-mail requests for medical advice on the World Wide Web. *Journal of the American Medical Association* 280: 1333–5.

Gallagher TH, Lo B, Chesney M, Christiansen K (1997) How do managed care physicians respond to patients' requests for costly, unindicated tests? *Journal of General Internal Medicine* 12: 663–8.

Impicciatore P, Pandolfini C, Casella N, Bonati M (1997) Reliability of health information for the public on the World Wide Web: Systematic survey of advice on managing fever in children at home. *British Medical Journal*: 1875–9.

Jonsen AR and Toulmin S (1988) *The Abuse of Casuistry: A History of Moral Reasoning*. Berkeley, CA: University of California Press.

Kao AC, Green DC, Zaslavsky AM, Koplan JP, Cleary PD (1998) The relationship between method of physician payment and patient trust. *Journal of the American Medical Association* 280: 1708–14.

Kravitz RL, Cope DW, Bhrany V, Leake B (1994) Internal medicine patients' expectations for care during office visits. *Journal of General Internal Medicine* 9: 75–81.

Levine RJ (1986) *Ethics and Regulation of Clinical Research*. Baltimore, MD: Urban & Schwarzenberg.

Mechanic D and Schlesinger M (1996) The impact of managed care on patients' trust in medical care and their physicians. *Journal of the American Medical Association* 275: 1693–7.

Miller TE (1997) Managed care regulation: In the laboratory of the states. *Journal of the American Medical Association* 278: 1102–9.

Minn Stat. §§144.335.3a (1997).

Nattinger AB, Hoffman RG, Shapiro R, Gottlieb MS, Goodwin JS (1996) The effect of legislative requirements on the use of breast-conserving surgery. *New England Journal of Medicine* 335: 1035–40.

Office of the Inspector General (1998) *Institutional Review Boards: Their Role in Reviewing Approved Research.* Washington, DC: Department of Health and Human Services.

Patrick K, Robinson TN, Alemi F, Eng TR (1999) Policy issues relevant to the evaluation of interactive health communication applications. *American Journal of Preventive Medicine* 16: 35–42.

Pellegrino ED and Thomasma DG (1988) *For the Patient's Good: The Restoration of Beneficence in Health Care.* New York: Oxford University Press.

Protection of Human Subjects 45 CFR 46 (1998).

Rind DM, Kohane IS, Szolovitis P, Safran C, Chueh HC, Barnett GO (1997) Maintaining the confidentiality of medical records shared over the Internet and the World Wide Web. *Annals of Internal Medicine* 127: 138–41.

Sage WM (1999) Physicians as advocates. *Houston Law Journal* 35: 1525–1630.

Soumerai SB, McLaughlin TJ, Ross-Degnan D, Casteris CS, Bollini P (1994) Effects of limiting Medicaid drug-reimbursement benefits on the use of psychotropic agents and acute mental health services by patients with schizophrenia. *New England Journal of Medicine* 331: 650–5.

Soumerai SB, Ross-Degnan D, Avorn J, McLaughlin TJ, Choodnovsky I (1991) Effects of Medicaid drug-payment limits on admission to hospitals and nursing homes. *New England Journal of Medicine* 325: 1072–7.

Spielberg AR (1998) On call and online: Sociohistorical, legal, and ethical implications of e-mail for the patient–physician relationship. *Journal of the American Medical Association* 280: 1353–9.

Sunnstein CR (1996) *Legal Reasoning and Political Conflict.* New York: Oxford University Press.

Terry NP (1999) Cyber-malpractice: Legal exposure for cybermedicine. *American Journal of Law & Medicine* 25: 327–66.

U.S. General Accounting Office (1996) *Continued Vigilance Critical to Protecting Human Subjects.* Washington, DC: Government Accounting Office.

Widman LE and Tong DA (1998) Requests for medical advice from patients and families to health care providers who publish on the World Wide Web. *Archives of Internal Medicine* 157: 209–12.

18

Ethical considerations in conducting health-care research: protecting privacy

LISA I. IEZZONI

What ethical values should inform future research about health care, especially relating to data privacy?[1] What gives somebody a right to ask about a person's health or health care and expect to get a valid answer?[2] This chapter examines this issue in the context of research about the health care system. Four specific questions frame the arguments:

- What is the role of person-specific information in research about health care, and how does it differ from other clinical research settings?
- What are the current characteristics of databases containing this person-specific information, and what will they be in the future?
- What are the political and social forces that shape not only the content of databases but also the availability of information for research about our health care system?
- What ethical values should inform future research about health care, especially concerning data privacy, and what research is needed to explore these ethical implications?

I argue here that the real and imagined risks of offering private information for health care research arise not only from fear of public exposure but also from the very context of that research: a fragmented health care system, riven by economic and physical barriers to care, with millions of people lacking insurance and countless others fearing its loss. The ethical challenge for health-care researchers is to ensure that the potential societal benefits of their studies are clearly articulated and that systems are implemented to minimize privacy risks to unknowing participants.

INFORMATION NEEDS OF HEALTH-CARE RESEARCH

Definitions and Distinctions

What is the role of person-specific information in research about health care, and how does it differ from other clinical research settings? Formulating an answer to this question first requires a definition of *health-care research* and a delineation of how it differs from other clinical research. Here, I use *health-care research* broadly to encompass health services, effectiveness, health policy, health systems, decision analysis and cost-effectiveness, quality measurement, quality improvement, and outcomes research. No single term has yet achieved consensus as capturing these varied perspectives.

The context for health-care research reaches back almost twenty years to policy concerns about unremitting escalation of health-care costs, unexplained wide variations in service use across geographic areas, and inappropriate provision of costly medical services. The "era of assessment and accountability" began in the mid-1980s (Relman, 1988) to quantify the health benefits from the dollars spent accruing not only to individuals but also to the American population. Research to address these issues, often known as "effectiveness" or "outcomes" studies, targeted the effects of services delivered by providers in communities or typical practice settings (U.S. Congress, Office of Technology Assessment, 1994).

This emphasis on usual care contrasts with prospective, controlled, clinical trials, in which treatments are administered by experts following highly specified protocols under ideal circumstances in closely monitored settings. Such tightly controlled clinical trials examine the "efficacy" of interventions, and the unit of observation is the individual.

Among the most notable differences between health-care research and clinical trials are the following constraints that operate upon the latter. Many clinical efficacy trials strictly limit their participants (e.g., eschewing people with comorbid conditions), ostensibly to avoid introducing unnecessary "noise"—extraneous clinical factors that could affect therapeutic outcomes. Some recruitment guidelines have had troubling consequences. The U.S. General Accounting Office (1992) discovered that 60% of clinical trials for new drugs under-represented women. Of 53 drug trials examined, only 25

(47%) specifically assessed whether men and women responded differently to the medication being tested. One study of clinical efficacy trials from the mid-1980s found that 15 out of 35 studies (43%) had no African American subjects, and almost two-thirds had a lower percentage of blacks than lived in the surrounding communities (Svensson, 1989). Because of such findings, federally funded research projects must now either explicitly include women and racial and ethnic minorities or make a cogent case for their exclusion.

In contrast, effectiveness and outcomes research typically embraces all comers, aiming to ensure broad representation and generalizability of results. As Donabedian noted, populations came into play, with accountability for the outcomes depending partially on how populations were defined:

> Outcomes are those changes, either favorable or adverse, in the actual or potential health status of persons, groups, or communities that can be attributed to prior or concurrent care. What is included in the category of "outcomes," depends, on how narrowly or broadly one defines "health" and the corresponding responsibilities of . . . practitioners or the health care system as a whole.
>
> Donabedian, 1985, 256

Health-care research also frequently encroaches on daily concerns about providing care, such as using evidence-based medicine, anticipating and preventing errors, and monitoring outcomes to continuously improve the quality of care. Unlike clinical trials that have clean boundaries (i.e., patients are either enrolled in specific, time-limited protocols or they are not), health care research can coexist with ongoing, longitudinal provision of care and its oversight. Paul Ellwood (1988) provides perhaps the strongest articulation of these concepts, proposing a "technology of patient experience." He touts outcomes evaluation and management as a way "to help patients, payers, and providers make rational medical care-related choices based on better insight into the effect of these choices on the patient's life." In his article Ellwood listed four basic components of outcomes evaluation:

1. Development of standards and guidelines;
2. routine, widespread measurement of disease-specific clinical outcomes and patients' functioning and well-being;
3. collection of clinical and outcome data "on a massive scale"; and
4. analysis and dissemination of findings from a continually expanding database.

As Ellwood envisioned it, data would flow from virtually every health care encounter, and these data could then be used to improve future care (e.g., by identifying effective clinical practices, deriving guidelines for care, targeting areas for improvement, and so on). His emphasis on patients' functioning and well-being introduced a new perspective, one that explicitly seeks patients' viewpoints.

Global self-assessments of health status and functioning increasingly became key outcome targets in health-care research and ongoing quality measurement programs. As Reiser (1993) wrote, the interest in outcomes gave new voice to patients:

> The modern outcomes movement, which developed in the 1980s and made the consequences of a medical intervention to its recipient a major criterion of determining its value, further enhanced the authenticity and authority of the patient's perspective. . . . The objective biological standards of evidence, which had formed the foundation of 20th-century medicine, were found to depict the effects of a medical procedure inadequately. Thus, the medical ethics and outcomes movements both drew their strength from the significance they gave to the patient's view of illness and therapy.
>
> Reiser, 1993, 1014

While seeking patients' views has inherent validity, it represents another key distinction from clinical trials. In many clinical trials patients are passive participants in assessing treatment successes or failures; researchers seek putatively "objective" endpoints, such as survival, tumor regression, or changes in a laboratory value. This has changed somewhat in recent years: Many clinical trials now look at symptom relief and participants' reports about pertinent aspects of their quality of life, but these are typically secondary outcome measures.

In contrast, the endpoints of patient-focused outcomes studies often require direct, conceptual input from the persons under study (e.g., filling out questionnaires, answering telephone surveys, etc.). The information is often considered by the subject to be deeply personal and self-revealing (e.g., persons' views of their health, social functioning, etc.), as opposed to being a disembodied number in the way that results from clinical trials can be (e.g., diastolic blood pressure, HbA_{1c}). While this approach brings health-care research closer to what people value in their daily lives, it heightens privacy concerns, literally by venturing into private spaces.

Thus, four major features distinguish much of health-care research from clinical trials and hold important implications for data requirements, privacy concerns, and ethical considerations:

- The focus on usual care in the community means that researchers can often, from an external vantage point, study what is happening without those being observed knowing they are under scrutiny. Health-care research has frequently relied on information collected for other purposes (e.g., claims submitted for reimbursement) in ongoing systems of care.

- The emphasis on populations or groups of people means that knowing the specific identities of individuals is often unnecessary. The law of large numbers can theoretically protect individual identities.
- Some health care studies, especially those targeting clinical practices (e.g., evidence-based medicine) and quality improvement (e.g., detection of medication errors) can affect on-going care, again without the populations involved necessarily knowing that they are participating in research. As such, the lines between practice and research blur.
- Studies that use patients' perspectives (e.g., about functioning, well-being, quality of life) capture absolutely critical information but do so at the risk of intruding into private lives.

Before moving on to consider further the implications of these factors, we should look at two other issues that arise.

Informed Consent

Voluntary consent has been central to the design and implementation of clinical trials since the Nuremberg Code was articulated in 1947 (Shuster, 1997). Although some controversy exists about whether all clinical trials require informed consent (Truog et al, 1999) and whether consent is truly "informed" (Daugherty et al, 1997), few disagree that clinical trial protocols must be scrutinized to identify potential risks to patients. Whenever any questions arise, requiring informed consent has been the ethical default.

Yet health-care studies that involve data gathered from records maintained in ongoing practice settings and for purposes that do not directly benefit the subjects—like the data taken from billing records—do not involve informed consent (Gostin and Hadley, 1998), for participants do not even know they are subjects of a research study. For example, when the Health Care Financing Administration (HCFA) gave me computer files containing almost 80 million Medicare claims (Iezzoni et al, 1999), persons whose claims were included had no idea that they were part of my study. To receive this file, I agreed to the confidentiality and data security policies of the HCFA regarding release of data to researchers, and individuals' health insurance claim numbers were encrypted.

Some might question why this situation raises concern. I could not identify individuals from my data set, so patient privacy was theoretically protected. Nonetheless, researchers can obtain data with identifiers sufficient to link information across data systems: for example, with the encrypted identification numbers, we linked Part A and B Medicare claims. Given the massive availability of electronic data on individuals these days and powerful probabilistic matching schemes (Roos et al, 1996), it is conceivable that ingenious people could use research data sets to identify individuals (Sweeney, 1997).

Even without probabilistic matching or sophisticated algorithms, one can winnow down data using simple descriptive techniques and thereby come close to discovering individual identities. Several years ago, a statistician colleague, skeptical of these arguments, experimented with a large administrative database containing information on several hundred thousand residents of her state. She lived in a densely-populated city and anticipated that dozens of people in her zip code would match her in age and sex, but she found only five women of her age in her zip code within this large database. In her view, that came perilously close to uncovering her identity.

These observations anticipate concerns of stringent privacy advocates, who argue against researchers having access to data without the specific informed consent of everyone represented. This requirement would essentially end health-care research: Obtaining consents would be a logistical nightmare and, moreover, would introduce inevitable bias, given that those who chose not to consent would likely skew the sample (Gostin and Hadley, 1998). To see this, we need only consider a strict privacy statute in Minnesota that has added considerably to the logistical complexities of conducting medical record research at the Mayo Clinic, an institution historically endowed with advanced information systems (Melton, 1997). If health-care research has important societal value, then it will be imperative to arrive at ways of balancing personal privacy concerns with researchers' access to information (Gostin and Hadley, 1998).

Implications of Personal Reports

The second issue concerning outcomes research is its patient-centered nature. As noted above, Ellwood (1988) argues that meaningful outcomes monitoring must examine the consequences of care on people's lives since people are the only authentic source of such experiential insight. Therefore, future outcomes research must either tap into large data sets containing patients' reports or newly gather this information. These efforts, however, will heighten concerns about privacy and confidentiality as well as those about data quality.

For example, the Health of Seniors measure has recently joined the Effectiveness of Care indicators promulgated through the Health Plan Employer Data Information Set (HEDIS). HEDIS, created by the National Committee for Quality Assurance (NCQA), has become the virtual standard for measuring performance of health plans nationwide (Iglehart, 1996). Version 3.0 of HEDIS describes the Health of Seniors measure as the "percentage of senior Medicare risk plan members whose self-reported health status has improved, stayed the same, or worsened. Change is measured over two years and has two components—mental and physical" (NCQA, 1996). This measure is based on mailed questionnaires to be completed twice, over time, by selected Medicare beneficiaries who belong to capitated health plans; the difference in self-reported health status between years 1 and 3 is the targeted outcome measure. At the core of the Health of Seniors questionnaire is the SF-36, a "short form" containing 36 questions from an instrument developed for the Medical Outcomes Study (Stewart et al, 1989; Stewart and Ware, 1992). This questionnaire asks not only about physical abilities, but also about social and emotional functioning.

This HEDIS initiative could potentially result in large databases of patients' self-reports ripe for outcomes research. Many persons may happily answer such questions openly and honestly, pleased that somebody cares enough to ask how they are doing. But what about someone who uses a wheelchair or people with other disabilities or potentially stigmatizing conditions? Without universal health insurance coverage in the United States, many may be fearful of being denied services or future health insurance. We all know about Americans without health care insurance—more than 40 million, and the numbers are growing (Carrasquillo et al, 1999). We have all heard about health plans leaving Medicare, setting their members adrift (Pear, 1998). Many know that capitated plans have generally enrolled beneficiaries who are healthier and less costly than average (Riley et al, 1996; Morgan et al, 1997; Medicare Payment Advisory Commission, 1998). In the six months prior to enrollment, new members of capitated plans have had 35% lower costs than Medicare's fee-for-service average (Medicare Payment Advisory Commission, 1998). Some plans specifically market to healthy persons (Neuman et al, 1998), profiting handsomely; Medicare overpaid capitated plans by 5% to 20% because of their healthy members (Greenwald et al, 1998). Despite assurances that their health status information will be held confidential, these fears could affect responses. People may report better functioning than they really have due to their worry about being denied future care. Although these fears may appear irrational to well-motivated data gatherers wanting to do good (e.g., by identifying the best health plans), these feelings can reflect lifetimes spent confronting disenfranchisement and discrimination. Against this real-world backdrop, even I, a wheelchair user, cannot guarantee that I would answer these functional status questions entirely honestly, regardless of promises about data confidentiality. As a researcher, I know that such skewed responses would bias data in a distinctly nonrandom way for an important subset of our population, but so be it!

Crispin Jenkinson (1999), deputy director of the Health Services Research Unit, University of Oxford, articulated similar concerns in an essay provocatively entitled Death by Questionnaire: Quality of Life Measurement Could

Seriously Damage your Health. The specific target of his commentary was the European EuroQol, a quality of life measurement technique (with questions on mobility, self-care, usual activities, pain/discomfort, and anxiety/depression), to derive judgments about resource allocation and outcomes of care. Nevertheless, many of Jenkinson's observations resonate with concerns within the U.S. health system:

> In many instances such data can be used benignly enough: to aid diagnosis, to assess competing treatment regimes in a trial, or to assess the burden of disease. However, such data can also be used to prioritise [sic], which, of course, is a modern day euphemism for rationing. The danger is that such a use threatens the outcomes movement, firstly in the eyes of patients and then in the eyes of clinicians and policy-makers. If patients believe that health status measures are being used in this way, then it is likely to affect their responses. . . .
>
> Researchers seem to have overlooked the fact that people are likely to react unfavorably when they realise [sic] that the act of asking patients about their health is not undertaken with a kindly and benign intention to increase the sum of human happiness but, instead, is a way of getting patients to indicate the (potentially limited) role treatment has played in their lives. Once patients have lost faith and decided either to withdraw help or to fill in questionnaires in any manner that so happens to entertain them, then any support the outcomes movement has gained from clinicians, managers, and politicians is likely to diminish pretty swiftly.
>
> Jenkinson, 1999, 129–130

Other health-care research methods can also be used to affect directly people's access to services. In the United States the closest we have come to the explicit rationing feared by Jenkinson was Oregon's Medicaid demonstration project, which ordered services in terms of their priorities. This use of health-care research methodologies to solve vexing health policy questions, such as that of how to allocate scarce resources, might further heighten public distrust of research.

Health-care research thus often resides at the cutting edge of health policy, in much the same way that it frequently accompanies clinical practice in the hospital or other health care settings. Just as health policy decisions carry ethical implications, the supporting research must also recognize these moral dimensions. The challenge is to build this recognition into research from its first conceptualization, as I will suggest at the end of this chapter.

DATABASES FOR HEALTH-CARE RESEARCH

What do health-care research databases containing this person-specific information currently look like, and what will they be like in the future?

Administrative Databases Today

As noted above, a hallmark of health-care research is its focus on usual care in communities. Researchers frequently can conduct their studies without knowing the specific identities of their research subjects and without those people knowing that they are under scrutiny. Health-care research has often relied on information collected for other purposes in ongoing systems of care, such as claims submitted for reimbursement or hospital discharge abstracts sent to states' regulatory agencies. The Patient Outcomes Research Teams (PORTs), the early flagship projects funded by the Agency for Health Care Policy and Research (AHCPR, renamed the Agency for Healthcare Research and Quality, or AHRQ, in 1999), used this approach (Mitchell et al, 1994; Lave et al, 1994). Even the legislation establishing the AHCPR (Section 6103 of Omnibus Budget Reconciliation Act of 1989, P.L. 101–239, December, 19, 1989) specified the use of large administrative files:

> For facilitating research, the Secretary shall . . . (1) conduct and support reviews and evaluations of existing methodologies that utilize large databases in conducting such research . . . (5) conduct and support research and demonstrations on the use of claims data . . . in determining the outcomes, effectiveness, and appropriateness of such treatment, and (6) conduct and support supplementation of existing databases, including collection of new information, to enhance databases for research purposes.
>
> Sec. 1142(c)

This strategy confers several advantages. First, the data exist, are frequently inexpensive to acquire, and are computer-readable. These practical advantages are significant. For example, in 1990, when California's Assembly debated mandating extensive clinical data collection for evaluating hospital outcomes, fiscal reality intervened. Since the annual costs for gathering new data were estimated at $61 million, the legislature balked, requiring the hospital outcomes project to use instead California's existing hospital discharge abstract database (Romano et al, 1995). Second, the inclusion of large groups of people, often entire populations (e.g., all residents in a state, all Medicare beneficiaries, etc.), enhances the generalizability of the findings. Thus, for example, women and racial and ethnic minorities are represented at the same proportions as they are present in the population. Third, if longitudinal patient-level data are available, administrative databases also minimize problems in tracking study subjects over time and remove the reliance on patients' recall of service use (Roos et al, 1987). Fourth, as suggested above, the large numbers can help hide individual identities.

Despite the advantages of large databases, and even after the AHCPR spent millions of research dollars using administrative data to evaluate patient outcomes, assessments of their value have been mixed. The former Office of Technology Assessment of the U.S. Congress (1994) offered the following blunt appraisal:

> Contrary to the expectations expressed in the legislation establishing AHCPR and the mandates of the PORTs, administrative databases generally have not proved useful in answering questions about the comparative effectiveness of alternative medical treatments. Administrative databases are very useful for descriptive purposes (e.g., exploring variations in treatment patterns), but the practical and theoretical limitations of this research technique usually prevent it from being able to provide credible answers regarding which technologies, among alternatives, work best
>
> Congress, 1994, 6

Tracing the roots of this disappointment leads quickly to the need for more specific information about individuals, their clinical characteristics, functioning, and views. The limited clinical content of administrative files severely circumscribes the questions that can be asked and answered meaningfully. While administrative data may be sufficient for some purposes, such as the examination of costs of care (Lave et al, 1994), they are inadequate to other goals, such as assessing quality or clinical outcomes of care (Iezzoni, 1997a).

Certainly, notable health-care research projects have gathered their own data on numerous patients receiving community-based care. Two leading examples are the Medical Outcomes Study (Stewart et al, 1989) and Phase I of SUPPORT, the Study to Understand Prognoses and Preferences for Outcomes and Risks of Treatment (Teno et al, 1994). But such studies are enormously expensive—the Robert Wood Johnson Foundation spent tens of millions of dollars on the two of them (Schroeder, 1999). With limited funds available for health-care research, large-scale studies involving primary data collection will be rare. Certainly, smaller projects gather their own data, but this small size inevitably limits the questions that can be asked and raises concerns about generalizability.

Thus, feasibility and cost concerns complete the circle, leading back to a reliance upon large, available data sets gathered for other purposes. As indicated below, this is not as bleak a prospect as it sounds, with the imminent electronic availability of extensive clinical information. But it again raises concerns about privacy and who should have access to sensitive information about health and health care.

Electronic Databases in the Future

The boundaries between traditional administrative data and more clinical information are blurring. In the future, merged electronic administrative and clinical information systems may become a mainstay of health-care research. Information generated during patient care or testing can already be transmitted automatically into central electronic data repositories, at least within institutions (Office of Technology Assessment, 1995). For example, the Regenstrief Medical Record System at Indiana University Medical Center networks data from three hospitals, 30 clinics, and other settings of care, capturing data from a clinician order-entry system, nursing notes, certain bedside monitors, laboratory, pharmacy, and various administrative sources. The Department of Veterans Affairs continuously updates central repositories containing data transmitted from health-care institutions nationwide (Meistrell and Schlehuber, 1996).

The trend toward entirely computerized, or "paperless," medical records offers almost endless research possibilities (Dick and Steen, 1991). Computerized medical records portend significant advantages, such as improved organization of massive quantities of data, easy access to individual data elements within records, the potential to organize data from diverse providers, the ability to insert pictorial representations (e.g., radiographs), legibility, and decreased space requirements for storage and processing. Although many technical, conceptual, and cultural challenges remain before computerized records will be widely used, they represent the wave of the future and appear inevitable.

Computerized records offer numerous potential advantages for improving care. For example, computerized rule-based alerts, reminders, and suggestions for care of specific patients in real time can be programmed into medical logic modules (Fitzmaurice, 1995). Some approaches have already been tested in health-care research projects, blurring the boundaries between practice and research. Rind and colleagues (1994), for example, sent computerized alerts to physicians about rising creatinine levels in their hospitalized patients receiving nephrotoxic or renally-excreted medications. Electronic laboratory reports and pharmacy records automatically generated the alerts, e-mailing them to the patient's doctor. The mean interval between an event and change or discontinuation of a medication was almost 22 hours shorter after institution of the alerts than it was before, with the relative risk of serious renal impairment falling to 0.45 compared to previously. Bates and colleagues conducted several studies using their hospitals' computerized clinical information systems to prevent serious medication errors (1998) and to minimize redundant test ordering (1999), again blurring the boundaries between practice and research.

One of the most advanced computerized hospital information systems, the HELP (Health Evaluation through Logical Processing) system at LDS Hospital in Salt Lake City, has integrated algorithms derived from health-care research (Kuperman et al, 1991). For intensive care unit (ICU) patients undergoing hemodynamic monitoring, for example, HELP periodically captures information directly from patients' physiologic probes on cardiac output, blood pressure, and pulmonary pressures, and from pumps administering intravenous medications. ICU rounds often start with reviews of computer printouts to see trends in physiologic parameters as well as drug administration. Embedded algorithms take data elements from HELP and automatically calculate Acute Physiology and Chronic Health Evaluation (Knaus et al, 1991) severity scores. Other decision rules alert physicians about such problems as nosocomial infections and adverse drug events. Thus, health care research and ongoing patient care explicitly converge through HELP.

Patients can also directly enter personal information into their electronic medical records. Wald and colleagues (1995), for example, designed a Health History Interview that asked patients about the medical review of systems, psychiatric symptoms, preventive health habits, and risk factors. New patients came early for their scheduled appointment and sat at terminals in the clinic waiting room. The information they entered was directly downloaded into their computerized medical record, and paper copies were printed for the patient and doctor. The computer interview averaged 27 minutes and, although 42% of the older patients had no prior keyboard experience, patients enjoyed it; 65% preferred a computer-administered survey to face-to-face interviews with their doctors. Patients conveyed fairly sensitive information: 13% reported domestic violence in the prior 12 months, and 16% reported suicidal ideation.

Nevertheless, electronic access to detailed clinical information has escalated concerns among privacy advocates. At one extreme is the sale of patient-level clinical information to health information vendors, pharmaceutical companies, credit record organizations, and other large data banks (Kolata, 1995). Often, those selling the records (e.g., health clinics, pharmacies, etc.) fail to remove patient names and other uniquely identifying information. At the other end are concerns about whether even doctors caring for individual patients should have access to portions of the record the patient wishes to keep confidential, such as mental health information (Page, 1996). For example, Harvard Pilgrim Health Care, a large managed care plan in Boston, has kept detailed clinical information in computer-based records for more than 20 years, sometimes including verbatim transcripts of psychotherapy sessions. Controversy erupted when a patient seeking treatment for a broken leg found that clinicians also had complete access to his mental health records.

There is no question that this brave new data world, with its clinical richness, will enhance the utility of the data for health-care research. The types of research questions and the clinical credibility of the answers will grow immeasurably. Nevertheless, with access to clinical information from electronic medical records, researchers could theoretically construct detailed portraits of individual patients, potentially disclosing their identities. Therefore, although these data sources offer a potential bonanza for future research, they must have strong strings attached. As discussed in the last section, especially when research merges with practice, important ethical concerns arise, and, regardless of the research design, appropriately protecting patients' confidentiality is the first priority.

POLITICAL AND SOCIAL FORCES AFFECTING INFORMATION FOR RESEARCH

What are the political and social forces that shape not only the content of databases but also the availability of information for research about our health-care system? Many political and societal forces affect the future course of health-care research and the associated ethical concerns. In the United States arguments have been ongoing for years about medical record privacy policies at both state and federal levels. Legislative resolutions are evolving. I touch briefly on three ongoing political debates that will shape the climate for health-care research.

Although these three areas pertain to specific laws or mandates, each raises general long-standing concerns with ethical implications. The first two relate to P.L. 104–191, the Health Insurance Portability and Accountability Act (HIPAA), signed by President Clinton on August 21, 1996. Widely viewed as an important, albeit modest, first step to protect health insurance for persons changing jobs and those with "preexisting" chronic conditions, two additional provisions of HIPAA could dramatically shape the content and scope of information available for health-care research studies.

Protecting Privacy of Health Information

HIPAA required the secretary of Health and Human Services to make detailed recommendations to Congress by August 1999 "with respect to the privacy of individually identifiable health information" (Gostin, 1997; Gostin and Hadley, 1998). These recommendations were required to address the rights of individuals regarding their own records, procedures needed to exercise these rights, and the uses and disclosures of information that should be authorized or required. The health records encompassed by these recommendations would have included health-care claims and other administrative transactions as well as medical charts. Given that Congress did not act by the specified August 1999 deadline, HIPAA stipulated that the president's privacy provisions would prevail. These provisions extended to a variety of data sources employed by health-care researchers, including private and public insurers' claims files and statewide administrative databases.

While these provisions were modified somewhat when the Patient Privacy Rule came into effect in April 2001, access to data by health-care researchers was nonetheless still restricted. Specifically, under this act consent must be obtained before a patient's information may be released for nonroutine uses and most non–health-care purposes, such as those sought by financial institutions or potential employers. The rule does, however, allow disclosure of health information without the individual's consent when doing so serves the nation's interest. As such, information may be released without consent for quality assurance or public health purposes, emergency circumstances, and so on. Even so, information released for the purposes of research is permitted only when a waiver of authorization is independently approved by a privacy board or institutional review board (IRB) (http://www.hhs.gov/news/press/2001pres/20010412.html).

As we can see, then, questions about "informed consent" figure prominently in debates about protecting privacy. As noted above, some privacy advocates argue against researchers' having access to such data sets without the specific informed consent of everyone represented. Obviously, these issues are very complex, and a complete airing of the arguments on both sides requires extensive discussion.

Suffice it to say that measures that prevent access to such databases without explicit consent from all persons included would significantly affect health-care research and, if broadly interpreted, possibly quality assurance and perhaps even delivery of health-care services. In the best-case scenario, these requirements would add tremendously to the costs and logistical complexities of conducting research and would result in biased samples due to the inability to obtain complete informed consent, for whatever reasons. In the worst-case scenario, such measures would stop altogether studies that use administrative or electronic databases and medical record reviews.

Privacy advocates, in some sense, have a "mom and apple pie" message—who can argue against protecting the privacy of medical information? Nevertheless, health-care researchers have only recently begun to make a compelling case about the value of their research and society's interest in supporting it. IRBs must also prove they are sensitive to potential privacy risks posed by large database research.

Administrative Simplification

Under the heading "Administrative Simplification," HIPAA also requires the adoption of standards for electronic interchange of various administrative health-care transactions, including health claims (or equivalent encounter information), enrollment and disenrollment in health plans, eligibility for health plans, health-care payment and remittance advice, referral certification and authorization, coordination of benefits information, and claims attachments. In addition, "supporting" standards must be designated, such as code sets and classification systems for data elements within the standard transactions; unique identifiers for individuals, employers, health plans, and health-care providers; security standards and safeguards for electronic information systems; and standards to ensure the privacy of electronic transactions. The standards apply nationwide to all public and private electronic health-care transactions.

Thus, the administrative simplification provisions will significantly affect databases used by health-care researchers. As noted above, standardization will increase the likelihood that data from diverse health-care settings will have comparable content and can be linked by a unique person-level identifier. Although probabilistic matching techniques have assisted health-care researchers in creating longitudinal person-level records (Roos et al, 1996), obviously a unique identifier would help.

But the possibility of a nationwide health-care identification number unleashed a maelstrom of dismay among numerous observers. Concerns arose not only about "big brother" watching patients wend through the health-care delivery system, taking potentially sensitive twists and turns, but also about the costs and logistical feasibility of assigning these numbers. In the summer of 1998, federal efforts to explore the person-level identifier were put on hold while Congress and the administration wrestled with privacy and security protections.

ACCESS TO RAW DATA FROM FEDERALLY FUNDED RESEARCH

On the evening of October 8, 1998, a one-line amendment was added to the 4000-plus-page appropriations bill approved by the U.S. Congress (Hilts, 1999). Requested by Senator Richard C. Shelby from Alabama, the amendment stipulated that, under the federal Freedom of Information Act (FOIA), anyone could request "all data produced" by published studies supported by any federal research dollars. The request could encompass the most minute information, including notebooks kept by scientists, e-mails, and details about patients. News reports indicated that the regulations to implement this law were being drafted by the Office of Management and Budget (OMB). Under a draft of the regulations, those who want data must ask for it under the FOIA by submitting a request to the agency that gave the grant to the scientist. The scientist must then turn over all the data, including names and addresses of patients and other private and commercially secret information, to the agency. Then the FOIA office of that funding agency must determine what must be given to the requester and what must be withheld. The information act carries protections against giving out some kinds of information, including commercial trade secrets, financial data, and private information such as medical records (Hilts, 1999).

The potential implications worried officials at the National Institutes of Health (NIH). Despite the legal strictures of the FOIA, they reportedly were nervous about implications for patients' confidentiality. "Even if they redact the name and address, there are other ways to identify the patients—if it was a female patient at a certain hospital with a particular diagnosis, that might be enough to identify them," noted an NIH official (Hilts, 1999). Obviously, even a hint that data could be given to outsiders would have a chilling effect on clinical trials. This type of regulation would also affect health-care researchers funded by federal agencies, such as AHRQ (the renamed AHCPR).

Although intellectually and philosophically Shelby's idea sounds reasonable and appropriate, the downstream practical implications are troubling. In addition to potentially frightening away research participants for studies that actively recruit subjects, two other concerns arise for health-care research. First, many investigations, especially of working-age adults and their young families, now turn to claims files from private insurers. Sometimes gaining access to these databases requires delicate negotiations and sensitivity to legitimate commercial interests, particularly in competitive environments. If these large databases from private sources could be obtained through FOIA requests, insurers would be unlikely to give their data to researchers. Since there is little other information for non-Medicare beneficiaries apart from the Medicaid files available in some states, this could substantially skew the populations included in health-care research.

A second, related issue involves intellectual property and ownership of data. In many studies using large databases, constructing the data file is 95% of the work. If an outside group obtains databases admittedly created with federal funds, should they nevertheless have the right to publish and thus claim some intellectual ownership of the data?

ETHICAL IMPLICATIONS FOR FUTURE HEALTH-CARE RESEARCH

Finally, what ethical values should inform future research about health care, especially concerning data privacy, and what research is needed to explore these ethical implications? The six points below summarize my recommendations, noting the research agenda raised by each.

Understand the Health Policy Context

Almost by definition, much of health-care research sits on the cutting edge of health policy and clinical practices. Some research has a more obvious, direct, human connection than does other research. For example, quality-adjusted life years and time trade-offs utility calculations are foreign concepts to some of us, while computerized approaches to prevent potential drug dosing errors feel more immediate and real. But, as witnessed by Oregon's Medicaid experiment and Europe's potential use of the EuroQol, even seemingly esoteric concepts can have direct policy relevance.

Researchers today obviously cannot anticipate fully how their work will be used tomorrow. Nevertheless, they must be aware of the health policy niche their investigations occupy. Applicants for investigator-initiated funding from the AHRQ are asked to delineate the significance of their work and its policy relevance. Unfortunately, our health-care system is still crisscrossed by cracks through which large numbers of people fall—the uninsured and underinsured; many with chronic health needs; and racial, ethnic, and linguistic minorities. Measuring quality, even for those within the system, remains an intractable conundrum (Eddy, 1998). The ethical imperative is to devise a research agenda that informs and directs the health policy agenda to fill these gaps.

When I served on a study section reviewing grants for the AHCPR in the early 1990s, I sometimes heard the following observation from my colleagues: "Oh, great! Another project that will tell us convincingly that poor people (or minorities or children or people with disabilities or some other disenfranchised group) don't get adequate care. So what if we prove that again, no matter how stellar the research methods? Who has the money or political willpower to fix it?" We need an answer to that question.

Justify the Need for Data on Personal Characteristics

Recognizing that it is infeasible to obtain informed consent for analyses using large, existing data files (and often medical record reviews), investigators must justify with a compelling conceptual rationale requests for each data element that could be used to identify specific individuals (Gostin and

Hadley, 1998). This would include information on the most basic variables, such as age, date of birth, sex, race, and ethnicity.

A parallel research agenda should consider what restrictions should be placed on such demographic variables before an investigator may obtain these data elements; statisticians should investigate the analytic consequences of making some variables less specific. For instance, except in the most unusual cases (e.g., the need to link the file of newborns with their mothers), I can think of few justifications for obtaining birthdate. Similarly, for the types of analyses performed with these large databases, having specific age is probably unnecessary. Age in five-year blocks (e.g., 40–44, 45–49, 50–54) is generally sufficient; broader blocks (e.g., 40–54, 55–64) might work in many instances.

Race especially needs justification. Williams (1994) examined 192 studies published between 1966 and 1990 in *HSR: Health Services Research.* He found that 63.0% included race and ethnicity; however, 54.5% made a black–white distinction only, and just 13.2% defined or justified using race in their research. Using racial variables in regression analyses may obscure important relationships, such as those involving education, socioeconomic class, culture, and health beliefs (Schulman et al, 1995). Evidence suggests that African American patients may receive worse quality care than white patients (Kahn et al, 1994; Ayanian et al, 1999). Examining outcomes adjusting for race could mask these important differences in health-care quality. Stratifying analyses by race (e.g., conducting separate analyses for African Americans and whites and comparing the results) could highlight differences that should be explored in greater depth (Iezzoni, 1997b).

A related research agenda should investigate the feasibility of secure data centers that could preprocess information to be given to investigators, stripping off data elements they have no need to know. These data centers could also potentially replace certain data elements with other information of greater utility to the researcher. For example, many investigators ask for patients' zip codes or census tracts, solely to later merge the file with census data containing sociodemographic characteristics of the area. A preprocessing center could perform that replacement before the data are ever released to researchers.

Justify the Need for Person-Reported Information

Asking people about their functioning, quality of life, and other perspectives injects the person's viewpoint front and center into health-care research. That is good, but it has a downside. While some people will welcome such questions, others will feel threatened by them. They will either not respond or answer the questions in the way least harmful to their interests. Global health policy problems alluded to above (e.g., lack of health insurance, inadequate access to care) could exacerbate these fears. As such, those asking about people's feelings and experiences are requesting an altruistic act of faith. Given that the information is unlikely to confer individual benefit, it must not hurt the informant.

From anecdotal reports, IRBs appear to deal inconsistently with studies requesting information from identified individuals. Some IRBs require signed, informed consent in situations, in which others do not (e.g., some IRBs view a person's answering a survey as de facto indicating their willingness to participate). An important part of the research agenda ought to be the examination of the ethical issues raised by asking people to participate in survey and questionnaire studies, especially focusing on populations particularly vulnerable to the ills of our current health-care system. New IRB guidelines must be feasible and practical to implement but recognize and respect the anxieties of some potential study participants.

Develop Fair Policies Concerning Ownership of Information and Methods

Who owns the information generated in health-care research? As suggested in the discussion of Senator Shelby's amendment, this question may become more complicated for federal grantees, but the question grows even more complex when individuals have given their informed consent to participate. The complexities expand again when focusing on electronic medical record or pharmacy information. Does the hematocrit value from my blood belong to me or to the entity settling the claim for the venipuncture? Who owns the information about prescriptions for potentially stigmatizing drugs?

Basic scientists have struggled with these issues for years. Millions of dollars ride on some laboratory research discoveries, especially those involving new pharmacotherapies. Debates around patenting the human genome raised troubling ethical implications that generated societal debates. Thus far, health-care research has sat on the sidelines of most of these discussions, but this is changing with the increasing fragmentation and competition in our health-care environment. Many insurers rely on in-house and other research to direct internal management decisions, quality oversight, and even patient care decisions (e.g., whether to cover a particular therapy). Some sell or contract their data to outside information vendors to generate revenue or meet other administrative needs.

An important part of the research agenda should thus involve exploring the ownership of health-care research data within the broader context of data generated through electronic information systems. When should information be allowed to be used for purposes other than direct patient care or administering that care? When and how should patients be told? Answers to these questions must consider federal legislation or administrative actions relating to the HIPAA mandates, including privacy protections.

Recognize the Blurring of Research with Real Life

This chapter repeatedly notes that health-care research often occurs in the context of daily practice. Making sure that IRBs understand the implications of this blurring should be an important part of the research agenda. In classic randomized, double-blinded clinical trials, the study is stopped if the oversight committee finds that patients in one arm of the trial are doing much better or worse than those in the other. If subjects getting the experimental therapy are doing much better, often those administered placebo or the control treatment will be switched to the new intervention.

Yet an analogous switch may be impossible in health-care research studies. For example, suppose a computerized drug order entry system is shown to be highly effective at minimizing dosage errors. Because of limitations in their information systems, control sites may be unable to implement that intervention. So in health-care research, everybody may not be able to receive the acknowledged superior treatment.

Somewhat more vexing are situations in which approaches are implemented on an operational basis that should rightly be viewed as experimental. Typically, these situations draw from tools developed in health-care research. The HEDIS Health of Seniors survey is a prime example. Nobody knows whether changes in SF-36 score over two years are a valid measure of health plan quality. The Health of Seniors survey is really an experiment that should be evaluated as such. The fact that it is a high-profile effort in a closely observed health policy setting (i.e., comparing performance of Medicare managed care plans) raises the stakes about the need for its validition.

The following interaction further highlights concerns raised when research confronts reality. At a recent meeting, a physician representing a large business coalition spoke warmly in favor of the Health of Seniors survey. He indicated that this was just the type of information about plan performance his business members sought. I asked him whether he thought there was really anything physicians could do to influence their patients' SF-36 scores. He replied enthusiastically and affirmatively, saying that if physicians took time to discuss functional issues with their patients, problems could be identified and addressed, preventing or minimizing future declines. I asked if the members of his business coalition would agree to increase payments to physicians so that they could have longer appointment times with their patients to discuss functional issues. After a moment's chagrined silence, he admitted they would not.

Who Has a Right To Ask?

Researchers should not automatically assume they have a right to ask about the most intimate details of other people's lives. Instead, researchers must first examine their motivations in conducting health-care studies and convince themselves that they have legitimate reason to know. They must be humble enough to recognize when their studies offer little direct benefit to their research participants.

An important part of the research agenda should thus involve developing a formal curriculum and other teaching approaches to educate health-care researchers about their responsibilities. Motivating this learning may be easier here than in other research fields, for the topics of health-care research and the related privacy concerns touch everybody directly, and it is not hard to imagine our families or ourselves as the research subjects.

NOTES

1. Here, "health-care research" encompasses health services, effectiveness, health policy, health systems, decision and cost-effectiveness analysis, quality measurement, quality improvement, and outcomes research.
2. I do not mean "right" in the legalistic sense of the word, but "right" in terms of legitimacy and appropriateness.

REFERENCES

Ayanian JZ, Weissman JS, Chasan-Taber S, Epstein AM (1999) Quality of care by race and gender for congestive heart failure and pneumonia. *Medical Care* 37:1260–9.

Bates DW, Leape LL, Cullen DJ, Laird N, Petersen LA, Teich JM, Burdick E, Hickey M, Kleefield S, Shea B, Vander Vliet M, Seger DL (1998) Effect of computerized physician order entry and a team intervention on prevention of serious medication errors. *Journal of the American Medical Association* 280:1311–6.

Bates DW, Kuperman GJ, Rittenberg E, Teich JM, Fiskio J, Ma'luf N, Onderdonk A, Wybenga D, Winkelman J, Brennan TA, Komaroff AL, Tanasijevic M (1999) A randomized trial of a computer-based intervention to reduce utilization of redundant laboratory tests. *American Journal of Medicine* 106:144–50.

Carrasquillo O, Himmelstein DU, Woolhandler S, Bor DH (1999) Going bare: Trends in health insurance coverage, 1989 through 1996. *American Journal of Public Health* 89:36–42.

Daugherty CK, Siegler M, Ratain MJ, Zimmer G (1997) Learning from our patients: One participant's impact on clinical trial research and informed consent. *Annals of Internal Medicine* 125:892–7.

Dick RS and Steen EB (eds) (1991) *The Computer-based Patient Record: An Essential Technology for Health Care.* Washington, DC: National Academy Press.

Donabedian A (1985) *The Methods and Findings of Quality Assessment and Monitoring. An Illustrated Analysis. Volume 3.* Ann Arbor, MI: Health Administration Press, 256.

Eddy DM (1998) Performance measurement: Problems and solutions. *Health Affairs* 17: 7–25.

Ellwood P (1988) Shattuck Lecture—Outcomes management. A technology of patient experience. *New England Journal of Medicine* 318:1549–56.

Fisher ES, Welch HG, Wennberg JE (1992) Prioritizing Oregon's hospital resources. An example based on variations in discretionary medical utilization. *Journal of the American Medical Association* 267:1925–31.

Fitzmaurice JM (1995) Computer-based patient records. In: JD Bronzino (ed) *The Biomedical Engineering Handbook*. Boca Raton, FL: CRC Press, Inc., 2623–34.

Gostin L (1997) Health care information and the protection of personal privacy: Ethical and legal considerations. *Annals of Internal Medicine* 127:683–90.

Gostin LO and Hadley J (1998) Health services research: Public benefits, personal privacy, and proprietary interests. *Annals of Internal Medicine* 129:833–5.

Greenwald LM, Esposito A, Ingber MJ, Levy JM (1998) Risk adjustment for the Medicare program: Lessons learned from research and demonstrations. *Inquiry* 35:193–209.

Hadorn DC (1991) Setting health care priorities in Oregon. Cost-effectiveness meets the rule of rescue. *Journal of the American Medical Association* 265:2218–25.

Hadorn DC (1992) The problem of discrimination in health care priority setting. *Journal of the American Medical Association* 268:1454–9.

Hilts PJ (1999) Law on access to research data pleases business, alarms scientists. *New York Times* July 31:A1.

Iezzoni LI (1997a) Assessing quality using administrative data. *Annals of Internal Medicine* 127:666–74.

Iezzoni LI (1997b) Dimensions of risk. In: Iezzoni LI (ed) *Risk Adjustment for Measuring Healthcare Outcomes, Second Edition*. Chicago: Health Administration Press.

Iezzoni LI, Mackiernan YD, Cahalane MJ, Phillips RS, Miller K (1999) Screening inpatient quality using postdischarge events. *Medical Care* 37:384–98.

Iglehart JK (1996) The National Committee for Quality Assurance. *New England Journal of Medicine* 335:995–9.

Jenkinson C (1999) Death by questionnaire: Quality of life measurement could seriously damage your health. *Journal of Health Services Research and Policy* 4:129–30.

Kahn KL, Pearson ML, Harrison ER, Desmond KA, Rogers WH, Rubenstein LV, Brook RH, Keeler EB (1994) Health care for black and poor hospitalized Medicare patients. *Journal of the American Medical Association* 271:1169–74.

Knaus WA, Wagner DP, Draper EA, Zimmerman JE, Bergner M, Bastos PG, Sirio CA, Murphy DJ, Lotring T, Damiano A, Harrell FE (1991) The APACHE III prognostic system: Risk prediction of hospital mortality for critically ill hospitalized adults. *Chest* 100:1619–36.

Kolata G (1995) When patients' records are commodities for sale. *New York Times* November 15:A1.

Kuperman GJ, Gardner RM, Pryor TA (1999) *HELP: A Dynamic Hospital Information System*. New York: Springer-Verlag.

Lave JR, Pashos CL, Anderson GF, Brailer D, Bubolz T, Conrad D, Freund DA, Fox SH, Keeler E, Lipscomb J, Luft HS, Provenzano G (1994) Costing medical care: Using Medicare administrative data. *Medical Care* 32:JS77-89.

Medicare Payment Advisory Commission (1998) *Report to the Congress: Medicare Payment Policy. Volume I: Recommendations*. Washington, D.C.

Meistrell M and Schlehuber C (1996) Adopting a corporate perspective on databases: improving support for research and decision making. *Medical Care* 34:MS91–102.

Melton LJ, III (1997) The threat to medical-records research. *New England Journal of Medicine* 337:1466–70.

Mitchell JB, Bubolz T, Paul JE, Pashos CL, Escarce JJ, Muhlbaier LH, Wiesman JM, Young WW, Epstein RS, Javitt JC (1994) Using Medicare claims for outcomes research. *Medical Care* 32: JS38–51.

Morgan RO, Virnig BA, DeVito CA, Persily NA (1997) The Medicare-HMO revolving door—the healthy go in and the sick go out. *New England Journal of Medicine* 337: 169–75.

National Committee for Quality Assurance (1996) *HEDIS 3.0 (Health Plan Employer Data Information Set)*. Washington, DC.

Neuman P, Maibach E, Dusenbury K, Kitchman M, Zupp P (1998) Marketing HMOs to Medicare beneficiaries. *Health Affairs* 17:132–39.

Page L (1996) Managed care files pose privacy risks. *American Medical News* June 10:3.

Pear R (1998) H.M.O.'s are retreating from Medicare, citing high costs. *New York Times* October 2:A17.

Reiser SJ (1993) The era of the patient. Using the experience of illness in shaping the missions of health care. *Journal of the American Medical Association* 269: 1012–17.

Relman AS (1988) Assessment and accountability: The third revolution in medical care. *New England Journal of Medicine* 319:1220–2.

Riley G, Tudor C, Chiang YP, Ingber M (1996) Health status of Medicare enrollees in HMOs and fee-for-service in 1994. *Health Care Financing Review* 17:65–76.

Rind DM, Safran C, Phillips RS, Wang Q, Calkins DR, Delbanco TL, Bleich HL, Slack WV (1994) Effect of computer-based alerts on the treatment and outcomes of hospitalized patients. *Archives of Internal Medicine* 154:1511–7.

Roos LL, Walld R, Wajda A, Bond R, Hartford K (1996) Record linkage strategies, outpatient procedures, and administrative data. *Medical Care* 34:570–82.

Roos LL, Nicol JP, Cageorge SM (1987) Using administrative data for longitudinal research: Comparisons with primary data collection. *Journal of Chronic Disease* 40: 41–9.

Romano PS, Zach A, Luft HS, Rainwater J, Remy LL, Campa D (1995) The California Hospital Outcomes Project. Using administrative data to compare hospital performance. *Joint Commission Journal on Quality Improvement* 21:668–82.

Schroeder SA (1999) The legacy of SUPPORT. *Annals of Internal Medicine* 131:780–1.

Schulman KA, Rubenstein LE, Chesley FD, Eisenberg JM (1995) The roles of race and socioeconomic factors in health services research. *Health Services Research* 30:179–95.

Shapiro P (1993) *No Pity: People with Disabilities Forging a New Civil Rights Movement*. New York: Times Books.

Shuster E (1997) Fifty years later: The significance of the Nuremberg code. *New England Journal of Medicine* 337:1436–40.

Stewart AL, Greenfield S, Hays RD, Wells K, Rogers WH, Berry SD, McGlynn EA, Ware JE Jr (1989) Functional status and well-being of patients with chronic conditions. Results from the Medical Outcomes Study. *Journal of the American Medical Association* 262:907–13.

Stewart AL, Ware JE Jr (eds) (1992) *Measuring Functioning and Well-Being: The Medical Outcomes Approach*. Durham, NC: Duke University Press.

Svensson CK (1989) Representation of American blacks in clinical trials of new drugs. *Journal of the American Medical Association* 261:263–5.

Sweeney L (1997) Guaranteeing anonymity when sharing medical data, the Datafly System. *Proceedings of the AMIA Annual Fall Symposium* 51–5.

Teno JM, Lynn J, Phillips RS, Murphy D, Youngner SJ, Bellamy P, Connors AF, Jr., Desbiens NA, Fulkerson W, Knaus WA (1994) Do formal advance directives affect resuscitation decisions and the use of resources for seriously ill patients? *Journal of Clinical Ethics* 5:23–30.

Truog RD, Robinson W, Randolph A, Morris A (1999) Is informed consent always necessary for randomized, controlled trials? *New England Journal of Medicine* 340: 804–7.

U.S. Congress, Office of Technology Assessment (1994) *Identifying Health Technologies that Work: Searching for Evidence*. Washington, DC: U.S. Government Printing Office, OTA-H-608.

U.S. Congress, Office of Technology Assessment (1995) *Bringing Health Care Online. The Role of Information Technologies*. Washington, DC: U.S. Government Printing Office, OTA-ITC-624.

U.S. General Accounting Office (1992) *FDA Needs To Ensure More Study of Gender Differences in Prescription Drug Testing*. Washington, DC.

Wald JS, Rind D, Safran C, Kowaloff H, Barker R, Slack WV (1995) Patient entries in the electronic medical record: An interactive interview used in primary care. *Proceedings Annual Symposium Computer Applications Medical Care* 147–51.

Williams DR (1994) The concept of race in health services research: 1966 to 1990. *Health Service Research* 29:261–74.

Afterword

LEWIS G. SANDY

The disparate yet complementary perspectives presented by the authors of this volume illustrate both the opportunity and the challenge of connecting the theory and practice of ethics to health policy. This unique compilation of topics and views elucidates issues in health, health care, and health policy from the perspectives of the ethicist, the social scientist, the policy analyst, and the policy maker.

Both the preceding chapters and the conference that initiated this volume highlight, in my view, four challenges in the examination and practice of ethics in the health policy realm.

THE STANDING OF ETHICS, ETHICISTS, AND ETHICAL ANALYSIS IN HEALTH POLICY

Clearly, there are myriad ethical facets to health policy, yet the standing of ethics in health policy varies as a function of the issue. The closer the health policy area is to traditional concerns of ethics, the greater the standing. For example, those concerned over medical privacy, confidentiality, and protection of research subjects can draw on existing ethical traditions and methods of analysis, as well as the human capital within the bioethics community.

On the other hand, the standing of ethics in the area of resource allocation is much less certain, competing for voice with the fields of political analysis, economics, and politics.

A second area for further deliberation for ethicists is the distinction between analysis and advocacy. This distinction is particularly problematic for a field that specializes in "oughts," in normative judgments. Most health policy analysts take the position that their role is to illuminate the likely effects of policy alternatives, not to provide their opinion as to a preferred approach. Ethicists making normative statements that flow from ethical theory will need to clarify whether these statements represent an ethical analysis or an ethical prescription. In health policy, the rules of engagement, while not always clear, do provide some bounds for the appropriate approach. This will need further explication if ethics is to provide a new perspective on health policy concerns.

THE CHALLENGE OF THE DETERMINANTS OF HEALTH TO HEALTH POLICY

Slowly but surely, evidence is emerging from social and behavioral science on the nonbiological determinants of health. From a population perspective, small changes to large numbers of individuals can have a greater impact on health than large changes to small numbers of people. We are learning that socioeconomic status, community and social structure, even the physical environment have major, independent effects on health status. As this evidence accumulates, traditional domains of health policy will need an enlarged perspective. In parallel, ethicists traditionally concerned with individualist perspectives will have an opportunity to explore new territory in a potentially receptive policy environment.

THE UPHILL BATTLE FOR PUBLIC EDUCATION

A third theme of this compilation is the importance of public opinion in spite of significant interpretive challenges. Ginzberg notes that the public is unaware of "who pays for what in health care," and Greenberg comments that the public has strong views, but little unanimity, when it comes to health care. Of particular note is the complexity of discerning public views. Many advocacy groups claim to represent both the public interest and the public's views, and few areas of public policy touch a citizenry so intimately as health care. These features of health care make "everyone an expert." Just as traditional medical ethics has invested significant energy in determining patient preferences, ethics and health policy will need to advance the science and practice of population-level preference determination.

THE NEED FOR INITIAL DIRECTIONS, OR "SOUND BITES FOR ETHICISTS"

Finally, if ethics is to take a seat at the health policy table, the ethics community will need to present a sharper image of its concerns, its approaches, and its areas of interest. This volume is a start in that direction, and, as a whole, presents an initial set of concepts and issues of importance in health policy. Although others may have a different set, mine include:

- Concerns over justice and equality of opportunity,
- The need to deal with limits in ways that go beyond economics, and
- The importance of process, deliberation, and accountability.

Health policy is the business of making choices that affect the costs, access, and quality of health care. As health care costs grow and continue to strain the national resources of virtually all countries, each nation seeks the ideal blend of public and private approaches that can achieve policy goals and concerns. In the United States in particular, health care has burgeoned into a $1.5 trillion industry. The lurching quality of American health policy reflects an almost unconscious "approach–avoidance" posture by the public and by policy makers concerning values and ethics in the face of overwhelming costs. As a result, although the health-care sector has undergone major market transformations in many countries, the body politic is scarcely better off in terms of understanding and deliberating the goals and mechanisms of the health-care system.

This volume, initiated by a public and private, academic and practitioner collaboration, is an attempt to make progress. If you, the reader, find herein ideas of interest and value beyond your core work, and if scholars and practitioners brought together to connect ethics and health policy can find new ways of working together, then we shall have succeeded.

Index

Page numbers followed by f indicate figures